Egyptology

The large-scale scientific investigation of Egyptian antiquities by Western scholars began as an unintended consequence of Napoleon's invasion of Egypt during which, in 1799, the Rosetta Stone was discovered. The military expedition was accompanied by French scholars, whose reports prompted a wave of enthusiasm that swept across Europe and North America resulting in the Egyptian Revival style in art and architecture. Increasing numbers of tourists visited Egypt, eager to see the marvels being revealed by archaeological excavation. Writers and booksellers responded to this growing interest with publications ranging from technical site reports to tourist guidebooks and from children's histories to theories identifying the pyramids as repositories of esoteric knowledge. This series reissues a wide selection of such books. They reveal the gradual change from the 'tomb-robbing' approach of early excavators to the highly organised and systematic approach of Flinders Petrie, the 'father of Egyptology', and include early accounts of the decipherment of the hieroglyphic script.

A History of Egyptian Mummies

First published in 1834, this work was an important early contribution to the emerging field of Egyptology in Britain. It united the twin passions of its author, the noted surgeon and antiquarian Thomas Joseph Pettigrew (1791–1865), who made a name for himself by unrolling and autopsying mummies: his London home was the scene of well-attended parties during which he would impress his guests with such displays. In the present work, Pettigrew delves into the history, technique and ritual of mummification in a depth that had never been attempted before, notably extending the coverage beyond ancient Egypt to other societies and eras. Describing the beliefs that informed these practices, the work also addresses the Egyptians' worship and embalming of animals such as bulls, dogs and hawks. Based on numerous examinations and years of study, this work stood as a landmark in the scientific and historical understanding of these funerary rites.

Cambridge University Press has long been a pioneer in the reissuing of out-of-print titles from its own backlist, producing digital reprints of books that are still sought after by scholars and students but could not be reprinted economically using traditional technology. The Cambridge Library Collection extends this activity to a wider range of books which are still of importance to researchers and professionals, either for the source material they contain, or as landmarks in the history of their academic discipline.

Drawing from the world-renowned collections in the Cambridge University Library and other partner libraries, and guided by the advice of experts in each subject area, Cambridge University Press is using state-of-the-art scanning machines in its own Printing House to capture the content of each book selected for inclusion. The files are processed to give a consistently clear, crisp image, and the books finished to the high quality standard for which the Press is recognised around the world. The latest print-on-demand technology ensures that the books will remain available indefinitely, and that orders for single or multiple copies can quickly be supplied.

The Cambridge Library Collection brings back to life books of enduring scholarly value (including out-of-copyright works originally issued by other publishers) across a wide range of disciplines in the humanities and social sciences and in science and technology.

A History of
Egyptian Mummies

*And an Account of the Worship and Embalming
of the Sacred Animals by the Egyptians*

Thomas Joseph Pettigrew

CAMBRIDGE
UNIVERSITY PRESS

CAMBRIDGE
UNIVERSITY PRESS

University Printing House, Cambridge, CB2 8BS, United Kingdom

Published in the United States of America by Cambridge University Press, New York

Cambridge University Press is part of the University of Cambridge.
It furthers the University's mission by disseminating knowledge in the pursuit of
education, learning and research at the highest international levels of excellence.

www.cambridge.org
Information on this title: www.cambridge.org/9781108066839

This edition first published 1834
This digitally printed version 2013

ISBN 978-1-108-06683-9 Paperback

HISTORY

OF

EGYPTIAN MUMMIES.

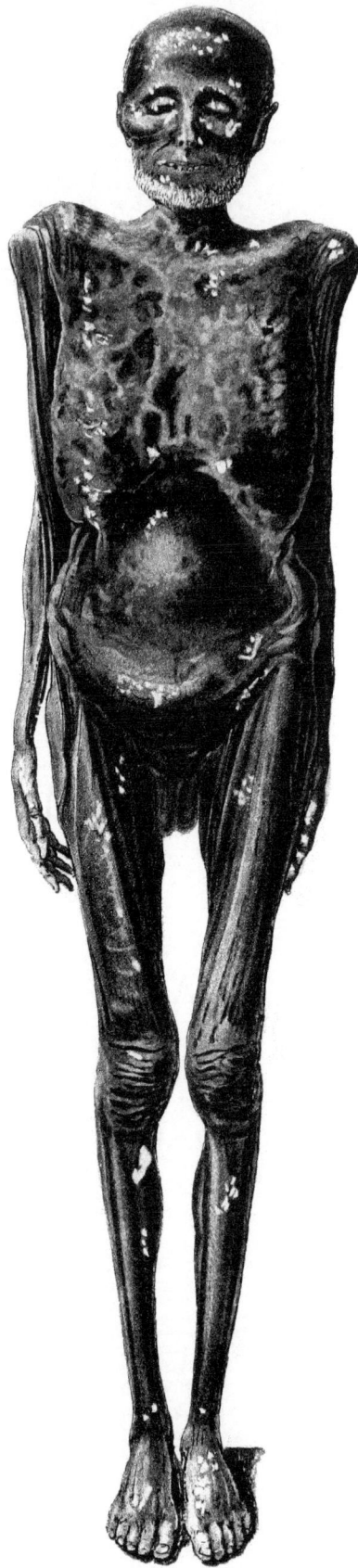

Geo Cruikshank del.^t

GRÆCO-EGYPTIAN MUMMY.

Unrolled April. 6.th 1833

Published by Mes.^{rs} Longman & Co Feb. 1. 1834.

A

HISTORY

OF

EGYPTIAN MUMMIES,

AND AN ACCOUNT OF

THE WORSHIP AND EMBALMING OF THE SACRED ANIMALS

BY

THE EGYPTIANS;

WITH

REMARKS ON THE FUNERAL CEREMONIES OF DIFFERENT NATIONS,

AND

OBSERVATIONS ON THE MUMMIES OF THE CANARY ISLANDS, OF THE ANCIENT
PERUVIANS, BURMAN PRIESTS, &c.

BY

THOMAS JOSEPH PETTIGREW, F.R.S., F.S.A., F.L.S.,

DOCTOR OF PHILOSOPHY OF THE UNIVERSITY OF GOTTINGEN, MEMBER OF THE ROYAL ASIATIC SOCIETY, CORRESPONDING
MEMBER OF THE ACADEMY OF ARTS, SCIENCES, AND THE BELLES LETTRES OF DIJON, AND OF THE SOCIÉTÉ
ACADEMIQUE DE MEDECINE DE MARSEILLE; SURGEON TO THE CHARING CROSS HOSPITAL,
THE ASYLUM FOR FEMALE ORPHANS, &c. &c. &c.

" Nec cremare aut fodere fas putant, verum arte medicatos intra penetralia collocant."
Pomponius Mela, lib. i. cap. 9.

LONDON:
LONGMAN, REES, ORME, BROWN, GREEN, AND LONGMAN,
PATERNOSTER ROW.

MDCCCXXXIV.

TO

HIS MOST EXCELLENT MAJESTY

KING WILLIAM IV.

SIRE,

DEEPLY impressed with gratitude for the most gracious permission afforded me to inscribe the following Work to Your Majesty, I avail myself of the high honour of laying the same at Your Majesty's feet; and I beg to be permitted to express the sentiments of devotion and attachment to Your Majesty's Person with which I am animated, and to have the honour of subscribing myself,

YOUR MAJESTY'S

Most loyal and devoted Subject and Servant,

THOMAS JOSEPH PETTIGREW.

SAVILLE STREET,
March 20, 1834.

LIST OF SUBSCRIBERS.

HIS MOST GRACIOUS MAJESTY. *Large Paper.*

His Royal Highness the Duke of Cumberland, K.G., G.C.B., K.S.P., G.C.H, F.R.S. *Large Paper.*

LIBRARY OF THE ROYAL COLLEGE OF SURGEONS.

Viscount Acheson, M.P.

Thomas Amyot, Esq., F.R.S., *Treasurer*, S.A.

Jasper Atkinson, Esq.

Benjamin Attwood, Esq.

William Ayrton, Esq., F.S.A.

Whitelaw Ainslie, M.D., F.R.A.S.

James Anderton, Esq.

— Andrews, Esq.

Le Comm Comte di Aceto.

His Grace the Duke of Bedford, F.S.A. *Large Paper.*

Viscount Boringdon, F.G.S.

Sir William Bolland, Baron of Exchequer

Sir William Beatty, M.D., F.R.S., F.L.S.

John Barrow, Esq., F.R.S., F.L.S.

William Beattie, M.D.

John Bayford, Esq., F.S.A.

J. T. B. Beaumont, Esq., F.S.A.

Rev. J. George Brett, M.A.

J. H. Bradshaw, Esq.

Henry Bosanquet, Esq., M.A.

Andrew Baird, M.D., F.R.S.

Henry Beaufoy, Esq., F.R.S., F.L.S.

Richard Bligh, Esq., M.A.

Edward Blore, Esq., F.S.A.

Gilbert Burnett, Esq. F.L.S., Prof. Bot. King's Coll.

William Hunter Baillie, Esq.

Thomas Bell, Esq., F.R.S., F.L.S.

George Lane Blount, Esq.

C. F. Barnwell, Esq., M.A., F.R.S., F.S.A.

Rev. Charles Parr Burney, D.D. F.R.S., F.S.A, F.L.S.

Colonel Hugh Baillie

Benjamin Guy Babington, M.D., F.R.S.

Edmund Beales, Esq.

John Baddeley, M.D.

John Barrow, Esq.

James Burton, Esq.

James Blundell, M.D.

William Behnes, Esq.

George Buckley Bolton, Esq.

E. S. Blundell, M.D.

Decimus Burton, Esq., F.S.A., F.G.S.

Mrs. Bowman

Bernard Brocas, Esq., F.S.A.

His Grace the Archbishop of Canterbury, D.D., F.R.S. F.S.A. *Large Paper.*

The Earl of Cadogan *Large Paper.*

Right Rev. Lord Bishop of Chichester, D.D., F.R.S., F.S.A.

Prince Cimitile *Large Paper.*

Sir George Cayley, Bart., M.P.

Sir Astley P. Cooper, Bart., F.R.S.

Sir Charles Mansfield Clarke, Bart., M.D., F.R.S.

Nicholas Carlisle, Esq., K.H., F.R.S., *Sec.*, S.A., M.R.I.A. *Two Copies, Large Paper.*

T. W. Coke, Esq.

Lieutenant General Calcraft

Miss Emily Fox Calcraft

James Copland, M.D., F.R.S.

Thomas Copeland, Esq., F.R.S.

Benjamin Bond Cabbell, Esq., M.A., F.S.A.

Adair Crawford, M.D.

George Cruikshank, Esq.

C. R. Cockerell, Esq., F.S.A.

Henry Clutterbuck, M.D.

John Cooke, M.D., F.R.S., F.S.A.

John Capel, Esq.

John Caley, Esq., F.R.S., F.S.A., F.L.S.   *Two Copies.*

Thomas Crofton Croker, Esq., F.S.A.

William Cubitt, Esq., F.R.S.

Miss Currer   *Large Paper.*

Edward J. Cooper, Esq., M.P.

William Coombes, Esq.

Francis Const, Esq.

Edward J. Cropper, Esq.

Alexander Copland, Esq.

Joseph Cholmondeley, Esq.   *Large Paper.*

William Chowne, M.D.

J. T. Coleridge, Esq., Serjeant at Law

George Capron, Esq.

H. S. Chinnock, Esq.

His Grace the Duke of Devonshire, K.G.

The Right Honourable Sir Thomas Denman, Lord Chief
  Justice of England

Captain Dillon, R.N.

Rev. Henry Drury, M.A., F.R.S., F.S.A. *Large Paper.*

Henry Davies, M.D.

John Davidson, Esq., F.S.A.   *Large Paper.*

Thomas Davidson, Esq.

George Darling, M.D.

Francis Douce, Esq., F.S.A.

Joseph Delafield, Esq., F.S.A.

George Drysdale, Esq.

Edward Downes, Esq.

George Dodd, Esq.

George Dollond, Esq., F.R.S., F.R.A.S.

Admiral Donnelly

James Dunlap, M.D.   *Large Paper*

Nicholas Dennys, Esq., F.G.S.

Miss Dyke.

The Earl of Egremont, F.R.S., F.S.A.

Sir Henry Ellis, K.H., B.C.L., F.R.S., *Sec.* S.A.

William Ewart, Esq., M.P.

John Easthope, Esq.

John Easthope, Jun., Esq.

James Evans, Esq.

William Esdaile, Esq.

The Earl Ferrers   *Large Paper*

Sir Francis Freeling, Bart., F.S.A.

Sir William B. Folkes, Bart., M.P.

Michael Faraday, Esq., D.C.L., F.R.S., M.R.I.A.,
  F.G.S.

Rev. Josiah Forshall, M.A., F.R.S., F.S.A.

Rev. —— Fiott, M.A.

George Fincham, Esq.

Rev. Charles Fletcher, M.A.

Rev. Dr. Fellowes

Charles F. Forbes, M.D., F.L.S.

John Richard Farre, M.D.

John Fearn, Esq.

William Frend, Esq.

Rev. Peter Fraser, M.A.   *Large Paper.*

Rev. William Victor Fryer, D.D.

James William Freshfield, Esq.

James William Farrer, Esq., F.S.A.

Sir Arthur Brooke Faulkner, M.D.

Earl of Gosford, M.A., F.R.S.

Viscount Gage   *Large Paper.*

Right Hon. Thomas Grenville, F.S.A.   *Large Paper.*

The Venerable George Glover, M.A., Archdeacon of
  Sudbury, F.R.S.

Hudson Gurney, Esq., F.R.S., V.P.S.A.

John Gage, Esq., F.R.S., *Director*, S.A., F.L.S.

John Lewis Guillemard, Esq., M.A., F.R.S., F.L.S.,
  F.G.S.

Gordon Gill, Esq.

Francis Goodwin, Esq.   *Large Paper.*

Isaac Lyon Goldsmid, Esq., F.R.S., F.S.A.

A. B. Granville, M.D., F.R.S., F.L.S.

Captain Robert Melville Grindlay, F.R.A.S.

G. J. Guthrie, Esq., F.R.S., Pres. Roy. Col. of Surgeons

A. W. Grant, Esq.

John Griffin, Esq.

R. H. Giraud, Esq.

Benjamin Golding, M.D.

Rev. Gilbert Gilbert, B.D., M.R.I.

George Glenny, Esq.

Fred. Alex. Grant, Esq.

His Grace the Duke of Hamilton and Brandon, F.R.S.,
  F.S.A.   *Large Paper.*

Earl of Hardwicke, K.G., LL.D., F.R.S., F.S.A.
                              Large and Small Paper.

Lord Howard, of Effingham

Lord Marcus Hill

Sir Henry Halford, Bart., G.C.H , M D., Pres. R. Col.
  of Phys., F.R.S., F.S.A.

Baron Heurteloup.

Rev. John Hailstone, M.A., F.R.S., F.L.S., F.G.S.

Rev. Thomas Power Hardwicke, M.A.

Chevalier J. B. Heath, F.S.A.

Rev. F. W. Hope, F.L.S.

Charles Hatchett, Esq., F.R.S., L. and E., F.S.A., F.L.S.
Large Paper.

Thomas Henry Hall, Esq., M.A., F.R.S.

Richard Heathfield, Esq.

Edmund Halswell, Esq., M.A.

John Henderson, Esq.

Massy Hutchinson, Esq.

Thomas Hadley, Esq.

Cæsar Hawkins, Esq.

Henry Heath, Esq.

John Hare, Esq.

Edward Harrison, M.D., F.R.A.S. Ed.

John Huntley, Esq.

Henry Thomas Hope, Esq., M.P.

Henry Philip Hope, Esq.

Alexander Copland Hutchison, Esq., F.R.S. Lond. and Ed.

J. D. Holm, Esq.

Philip Hardwick, Esq., F.R.S., F.S.A.

Miss Hamilton

— Harding, Esq.

James Patten Heath, M.D.

John Iggulden, Esq.

Hon. H. Stafford Jerningham, M.P.

Sir Richard Paul Jodrell, Bart.

John T. Justice, Esq.

James Johnson, M.D.

William Cornelius Jourdain, Esq.   *Large Paper.*

Charles Konig, K.H., For. Sec. R. S., F.L.S.

James Lewis Knight, Esq., K.C., F.R.S., F.S.A.

John Kidd, M.D., Reg. Prof. Med· Oxford, F.R.S., F.G.S.   *Large Paper.*

Rev. William Kirby, M.A., F.R.S., F.L.S., F.G.S.

William Kingdon, Esq.

Daniel Keane, Esq.

R. M. Kerrison, M.D.

William King, Esq.

A. Keightly, Esq.

Leonard Koecker, Esq.

His Grace the Duke of Leinster

The Most Noble the Marquis of Lansdowne, D.C.L., F.R.S.

The Earl of Lonsdale, K.G., F.S.A.

The Right Honourable the Lord Bishop of London, D.D.

Lieut. Col. W. M. Leake, F.R.S.

Thomas Lane, Esq.

William Thomas Luxmoore, Esq.

Sir Peter Laurie.

Rev. Samuel Lee, D.D., Reg. Prof. of Hebrew, Cambridge

John Gibson Lockhart, Esq. LL.B.

John Lee, LL.D., F.R.S., F.R.A.S.

Robert Lemon, Esq., F.S.A.

Rev. John Lindsay, M.A., F.S.A.

William Linley, Esq.

G. J. Letton, Esq.

John Lawrie, Esq.

Robert Peter Laurie, Esq.

Hugh Ley, M.D.

E. A. Lloyd, Esq.

W. Nanson Lettsom, Esq.

Charles Morgan Lemann, M.D., F.L.S.

Thomas Le Blanc, Esq., LL.B., F.S.A.

H. R. Lewis, Esq.

The Earl of Munster, G.C.H., F.R.S., F.R.A.S.

Honourable Charles Augustus Murray

Count Mortara

Sir James Mac Grigor, Bart., F.R.S, Lond. and Ed.

Sir Samuel Rush Meyrick, K.H., LL.D., F.S.A.

Sir Frederic Madden, K.H., F.R.S., F.S.A.

G. W. Maton, M.D., V.P.R.S., F.S.A., V.P.L.S.

Thomas Moore, Esq., F.S.A.

J. M. Mathew, Esq., F.S.A.   *Large Paper.*

W. A. Mackinnon, Esq., F.R.S., F.S.A.

Basil Montagu, Esq.

Joseph Moore, M.D.

James Heywood Markland, Esq. F.R.S., F.S.A.

George Macilwain, Esq.

Samuel Merriman, M.D., F.L.S.

R. Maugham, Esq.

William B. Maurice, Esq., F.L.S.

William Meyrick, Esq.

Joshua Mayhew, Esq.

J. M. Morgan, Esq.

Alexander Mundell, Esq.

James Morrah, Esq.

C. P. Magra, Esq.

b

Lady Montfort.
W. H. Merle, Esq.
Captain James Mangles, R.N., F.R.S.

Joseph Neeld, Esq., M.P., F.S.A., F.L.S. *Large Paper.*
John Nicholls, Esq.
T. V. Nugent, Esq.

The Earl of Ormelie, M.P.
Viscount Ossulston, M.P.
Right Hon. Sir Gore Ouseley, Bart., G.C.H., F.R.S., F.S.A., F.R.A.S.
William Young Ottley, Esq., F.S.A.
B. F. Outram, M.D.
Benjamin Oakley, Esq.

Honourable William Ponsonby, M.P., F.R.S.
Count Ferdinand dal Pozzo.
Sir Francis Palgrave, K.H., F.R.S., F.S.A. Lond. & Ed.
Thomas Phillips, Esq., R.A., F.R.S., F.S.A.
John Story Penleaze, Esq., M.P.
Rev. George Peacock, M.A., F.R.S. *Large Paper.*
David Pollock, Esq., K.C., F.R.S., F.S.A. *Large Paper.*
Henry Perkins, Esq. *Large Paper.*
Right Hon. Lord Prudhoe, F.R.S., F.S.A.
Frederick Perkins, Esq. *Large Paper.*
George Henry Pettigrew, Esq. *Large Paper.*
Richard Percival, Jun., Esq., F.S.A.
James Prior, Esq., F.S.A.
Louis Hayes Petit, Esq., M.A., F.R.S., F.S.A.
Thomas Ponton, Esq., F.S.A.
Charles Pugh, Esq.
Samuel Poynder, Esq. *Large Paper.*
James Cowles Prichard, M.D., F.R.S.
John Propert, Esq.

The Earl of Rosebery, D.C.L., F.R.S.
R. Richardson, M.D.
H. S. Roots, M.D.
George Rennie, Esq., F.R.S.
Samuel Rogers, Esq., F.R.S., F.S.A.
John Rouse, Esq., F.S.A.
J. Evans Riadore, Esq., F.L.S.
William Reid, Esq.
Cuthbert Rippon, Esq. *Large Paper.*
Captain Robert Richardson.
Joseph Rumer, Esq.
Mrs. Anne Russell.

Edward Rudge, Esq., F.R.S., F.S.A., F.L.S.
Large Paper.
Sir William Rawlins, Knt.

His Grace the Duke of Somerset, D.C.L., F.R.S., F.S.A. P.R.I., F.L.S.
Earl Spencer, K.G., F.R.S., F.S.A.
Sir George Thomas Staunton, Bart., D.C.L., F.R.S., F.S.A., F.L.S.
Sir John E. Swinburne, Bart., F.R.S., F.S.A.
Sir Walter Stirling, Bart.
Sir Martin Archer Shee, P.R.A., F.R.S.
E. Ayshford Sanford, Esq., M.P., F.R.S. *Large Paper.*
A. R. Sutherland, M.D., F.R.S., F.G.S.
James Craig Somerville, M.D., F.G.S.
William James Smith, Esq.
Thomas Field Savory, Esq.
Philip J. Salomons, Esq., F.S.A.
John Spurgin, M.D.
Sutton Sharp, Esq. F.S.A.
R. A. Stafford, Esq.
B. G. Snow, Esq.
Henry Sass, Esq.
Samuel Smith, Esq.
T. A. Stone, Esq.
John Smirnove, Esq., F.R.S., F.L.S.
John Shakespear, Esq., F.R.A.S.
Thomas R. Smith, Esq.
Thomas Snodgrass, Esq., F.R.S. *Large Paper.*
Thomas Saunders, Esq., F.S.A. *Large Paper.*
John Sweatman, Esq.
J. S. Stevens, Esq.
Joseph Sams.
A. J. Stephens, Esq., F.R.S.
Samuel Sotheby, Esq.
R. C. Scarlett, Esq.
Christopher Stanger. M.D.

Right Honourable Lord Tenterden.
Sir Matthew Tierney, Bart., M.D., K.C.H.
J. Ruddell Todd, Esq., M.P., F.R.A.S.
Dawson Turner, Esq., F.R.S., F.S.A., M.R.I.A.
Large Paper.
Charles Hampden Turner, F.R.S., F.L.S., F.G.S.
Augustus U. Thiselton, Esq.
E. W. Tuson, Esq., F.L.S.
Honoratus Leigh Thomas, Esq., F.R.S.
P. P. Thoms, Esq.

William Thomson, Esq.
Martin Tupper, Esq.
Lieut. General Thornton
Charles Kemeys Tynte, Esq., M.P.
Colonel Tuffnel.
William Tite, Esq., Sec. Lond. Inst.

David Uwins, M.D.
Edward V. Utterson, Esq., F.S.A.

George Vance, Esq.
B. L. Vulliamy, Esq.
Lewis Vulliamy, Esq.
James Veitch, M.D.

Right Hon. and Rev. Lord Ward.   *Large Paper.*
Richard Westmacott, Esq., R.A., F.S.A.
David Wilkie, Esq., R.A.
Lieutenant Colonel Thomas Wildman.
Charles Winn, Esq.   *Large Paper.*

Frederick Webb, Esq., F.R.S., F.S.A.   *Large Paper.*
Martin Ware, Esq.
Edwin Wheatley Wight, Esq.
George Wallace, Esq.
J. G. Wilkinson, Esq., M.A.   *Large Paper.*
Sir William Woods, F.S.A.
James Wigram, Esq., F.S.A.
George Walford, Esq.
Thomas Walshman, M.D.
Lawrence Walker, Esq.
Isaac Wilson, M.D., F.R.S.
John Warburton, M.D.   *Large Paper.*
George Woodfall, Esq., F.S.A.
Bowes Wright, Esq.
Ralph Watson, Esq., F.R.S., F.S.A.
Samuel Weld, Esq.

George William Young, Esq.
Charles M. Young, Esq.

CONTENTS.

———

			Page
INTRODUCTION	.	.	xv
CHAP. I.	On Mummy	.	1
II.	On Mummy as a Drug	.	7
III.	On the Theology of the Ancient Egyptians, and Funeral Ceremonies of Different Nations	.	13
IV.	On Egyptian Tombs	.	23
V.	On Embalming	.	43
VI.	On the Medicaments employed in Embalming	.	75
VII.	On the Bandages	.	89
VIII.	On the Egyptian Idols, Amulets, Ornaments, &c.	.	103
IX.	On the Cases and Sarcophagi	.	115
X.	On the Papvri Manuscripts	.	131
XI.	On the Physical History of the Egyptians	.	155
XII.	On the Sacred Animals embalmed by the Egyptians	.	169
XIII.	On the Sacred Animals—the Mammalia	.	183
XIV.	——————————the Aves	.	202
XV.	——————————Amphibia—Pisces—Insecta	.	211
XVI.	On Deceptive Specimens of Mummies	.	227
XVII.	On the Guanches—the Mummies of Peru—the Desiccated Bodies at Palermo—the Burman Embalmings	.	231
XVIII.	On Modern Embalmings	.	252
	Explanation of the Plates	.	261

INTRODUCTION.

WITHIN the range of archæological enquiry there can scarcely be a subject of greater curiosity or interest than that which relates to the preservation of the remains of mankind of so early a period as were the first inhabitants of Egypt. The practice of embalming the dead is deeply interesting, were it to rest upon its antiquity alone; but when it is considered in relation to the history of the human species, and to the condition of the arts and sciences of so remote a period, it rises in importance, and it is remarkable that there should not exist in any language, as far as I have been able to ascertain, any work devoted expressly to the treating of this subject in all its branches. The matter to be gleaned from various travellers and enquirers is most extensively diffused, and I trust I am neither trifling with my own time nor that of my readers in having endeavoured to collect together all that I could rely upon in connexion with every branch of the enquiry, and making such humble additions as the objects of research and investigation, which have chanced to fall in my way, have afforded me an opportunity of doing.

I had the gratification of knowing the lamented Belzoni, that most intrepid and enterprising traveller, and by his kindness I was present at the opening of three mummies. I also witnessed the unrolling of a mummy at the Royal Institution, which was presented to the Royal Asiatic Society by the late Sir John Malcolm, and I have lately examined several mummies. The finest and most interesting specimen I have met with is accurately pourtrayed in the frontispiece to this work, and was brought from Egypt (Thebes, I think) for the purpose of sale, without any history whatever being attached to it, and enclosed in a case not coeval with the mummy, but made up, as I believe, merely for the convenience of transportation into this country. This specimen had even been deprived of its outer rollers and bandages; but the dry state of those that remained, together with the evidences of their being genuine, induced me to become the purchaser of the mummy, and to be sanguine as to the result of its examination. In this I have certainly not been disappointed; for, of all the instances on record, there is nothing to compare with it in point of perfection or interest. The particulars of the examination will be recorded in various parts of this work; but it may be as well here just to premise a few remarks.

For the convenience of accommodating a few friends whom I had invited to witness the interesting exhibition of bringing to light the form which had been hidden for perhaps two or three thousand years, I undertook the task at the Charing Cross Hospital on the 6th of April, 1833, in the presence of Prince Cimitile, Viscount Boring-don, Lord Hotham, Lord Henley, Sir Henry Halford, Bart., Sir David Barry, Drs. Shearman, Copland, Sayer, Crawford, Richardson, Elliotson, Clutterbuck, Golding, &c., Messrs. Barrow, Lockhart, Gage, Hawkins, Barnwell, H. Bosanquet, L. H. Petit, Cabbell, Ottley, Douce, Delafield, Lemon, Westmacott, Howard, &c. &c. The more immediate envelopes of the mummy, as I have stated, alone remained; I was therefore unable to observe those peculiarities in the mode of bandaging which have been noticed by M. Jomard, Dr. Granville, and some other writers. It was a task of no little difficulty, and required considerable force to separate the layers of bandage from the body. These consisted of envelopes of cloth extending from the head to the feet, under the soles of which they were wrapped up, and there presented a fringed appearance. Between the cloths, a quantity of pitchy matter had been applied in a heated state, so that it was impossible to separate them from each other, and levers were absolutely necessary to raise the bandages, and develope the body. This, however, was most effectively and perfectly done—the feet were first made out, the soles of which were perfectly soft and yielded to the impression of my nails. The nails of the toes were all entire, and the upper surfaces of the feet were found to have been gilt— the same occurred on the legs, thighs, abdomen, chest, and head. The specimen was ascertained to be that of a male, and from its appearance rather of an advanced age— the beard was perfect and full, the hairs being about half an inch in length. It was of a reddish-brown colour, and similar in appearance to the hair of the head, which was scanty in quantity. The colour of the whole body was of a brownish black, and on various places it could be perceived that a quantity of resinous varnish had been smeared and applied while hot.

By the kindness of Thomas Saunders, Esq., I opened a mummy purchased by him at the same time that I obtained the previous specimen. This was enclosed in two cases. The mummy, a female, was destroyed by the excessive heat with which the applications had been made, and the bandages were literally burnt to tinder.

My excellent friend Dr. John Lee, of Doctors' Commons, also purchased a specimen at the same sale as the former had been obtained at, and with great kindness gave me liberty to do whatever I thought proper with it. Accordingly, on the 24th of June, 1833, and in the presence of Dr. Lee, M. Rifaud, Mr. Fisher, Mr. Bowes Wright, Dr. Forbes, Dr. Richardson, Mr. Davidson, and Mr. Burgon, all of whom had visited

Egypt, and honoured also by the attendance of the Bishop of Chichester, Viscount Ossulston, Mr. Phillips, R. A., Mr. Douce, Mr. Renouard, Mr. Dawson Turner, Mr. Hawkins, Mr. Barnwell, Captain Dillon, the Rev. Mr. Baber, and a few other friends, I examined this mummy. I should premise that it was enclosed in two cases (represented in Plates IX and X), and was in a very sound and dry condition. The bandages were very neatly applied, and were of a fine texture. The unrolling was a work of great ease. Every variety of form best adapted to preserve the shape of the body and fill up all spaces was adopted.   Occasionally a whole length would be found passing from the feet along one side, over the head, down the other side, and crossing into the previous fold at the feet. Two portions were even split to allow of the feet passing through them. Between the legs and thighs large portions which surgeons would call compresses were placed, and the two limbs were then bound closely together. In this, as in all the instances I have witnessed, as you approach nearer to the body the bandages become of a coarser texture, and that immediately in contact with the body is the coarsest of all. The body was that of a female, and the mode of embalming by incision into the left flank was apparent.

On the 13th of July, 1833, I assisted my friend John Davidson, Esq., to unroll a mummy that had been brought from Thebes by Mr. Henderson. This was done at the Royal Institution in the presence of the Duke of Somerset, the President, and a very large attendance of the members of the Institution and other literary and scientific characters. Mr. Davidson delivered an exceedingly interesting lecture* on the occasion, to which I shall feel it necessary to refer in the course of this work. The mummy was that of a female, and enclosed within a very highly ornamented case. The bandages were more abundant than in any I had previously seen, and of a fine texture: they were indeed so pure, so dry, and had altogether such an air of freshness about them, that many were disposed to suspect the genuineness of the specimen; of this, however, there can be no doubt, as the references I shall make to it will abundantly show.

A few years since I purchased at a sale by auction a fine specimen of a sycamore sarcophagus, which contained the remains of a mummy. This formerly belonged to that ingenious but eccentric artist Mr. Cosway, R. A., and I have since found that it was the specimen brought into this country by Dr. Perry, and particularly described and figured by him in his Travels in the Levant. † Of this mummy he gives an elaborate account. It was found by the Arabs of Saccara in the catacombs of the adjacent mountain two months before he and his fellow-travellers left Cairo, and was looked

---

* Since printed but not published. It is entitled " An Address on Embalming generally."

† View of the Levant, particularly of Constantinople, Syria, Egypt, and Greece, by Charles Perry, M. D. fol. Lond. 1743.

c

upon by some of the oldest dwellers there, who were familiar with the various objects of antiquity, to be the most curious of the kind ever obtained, with but one exception Dr. Perry resolved upon purchasing it, and it was sent to London in the year 1741. I have reduced the 18th Plate in Dr. Perry's work, and corrected the hieroglyphics upon the sarcophagus, in order to give a representation of this truly magnificent case, and to enable the reader to comprehend the references I shall have occasion to make to it. (See Plate VI., *fig.* 4.) Having removed the mummy from the case, I found it in a very decayed state. The flesh had been burnt up by the rapidity with which the process of embalming had been conducted, and the bones were rendered exceedingly brittle. I have obtained only the skull and the vertebræ of the neck entire. The former is remarkable from having a bony tumour (an exostosis) extending along the outer side of the right orbit, and affecting even the cheek (malar) bone.

I have also had the opportunity of witnessing, at the Mechanics' Institution, the unrolling of an adult female mummy belonging to Mr. Reeder, in which the process of desiccation appears to have been adopted previously to the application of the bandages, as there literally remained nothing beyond the dry skin and bones; and, to show that the body had been subjected to heat, I may mention that the bones had all their fatty matter withdrawn from them, and were rendered exceedingly brittle and quite white. The inside of the body was filled with earthy matter. Each limb had been separately bandaged.

In addition to these I have had, through the kindness of Mr. Wilkinson, the opportunity of examining three heads brought from Thebes; and I owe to the liberality of the President and Council of the Royal College of Surgeons the permission to examine a mummy brought from Thebes in 1820 by Mr. Henderson, at the same time as that of Mr. Davidson, and, I believe, taken from the same tomb. I notice this circumstance here in order to remark that the mode of preparation adopted in both these instances was precisely similar: both were furnished with artificial eyes, had necklaces of the same materials, and a scarabæus on the breast. They were also unfortunately both much injured by the heated state of the embalming material when applied to them. The cases containing these mummies were also of a similar description. Mr. Davidson has done ample justice to that which contained his specimen. That of the College naturally attracted my attention, and when, from an examination of the hieroglyphic characters marked upon it, I declared its inhabitant to have been a priest of the temple of Ammon, I was assailed by not a few with ridicule, the face painted upon the case being so delicate and strongly resembling that of a female. To satisfy myself upon this subject, I solicited from the council of the College the loan of some drawings of the case which had been some years since very carefully executed by Mr. Clift, jun., under the inspection of his father, William Clift, Esq., the very respected and intelligent conservator of the Museum. By the assistance of Mr. Wilkinson I was enabled to make out very satisfactorily, not only that the mummy contained within the case was that of a priest of the temple I have mentioned, but that he was of an inferior order of the priesthood (an incense bearer), and that his name was Horseisi, and the son of Naspihiniegori of the same grade and profession; and, having ascertained this, I was desirous not only on account of my own reputation, but for the verification of hieroglyphical literature, to have the case opened and the matter determined. The council of the College most liberally assented to my request,* and honoured me by their invitation to perform this in the theatre of the College in the presence of the members and a large assemblage of distinguished literary and scientific characters, who did me the honour to attend upon the occasion. One circumstance only dwelt upon my mind as likely to cause a possible disappointment—the occurrence of, by any accident, a body having been substituted for the one originally intended. Upon opening the case, however, the first thing that presented itself was a singular identification of the individual, by having a fillet of linen loosely folded round the legs, on which were inscribed the hieroglyphical characters denoting the name and profession of the deceased. In the course of the unrolling of the mummy I found this inscription repeated, with slight variations, no less than four times; and it is worthy of remark, as showing the hieroglyphics to have been used with great freedom and as a kind of tachygraphy, that in one instance the hieroglyphics denoting some of the letters were left out, thus abridging the name, as would be likely to occur in any rapid writing of the present day. It is sufficient to observe that the result of the examination justified the prediction I had given—the particulars of the investigation will be found in their proper places in this work. †

Although I believe I have acknowledged the obligations I owe to many friends in the different parts of this work for various information they have been so kind as to favour me with, I cannot omit here to express my most sincere thanks in an especial manner to J. G. Wilkinson, Esq., whose knowledge of Egyptian antiquities and hieroglyphical literature exceeds, I believe, that of any other individual of the present day, for many valuable observations and suggestions he has favoured me with. Nor am I less indebted to Dr. Richardson, Mr. Davidson, Dr. Lee, Captain Mangles, Captain

---

* I regret to have here to state conduct of an opposite nature on the part of the Trustees of the British Museum, to whom I made application to be permitted to examine one or two of the specimens contained in that *national* establisment. The Trustees were of opinion that it would destroy the *integrity* of the collection!

† I wish here to correct one point mentioned in the Postscript to Chapter V., in which it is stated that the viscera were found wrapped up in three portions in the cavity of the belly. After I had drawn up the account, a fourth portion was found imbedded in some of the earthy matter with which the body was filled. These are all preserved in the Museum of the College.

Henvey, and others who have travelled in Egypt; to Dr. Ure for the communication respecting the textile fibre of the bandages; to the Rev. W. F. Hope for his illustrations of the new species of insects I found in the head of a mummy; to Captain Coke for the (I believe hitherto undescribed) account of the embalming of the Burman priests; and to Mr. Kirkmann and Mr. Burgon for information relative to the medals found in and upon Egyptian and Græco-Egyptian mummies. I am also indebted to the curators of the Royal College of Surgeons for their permission to figure the Peruvian mummy contained in the College Museum, and to the Trustees of the British Museum for the copy of the Portrait in Plate VII. To Samuel Rogers, Esq., my best thanks are due for permitting me to represent the Funereal Tablets and the interesting figures of Isis and the infant Horus in Plate VIII. To Dr. Lee I am indebted for Plates IX. and X. representing the inner and outer cases of his mummy, and to Mons. Passalacqua for the drawings of the Sacred Barge in Plate III., various embalmed animals in Plates XII. and XIII., all taken from the Collection at Berlin; and I must here also acknowledge my obligations to my friend Dr. Alexander Henderson for his kind superintendance of this matter. I am also glad to have an opportunity of expressing my satisfaction at the fidelity with which my very ingenious and talented artist Mr. George Cruikshank has executed the various drawings for the work, and the great spirit with which he has etched them.

After the preceding pages of this introduction had been committed to the press, I received an obliging invitation to attend the unrolling of a male Egyptian mummy in the Museum of the London University, to which collection it was presented by James Morrison, Esq., M. P. The body had not been embalmed in the best manner, but sufficient attention had been paid to its preservation to display the form and features of the individual. According to the hieroglyphics on and within the case in which it was contained, it appears to have been the mummy of KANNOPOS or CANNOPUS, the son of Osiri-Pasht, and Tatiosiri or Tattiosiri or Tattosiri. The name Cannopus has no relation to the word NOUB (gold), but is taken from the word CANOP, which appears to signify *strength* or *power, victory,* or something of similar import, being among the beneficent gifts of the gods to the kings mentioned in the hieroglyphics: nor is this name Cannopus related to the city of that name in the Delta. The bandages of the mummy were in good preservation; but presented nothing remarkable, with the exception of the name of the individual, which was repeated in five or six places in various ways, and giving a date of the seventeenth year; but the application of this, either to the age of the individual embalmed, or to the sovereign during whose reign he lived, is uncertain; the latter conjecture I believe to be the most probable. No cartouche to show under what dynasty the Egyptian had his existence appears upon the case to guide us in the enquiry. One of the names on the bandages was written KANNOP, on another

KNNP, and on another *Knps* or *Kanopos* (the final *s* is the Greek termination), followed by the figure of a man. This mode of abbreviating the name agrees with that noticed on the bandages of the mummy of Horseisi, and appears to me to prove very satisfactorily the stages of the preparation of the mummy. Different series of rollers were applied at different times; and, to prevent mistakes, at the end (for it is always at the termination of the bandage), the name of the individual is inscribed either at length or curtailed, to denote the individual subject contained.

In this mummy the intestines and other viscera had been removed by the usual incision in the left flank, and portions of the viscera imbedded in some embalming material were found enclosed within the enveloping bandages both upon the legs and thighs. I have never before met with this. In the mummy of Horseisi at the College of Surgeons, and that of Mr. Davidson (now by the kindness of that gentleman deposited in my collection), the viscera had been returned into the cavity of the abdomen in four distinct portions, each separately enveloped in its proper bandages. The inside of the body of Kannopus was filled with the dust of some wood, probably cassia. The brain had not been extracted through the nostrils, but the residue of it was found as a mass lying at the hind part of the skull. The head had been shaved. The cavities of the external ears were filled with portions of linen cloth, by which their shape was well preserved. The orbits were also filled with linen, and in one it was observed that the transparent part of the eye was attempted to be represented. No amulet, necklace, or ornament of any kind was discovered, nor were there any marks by which the character or profession of the deceased could be ascertained. The body measured five feet two inches.

A

HISTORY OF MUMMIES.

CHAPTER I.

ON MUMMY.

Etymology of the term Mummy—allusions to its Qualities—Abd'Allatif's description of natural Mummy—the opinions of Dioscorides, Serapion, Bomare, Sir William Ouseley, and Kæmpfer on this subject.

THE word MUMMY has been variously derived. Bochart, Menage, Vossius, and others have derived it from the Arabic noun موم *mum*, meaning wax; and Avicenna defines it thus: "Mum purum est parietes domorum apum in quibus faciunt ova et pullos et advenit in eis mel."* But Salmasius derives it from *amomum*, a kind of perfume. Some authors believe the Arabic word مومیا, *mumia*, to signify a body embalmed or aromatised.

The Persian word مومیا, *múmiyà*, means bitumen, or mineral pitch, the

---

* Avicennæ Opera, lib. ii., tract. 2, cap. 473.

B

PISSASPHALTOS, which is generally found in the bodies embalmed by the ancient Egyptians.

The term mummy is mostly applied to the body embalmed, not to the embalming ingredients, and in such sense I shall employ it throughout this work.

Vossius explains mummy to mean the flesh of man preserved against corruption in balsam or myrrh, and aloes, and asphalt. Turton describes it as a bituminous liquor of the consistence of wax, found in sepulchres in which bodies have been embalmed.

In allusion to its qualities of softness, durability, power of preservation, &c., it has been employed by many writers in various ways.

As implying *softness* :

> *Tib.*—" You shall grow *mummy*, rascals."
> > *Beaumont and Fletcher.   The Sea Voyage, Act III., Scene 1.*

> " Let some soft *mummy* of a peer, who stains
> > His rank, some sodden lump of ass's brains,
> > To that abandon'd wretch his sanction give ;
> > Support his slander, and his wants relieve !"

> > > *Falconer.   The Demagogue.*

> *Falstaff.*—" I had been drown'd, but that the shore was shelvy and shallow ; a death that I abhor ; for the water swells a man ; and what a thing should I have been, when I had been swell'd !   I should have been a mountain of *mummy*."
> > *Merry Wives of Windsor.   Act III., Scene 5.*

As denoting *permanency—durability* :

> " Thy virtues are
> The spices that embalm thee ; thou art far
> More richly laid, and shalt more long remain
> Still *mummified* within the hearts of men,
> Than if to lift thee in the rolls of fame
> Each marble spoke thy shape, all brass thy name."

> > *J. Hale's Poems* (1646), p. 50.

Probably in the sense of *durability* or *preservation*, it is used by Shakspeare when he makes Othello to describe the charmed handkerchief.

" A sibyl, that had number'd in the world,
The sun to make two hundred compasses,
In her prophetick fury sew'd the work :
The worms were hallow'd, that did breed the silk ;
And it was dy'd in *mummy* which the skilful
Conserv'd of maiden's hearts."

The Moor of Venice. Act III., Scene 4.

Abd'Allatif, an Arabian physician who flourished in the twelfth century, describes mummy, properly so called, to be a substance that flows down from the tops of mountains, and which, mixing with the waters that carry it down, coagulates like mineral pitch, and exhales an odour resembling that of white (Burgundy) pitch and bitumen. " Quant à la momie," says this author, as translated by Silvestre De Sacy, " proprement dite, c'est une substance qui découle du sommet des montagnes, mêlée avec les eaux qui l'entraînent ; elle se coagule ensuite comme la poix minérale, et exhale une odeur de poix blanche mêlée avec du bitume. Suivant Galien, la momie sort de source comme la poix minérale et la naphte ; d'autres disent que la momie est une variété de poix minérale, et on la nomme *menstrues des montagnes*. Cette momie qu'on trouve dans les cavités des cadavres en Egypte, s'éloigne peu de la nature de la momie minérale, et l'on peut en substituer l'usage à celui de la momie minérale, quand on a de la peine à s'en procurer."* But the learned translator in a note,† expresses his doubts as to the correctness of the reference to Galen, and hints that the description may have been taken from Dioscorides. This most likely has been the case ; for in looking into the writings of Serapion, who compiled his *Historia Simplicium Medicamentorum*‡ from the works of the Arabian and Greek physicians, especially those of Paulus Ægineta, Dioscorides, and Galen, I find the following citation from Dioscorides, under the head *De Pissasphalto*. " Vocatur et in bituminis genere Pissasphaltus, quasi pici-bitumen dicas composita ex pice et bitumine re et rei appellatione. Nascitur ad Apolloniam quæ in Epiro est, fluminumque impetu ex Cerauniis montibus delatum in litora eructatur, glebarum modo concretum, odore picis bitumini mistæ. Potest Picibitumen omnia quæ

* Relation de L'Egypte, 4to. Paris, 1810. Page 201.　　† No. 133, p. 271.
‡ Edit. fol. Venet. 1552.

possunt mista simul Pix et Bitumen."* Again, in another work of the same author, *De Simplici Medicina*,† I find the following extract from Dioscorides under the head *Mumie*. "Mumia est in terris Apolloniæ: descendit namque ex montibus, qui ducunt flumina cum aqua, et ejicit eam aqua fluminis in ripis, et est coagulata, et fit sicut cera, et habet odorem picis mixtæ cum asphalto cum aliquo fœtore: et virtus ejus est, sicut picis, et asphalti mixtorum.‡

Ibn Baïtár says that "the Múmiyá of the tombs, found in great quantities in Egypt, is nothing more than the amalgam anciently used by the Greeks to preserve their dead bodies from putrefaction." He says also that the term Múmiá is given to a kind of light black stone found near Sen'á in Yemen, and which contains a black fluid substance in a small cavity.

Bomare§ gives an interesting note on the subject of liquid pitch from the mountains: " Gemelli Carreri dit que sur la route de Schiras à Bender-Congo, l'on voit la montagne de Darap, toute de pierre noire, d'où distille le fameux *baume-momie*, lequel devient noir en s'épaississant (du Pissasphalte, ou Asphalte). C'est le plus réputé en Perse; la montagne est gardée par ordre du Sophi; tous les ans les Visirs de Geaxoux, de Schiras et de Lar, vont ensemble ramasser le *baume-momie* qui coule et tombe dans une conque où il se coagule; on n'en tire pas plus de quarante onces chaque année; ils l'envoient au Sophi sous leur cachet. On voit au Cabinet du Roi les deux boîtes d'or remplies de ce bitume ou *baume-momie* que l'Ambassadeur de Perse apporta et presenta à *Louis XIV*; une autre boîte en argent, pleine de ce même bitume, fut donnée au Prince de Condé, on la voit dans le Cabinet de Chantilly. Ce présent n'avoit de mérité que dans l'opinion de ceux qui l'ont offert. L'ambassadeur de Perse dit a *Louis XIV*, que le *baume-momie* étoit un spécifique pour les fractures des os, et généralement pour toutes les blessures; qu'il étoit employé pour les maladies et ulcères tant internes qu'externes; en un mot, qu'il avoit la propriété de faire sortir le fer qui pourroit être resté dans les blessures. Ce fameux *baume-momie* qui est une espéce de *poix minérale*, distille des rochers en beaucoup d'autres contrées."

* Page 101.   † Fol. Venet. 1503.   ‡ Page 138.   § Dictionnaire
d'Histoire Naturelle, 8vo., Lyon, 1791. tom. VIII. p. 542.

The account given by Sir William Ouseley* confirms in many particulars that just quoted. Sir William visited the Mummy Mountain (Kíeh Múmiáy) in the territory of Darábgerd in Persia. He fancied that it presented a darker appearance than the mountains adjacent to it. He says the mummy is a blackish bituminous matter, which oozes from the rock, and is considered by the Persians as far more precious than gold; for it heals cuts and bruises, as they affirm, almost immediately, causes fractured bones to unite in a few minutes, and, taken inwardly, is a sovereign remedy for many diseases. Sir William informed some of those who were thus describing to him the miraculous efficacy of the mummy that, after an experiment made on the broken leg of a fowl at Shiráz, Mr. Sharp, the surgeon, had declared that in his opinion the application of any common bitumen would have been attended with the same effect; but this they disbelieved, and asserted that mummy of an inferior quality might have been employed. Sir William quotes from a manuscript work of the tenth century (Súr al beldán) in which the mountain is described, and states that the mummy was gathered for the king, and that numerous officers were commissioned to guard it; that once in every year they opened the door of the cavern, in which was a stone, perforated with a small hole, and in this the mummy was found collected. The produce of the year amounted only to a portion of the size of a pomegranate, and it was sealed up in the presence of priests, magistrates, &c., and deposited in the Royal Treasury. This substance is also alluded to by other oriental writers, referred to by Sir William Ouseley, who concludes his account by stating that the eastern princes, both the giver and receiver, esteem a very small portion as a present of considerable value.

Mirza Abu'l Hassan brought to the Queen of England, in 1809, a portion of this mummy as a present from the King of Persia. The Empress of Russia received a like present, about an ounce, in a gold box.† A man at Isfáhán demanded nine tománs (about eight pounds sterling), and would not accept less, from a gentleman of Sir William Ouseley's party, for as much as could be contained within a common-sized walnut shell.‡

* Travels, vol. II. p. 117.

† See M. de Ferrières Sauvebœuf Mem. Hist. &c., des Voyages., tom. II. p. 33. Paris, 1790.

‡ For further information on this subject, the reader may consult Kæmpferi, Amœnitates

Kæmpfer states it as a popular opinion that the ancient Egyptians preserved the bodies of their Princes and chief personages by means of the
natural mummy; for which they afterwards substituted, under the same
name, a compound aromatic balsam.*

The resemblance and supposed identity of the natural Mummy to the
bituminous preparation found in the embalmed bodies of the Egyptians
doubtless contributed to maintain its character and to enhance its value in
the estimation of the Arabs.

Exoticæ, pp. 517, 519. Chardin's Travels. Voyages de Corneille Le Brun, Tom. I. p. 231.
fol. Amst. 1718. Fryer's Travels, p. 318, and Father Angelo (Gazophylac. Pers.) p. 234.

* Amœnit. Exot. p. 520.

CHAPTER II.

ON MUMMY AS A DRUG.

Its use as a Drug—its introduction by Elmagar, a Jewish Physician—deceptions practised —Guy de la Fontaine's enquiries as to the supply of real Mummy—the demand for it, especially in France—Superstition of François I.—Opinions of various Authors as to the virtues of Mummy—Avicenna—Lord Bacon—Boyle—Olaus Wormius—Grew—Lemery —Ambrose Paré—Anecdote from Guyon, to account for the suspension of the traffic and cessation of the employment of Mummy in Medicine.

In the sixteenth and part of the seventeenth centuries, mummy formed one of the ordinary drugs, and was to be found in the shops of all apothecaries, and considerable sums of money were expended in the purchase of it, principally from the Jews in the East. No sooner was it credited that mummy constituted an article of value in the practice of medicine than many speculators embarked in the trade; the tombs were searched, and as many mummies as could be obtained were broken into pieces for the purpose of sale. The demand, however, was not easily supplied; for the government of Egypt was unwilling to permit the transportation of the bodies from their sepulchral habitation; too great temptation was thus created to the commission of fraud, and all kinds of impositions were in daily practice. According to the " Leçons de Guyon," as early as the year 1100, or as others say 1300, an expert Jewish physician named Elmagar, a native of Alexandria, was in the habit of prescribing mummy both for the Christians and the Mahometans, then in the East contending for the possession of Palestine. From that time, following the example thus set, physicians of all nations commonly prescribed it in cases of bruises and wounds. The asphalt and the bitumen it was contended consolidated and healed the broken and lacerated veins, and, its piquancy occasioning sickness, it was said to have the power of throwing off from the stomach collections of congealed blood. Some Jews entered upon a speculation to furnish the mummy thus brought into demand as an article of commerce, and undertook to embalm dead bodies and to sell them to the Christians. They took all the executed criminals, and bodies of all descriptions that could be obtained, filled the head and inside of the bodies with simple asphaltum, an article of very small price, made incisions into the muscular parts of the limbs, inserted into them also the asphaltum and then bound them up tightly. This being done, the bodies were exposed to the heat of the sun ; they dried quickly, and resembled in appearance the truly prepared mummies. These were sold to the Christians.

Guy De la Fontaine, physician to the king of Navarre, took a journey into Egypt, and being at Alexandria in 1564 he made enquiries as to the supply of mummy as a drug. He communicated the result of his enquiries to his friend Ambrose Paré, the celebrated French surgeon, who made known the particulars to the public through the medium of his works. It appears that De la Fontaine sought out the principal Jew concerned in this traffic, and requested to see his collection of mummies. This was very willingly granted, and several bodies heaped one on the other were speedily shown to him. Enquiring as to the places whence they had been obtained, and anxious to know whether that which the ancients had written respecting the treatment of the dead and their mode of sepulture could be confirmed, the Jew laughed at him and hesitated not to say that all the bodies then before them, amounting to between thirty and forty, had been prepared by him during the last four years, and that they were the bodies of slaves or other persons indiscriminately collected. De la Fontaine then enquired as to what nation they belonged, and whether they had died of any horrible disease, such as leprosy, the small pox, or the plague, to which the Jew replied that he cared not whence they came, whether they were old or young, male or female, or of what disease they had died, so long as he could obtain them, for that when embalmed no one could tell, and added that he himself marvelled how the Christians, so dainty mouthed, could eat of the bodies of the dead. The Jew then detailed to De la Fontaine the mode of embalming adopted by him, which was in agreement with that just alluded to by M. Guyon.

The demand for mummy was greater in France than in any other country, and François I. is stated by Belon* to have been in the habit o always carrying about with him a little packet containing some mummy mixed with pulverised rhubarb, ready to take upon receiving any injury from falls, or other accidents that might happen to him. Armed with this universal remedy, François I. thought himself secure against all danger.

The medicinal use of mummy is alluded to by Shirley the dramatist :—

" Make *mummy* of my flesh, and sell me to the apothecaries."

The Bird in a Cage (1633).

" That I might tear their flesh in mammocks, raise
My losses, from their carcases turn'd *mummy*."

The Honest Lawyer (1616).

Avicenna, one of the most celebrated physicians of antiquity, treats of the use of mummy in medicine. He describes it thus : " Mumia calida est in fine [tertii] sicca prout creditur in primo. Inest autem ei proprietas omnem spiritum confortandi (quod adijuvat continuativa viscositas)."† He says it is subtle and resolutive, useful in cases of abscesses and eruptions, fractures, concussions, paralysis, hemicrania, epilepsy, vertigo, spitting of blood from the lungs, affections of the throat, coughs, palpitation of the heart, debility of the stomach, nausea, disorders of the liver and spleen, internal ulcers, also in cases of poisons.‡ For contusions he speaks of it as the best of all remedies. " De medicinis autem quas oportet sumere illum, qui patitur contusionem, aut offensionem, aut casum melior, et antecedens est mumia pura cum oleo nominato sambacino et vino."§ It is prescribed to be taken in decoctions of marjoram, thyme, elder, barley, roses, lentils, jujubes, cummin seed, carraway, saffron, cassia, parsley, with oxymel, wine, milk, butter, castor, syrup of mulberries, &c.

Lord Bacon says,‖ " Mummy hath great force in staunching of blood ;

* Observations de Plusieurs Singularitez, et Choses Memorables, &c. p. 261.
† De Viribus Cordis. Tom. II. p. 348, fol. ed. Venet. apud Juntas, 1608.
‡ Tom. I. lib. ii. p. 357.   § Tom. I. lib. iv. p. 151.
‖ Sylva Sylvarum, Cant. X. s. 980.

which, as it may be ascribed to the mixture of balmes that are glutinous, so it may also partake of a secret propriety, in that the blood draweth man's flesh."

"Mummy," says Boyle, "is one of the useful medicines commended and given by our physicians for falls and bruises, and in other cases too."*

Olaus Wormius speaks of mummy as beneficial in contusions, clodded blood, hard labour, &c.† But the sagacious Grew says, "Let them see to it, that dare trust to old gums, which have long since lost their virtue."§

Lemery‖ describes mummy as detersive, vulnerary, and resolutive, capable of resisting gangrene, good for contusions, and preventing the blood from coagulating in the body. He was alive to the deceptions practised in this article during his time, and gives directions for the choice of the " véritable mumie d'Egypte."

In the Pharmacopœia Schrodero-Hoffmanniana¶ are several formulæ of mummy as a drug, such as 1. Tinctura s. extract. mumiæ Quercetan. 2. Tinct. s. extr. mumiæ Crollii. 3. Tinct. alcalisata s. elix. mumiæ. 4. Alia tinct. seu arcan. carnis humanæ. 5. Ol. oliv. mumat. 6. Ol. exaltatum.

Ambrose Paré has a chapter expressly upon " Mummie," under the division of Contusions and Gangrenes. He speaks of mummy as the means upon which most dependence was placed in his time ; but he states that neither the physicians who prescribe mummy, nor the authors that have written of it, nor the apothecaries who sell it, know any thing of certainty respecting it. After enumerating the opinions of Serapion, Avicenna, Dioscorides, his commentator Mathiolus, and Thevet, and showing the diversity of conjectures relative to it, he condemns its use in the following terms :—" This wicked kinde of drugge, doth nothing helpe the diseased, in that case, wherefore and wherein it is administered, as I have tryed an hundred times, and as *Thevet* witnesses, he tryed in himselfe when

---

* Boyle's Works, vol. II. p. 451.

† " Magnus ejus usus est ad contusiones, sanguinis grumos dissolvit, partum facilitat, spasmum et convulsiones juvat, omnia interna et externa vulnera, exulcerationes, aliaque ejus generis curat. Permiscent aliis, vel seorsim, drachmam dimidiam exhibent." Museum Wormianum, fol. Amst. 1655, p. 344.

§ Museum Regalis Societatis, fol. Lond. 1681, p. 3. ‖ Lemery (N.) Dictionnaire des Drogues Simples, 4to. Amst. 1716, p. 362. ¶ Fol. Genev. 1687, p. 609.

as hee tooke some thereof by the advice of a certaine Jewish physition in Egypt, from whence it is brought; but it also inferres many troublesome symptomes, as the paine of the heart or stomacke, vomiting, and stinke of the mouth." "I, perswaded by these reasons, doe not onely myselfe prescribe any hereof to my patients, but also in consultations, endeavour what I may, that it bee not prescribed by others."* It would be easy to multiply authorities in favour and against the use of mummy in medicine;† but it is time to draw this part of my subject to a close, and I shall do this by relating an anecdote upon the authority of Guyon to account for the suspension of the nefarious traffic in mummy. A Jew of Damietta, who was principally concerned in the manufacture of false mummies, had a Christian slave, for the safety of whose soul he appears to have entertained more concern than for his own, repeatedly urging him to abjure his religion and embrace that of the true faith; he at last insisted upon the slave submitting to the operation of circumcision as the evidence of his sincerity: this the slave resisted, and in consequence of his perverseness was very ill treated by his master. The slave represented to the pacha the practices of his master, and denounced him for the frauds he was committing in the making of mummies. The Jew was thrown into prison, from which he obtained his release on condition of the payment of no less a sum than three hundred sultanins of gold. When intelligence of this reached the governors of Alexandria, Rosetta, and other cities of Egypt, and the city of Aleppo, delighted with the prospect of readily obtaining so much money, they exacted a ransom from all those Jews who were merchants of mummies. From this time the traffic ceased; the Jews, fearful of being subjected to a new oppression, dared no longer to continue their trade.

It will thus be seen that the employment of mummy in medicine did not cease from any discovery of its inefficacy in the relief or cure of disease; but merely from the hazard with which the traffic in the substance must be

---

* The Workes of that famous Chirurgion Ambrose Parey, fol. Lond. 1634, p. 448.

† See a very sensible thesis on this subject by J. A. Gladbach, entitled "Diss. Inaug. de Mumiis in praxi Medica, 4to. Helmstad. 1735.—Also Lanzoni (I.) Tractatus de Balsamatione Cadaverum, 12mo. Genev. 1696.

carried on. The desiccated bodies of travellers lost in the desert, and buried beneath the sands, were equally with the mummies employed in medicine; and Roquefort tells us that the bodies of young girls were considered more efficacious than others, and therefore produced a larger price.

The Arabs to this day make use of mummy powder for a medicine. They mix it with butter and call it *mantey*.* It is esteemed as a sovereign remedy for bruises both external and internal.

* Madden's Travels in Turkey, Egypt, Nubia, and Palestine, vol. II. p. 90.

CHAPTER III.

ON THE THEOLOGY OF THE ANCIENT EGYPTIANS, AND FU-NERAL CEREMONIES OF DIFFERENT NATIONS.

The perfection of the art of embalming, as practised by the Egyptians, to be traced to their theology—Immortality of the soul—the Egyptians the first, according to Hèrodotus, to lay down this principle—transmigration of souls—Servius's Commentary on a passage of Virgil in relation to this subject—St. Augustine's opinion—Cicero on the Egyptian embalmings—Allusions to the practice by Sextus Empiricus—Pomponius Mela—Athanasius—Silius Italicus—Lucian—Mummies as a security—confirmation of this by Herodotus and Diodorus Siculus—practice of embalming by the Persians, Arabs, Jews, and Ethiopians—also by the Christians—embalming of Jacob—sepulture in the earth the most natural mode of disposing of the dead—funeral ceremonies of different nations—mode of preserving the bodies among the Persians, Syrians, Ancient Arabians, the Brazilians, Chinese, and Ethiopians.

THE desire of immortality is most strongly rooted in the mind of man, and innumerable means have in all ages, and under all circumstances, been devised to perpetuate his memory after death. In no part of the world does this principle appear to have acted so strongly as in Egypt, and its ancient inhabitants have not only built huge pyramids, and erected mighty temples and obelisks, covered with symbols, expressing, in hieroglyphical language, characters and events; but they have succeeded beyond all other ages and people in preserving from decay the remains of their own fragile frames. The extraordinary perfection to which they carried the art of embalming the dead is, perhaps, alone to be accounted for by referring to their theology. Believing in the immortality of the soul, the ancient Egyptians conceived that they were retaining the soul within the body as long as the form of the body could be preserved entire, or were facilitating the reunion of it with the body, at the day of resurrection, by preserving the body from corruption.

According to Herodotus :

" Πρῶτοι δὲ καὶ τόνδε τὸν λόγον Αἰγύπτιοί εἰσι οἱ εἰπόντες, ὡς ἀνθρώπου ψυχὴ ἀθάνατός ἐστι· τοῦ σώματος δὲ καταφθίνοντος, ἐς ἄλλο ζῶον αἰεὶ γινόμενον ἐσδύεται· ἐπεὰν δὲ περιέλθη, πάντα τὰ χερσαῖα καὶ τὰ θαλάσσια καὶ τὰ πετεινὰ, αὖτις ἐς ἀνθρώπου σῶμα γινόμενον ἐσδύνειν· τὴν περιήλυσιν δὲ αὐτῇ γίνεσθαι ἐν τρισχιλίοισι ἔτεσι. τούτῳ τῷ λόγῳ εἰσὶ οἳ Ἑλλήνων ἐχρήσαντο, οἱ μὲν, πρότερον, οἱ δὲ, ὕστερον, ὡς ἰδίῳ ἑωυτῶν ἐόντι· τῶν ἐγὼ εἰδὼς τὰ οὐνόματα, οὐ γράφω."

Herod. Hist. lib. ii. § 123.

" The Egyptians are also the first that laid down the principle of the immortality of the human soul ; and that, when the body is dissolved, the soul enters into some other animal which is born at the same time ; and that, after going the round of all the animals that inhabit the land, the waters, and the air, it again enters the body of a man which is then born. This circuit, they say, is performed by the soul in 3000 years. There are several among the Greeks who have adopted the above opinion as though it were an invention of their own, some in former and others in later times, whose names I do not mention, although I am not unacquainted with them."

Laurent's Translation.

Upon this passage the ingenious Larcher has the following comment : " Hérodote ne dit pas que les Egyptiens soient les premiers qui aient cru à l'immortalité de l'ame, mais qu'ils sont les premiers qui aient avancé que l'ame, étant immortelle, passoit après la destruction du corps dans celui de quelque animal. Je ne doute pas que les Egyptiens n'aient cru de tout temps à l'immortalité de l'ame. Il seroit aisé de prouver que Noë y croyoit. Ce dogme se perpétua dans sa famille. Mesraïm, son petit-fils, peupla l'Egypte. Ainsi l'immortalité de l'ame fut connue de tout temps dans ce pays."*

Those who held the doctrine of transmigration of souls would take extraordinary pains to preserve the body from putrefaction, in the hope of the soul again joining the body it had quitted. Servius, in his Commentary

---

* Histoire d'Hérodote, par Larcher, Tom. II. pp. 426, 427.

upon a passage of Virgil descriptive of the funeral of Polydorus, in the third Book of the Æneid.

> " animamque sepulchro
> Condimus,"

takes occasion to remark, on this subject, that " the Egyptians, skilful in wisdom, do keep their dead embalmed so much the longer, to the end that the soul may for a long while continue and be obnoxious to the body, lest it should quickly pass to another. The Romans, on the contrary, burned their dead, that the soul might speedily return into its own nature."*

Upon the practice of the Egyptians, St. Augustine† asserts that they alone believed the resurrection, because they carefully preserved their dead bodies; for (says he) *they have a custom of drying up the bodies and rendering them as durable as brass.* The account of Herodotus respecting the depositing of the embalmed bodies of their relatives in the habitations of the Egyptians is confirmed by various authors. Cicero says, they embalmed their dead and kept them at home.

> " Condiunt Ægyptii mortuos, et eos domi servant."
>
> *Tuscul. Quæst.* lib. i.

" Amongst themselves, and above ground," says Sextus Empiricus.

" Inter penetralia" (Pomponius Mela, lib. i., c. 9.)

" In lectulis," says Athanasius.

So also Silius Italicus, (lib. iii Punicorum.)

> Ægyptia tellus
> Claudit odorato post funus stantia saxo
> Corpora, et a mensis exanguem haud separat umbram.

---

* "Unde Ægyptii periti sapientiæ condita diutius reservant cadavera, scilicet ut anima multo tempore perduret, et corpori sit obnoxia, ne citò ad aliud transeat. Romani contra faciebant, comburentes cadavera, ut statim anima in generalitatem, id est, in suam naturam rediret."—*Servii Comment. in* lib. iii., *Æneid.*

† Augustini (Sti.) Sermones 120 de Diversis, cap. 12, thus :—" Ægyptii soli credunt resurrectionem, quia diligenter curant cadavera mortuorum : morem enim habent siccare corpora et quasi ænea reddere, *Gabbaras* ea vocant."

But Lucian goes further, and says, in his tract *De Luctu*,* that he speaks what he has seen, and that they bring the dried body as a guest to their feasts and invitations ; and oftentimes one necessitous of money is supplied by giving his brother or his father in pledge, which practice is fully confirmed by Herodotus, who says,—

"Ἐπὶ τούτου βασιλεύοντος, (Ασυχιν) ἔλεγον, (οἱ ἱρεές) ἀμιξίης ἐούσης πολλῆς χρημάτων, γενέσθαι νόμον Αἰγυπτίοισι, ἀποδεικνύντα ἐνέχυρον τοῦ πατρὸς τὸν νέκυν, οὕτω λαμβάνειν τὸ χρέος· προστεθῆναι δὲ ἔτι τούτῳ τῷ νέμῳ τόνδε, τὸν διδόντα τὸ χρέος καὶ ἀπάσης κρατέειν τῆς τοῦ λαμβάνοντος θήκης· τῷ δὲ ὑποτιθέντι τοῦτο τὸ ἐνέχυρον, τήνδε ἐπεῖναι ζημίην, μὴ βουλομένῳ ἀποδοῦναι τὸ χρέος, μηδὲ αὐτῷ ἐκείνῳ τελευτήσαντι εἶναι ταφῆς κυρῆσαι μήτ' ἐν ἐκείνῳ τῷ πατρῴῳ τάφῳ, μήτ' ἐν ἄλλῳ μηδενὶ, μήτε ἄλλον μηδένα τῶν ἑωυτοῦ ἀπογενόμενον θάψαι."

Herod. Hist. lib. ii. § 136.

" In his (Asychis') reign, according to their (the priests') account, money circulating very slowly, a law was enacted for the Egyptians, that, by giving his father's body as a pledge, a man might borrow money ; and to this law was added another, that the person who lent the money should be put in possession of the whole sepulchral repository of the borrower ; that if, after giving this pledge, any one refused to refund, the following punishment should be inflicted on him, that, in the case of his own death, he should have no right to be interred either in the tomb of his forefathers or in any other, neither should he be at liberty to entomb any of his relations that departed this life."

Laurent's Translation.

And Diodorus Siculus (lib. i.) also writes, " they have a custom of depositing for a pledge the bodies of their dead parents. It is the greatest ignominy that may be not to redeem them ; and, if they do it not, they themselves are deprived of burial." And, in another place, he says, " such as for any crime or debt are hindered from being buried, are kept at home without a coffin, whom afterwards their posterity, growing rich, discharging their debts, and paying money in compensation of their crimes, honourably

* Ὁ μὲν Ἕλλην ἔκαυσεν· ὁ δὲ Πέρσης ἐθαψεν· ὁ δὲ Ινδος ὕαλῳ περιχρίει ὁ δὲ Σκόθης κατεσθίεις. ταριχεύει δὲ ὁ Αἰγύπτιος.

bury. For the Egyptians glory that their parents and ancestors were buried with honour." Greenhill conjectured that the law of Asychis was framed to restrict the practice of borrowing; attaching an infamy to it, by connecting it with the pledge of the debtor's most sacred possession.*

The practice of embalming, although originally and in the most perfect manner adopted by the ancient Egyptians, was not entirely confined to their use; for the Persians, the Arabs, the Jews, the Ethiopians, and even the Christians in some degree employed these ceremonies. Thus we read in the book of Genesis† that the body of the father of Joseph was, according to his commands, embalmed by the physicians :—" And Joseph commanded his servants the physicians to embalm his father: and the physicians embalmed Israel. And forty days were fulfilled for him; for so are fulfilled the days of those which are embalmed: and the Egyptians mourned for him threescore and ten days."

In the New Testament we read that Nicodemus carried 100 lbs. of myrrh and aloes to embalm the body of Jesus and to envelop it in linen with aromatics according to the manner of the Jews : " And there came also Nicodemus, which at the first came to Jesus by night, and brought a mixture of myrrh and aloes, about an hundred pound *weight*. Then took they the body of Jesus, and wound it in linen clothes with the spices, as the manner of the Jews is to bury."‡

All civilized nations have practised the same on the bodies of their kings or rulers, or persons of great distinction. Sepulture in the earth, however, has been the most ordinary mode of disposing of the dead; but many nations committed the bodies to the action of fire, and even reduced their frames to a state of powder, which was taken either in their drinks or dispersed to the winds. Erasmus Franciscus reports of a nation of the kingdom of Guinea (Arvvacæ vocantur) that they pulverise the bones of their lords, ladies, relations, &c., then mix the dust in their ordinary drink, and so absorb it. " Pulverem hunc miscet potui ordinario, et bibendo ita absorbet."§

---

* Art of Embalming, p. 303.   † Chap. i. 2, 3.   ‡ John xxix. 39, 40.
§ See Clauderi, Methodus Balsamandi Corpora Humana, &c. 4to. Altenb. 1679, p. 31.

Interment in the earth appears to have been the earliest, as it is certainly the most natural,* way of disposing of the dead ; and the first instance on record of this mode of burial, though there can be little doubt but that the practice existed anterior to the record of it, is that of Sarah the wife of Abraham.† The burning of the bodies of the dead had probably its origin in the endeavour to prevent any insult or ill treatment being offered to them; and we find that this custom prevailed among the ancient Greeks, Romans, Germans, Gauls, and others. The people of Chios and the old Romans not only burnt their dead, but beat the bones in a mortar, and when thus reduced to powder sifted it through a sieve, and scattered the dust abroad by the winds. The ancient Romans also washed the body and rubbed it with perfumes, as we learn from the poet Ennius :

" Tarquinii corpus bona fœmina lavit et unxit;"

and Tacitus, speaking of Poppœa, the wife of Nero, says, " Corpus non igni abolitum, ut Romanus mos ; sed regum externorum consuetudine, differtum odoribus conditur."—*Annales*, xvi. 6. This latter mode approaches nearer to that of the Egyptians than the former; though they were both probably derived from that people. Pliny‡ relates that it was customary among the northern people near the Riphæan Mountains to bury the bodies in water. So indeed in Scythia, they formerly kept the dead bodies of their parents affixed

---

* " For dust thou art, and unto dust shalt thou return."—Gen. iii. 19.
" His breath goeth forth; he returneth to his earth."—Psalm cxlvi. 4.
And Euripides, in his Supplicants, introduces Theseus thus speaking :

" Εασατ' ηδη γη καλυφθηναι νεκρους
Οθεν δ' εκασον εις το σωμ' αφικετο
Ενταυθ' απηλθε, πνευμα μεν προς αιθερα,
Το σωμα δ' εις γην."

" Now they are dead, permit them in the earth
To rest concealed. For whence at first proceeds
Each portion of our frame, thither again
Must it return: the spirit flies aloft,
And with its native æther claims alliance;
The body mingles with the dust below."
† Gen. xxiii. 19, 20.   ‡ Hist. Natural. lib. iv cap. 12.

to the trunks of trees in the snow and ice. Blasius Viginerus reports that the Macrobians and Ethiopians, having emptied and deprived the bodies of the dead of their flesh, covered the remains with plaster, on which a kind of fresco painting was laid, so as to represent as nearly as possible the natural body. This done, it was put into a glazed case or coffin. The nearest relatives kept it in their possession for one year, making offerings and oblations to it during that time, at the expiration of which the body was removed to the environs of the city, and there buried. The Tranzianes * removed the heart and intestines from their dead, bathed them in aromatic and spicy liquors, and then burnt them in honour of their gods. The ashes were carefully collected together and replaced in the body, that no part might be found wanting at the day of resurrection. The Colchians and Tartars suspended their dead upon the trees for three years, to be dried by the sun. When the desiccation was complete, they took down the bodies and burnt them entire.

The Persians, as also the Syrians and the ancient Arabians, covered their dead with honey or wax, and so preserved them. Erasmus Franciscus reports† that a certain people of the kingdom of Guinea (Tivitivæ) dwelling about the river Orenoque, mourn their dead with great wailing, and bury them. When it is suspected that the flesh, through the process of putrefaction, has become separated from the bones, they dig it up afresh, hang up the skeleton in the house, decorate the skull with different coloured-feathers, and affix plates of gold to the arms and thighs. A certain nation of the Brazils mourn the death of their kindred with extraordinary sorrow and weeping; then paint the body with various colours, and afterwards roll it in silk, lest it be rudely touched by the earth in which it is placed.‡ The same authority § acquaints us that it often happens among the Chinese that the children preserve the bodies of their parents for three or four years in the house, as a token of their devoted love and adoration. But the chinks of the coffin are so firmly glued up that no noisome sense of putrefaction can offend the nostrils.

* Erasmus Franciscus de Sepulturis et honoribus Sepulchralibus, p. 1502.

† p. 1486.   ‡ p. fol. 1488.   § p. 1509.

Mr. Thoms, who resided some years at Macao and at Canton, informs me that he has often seen coffins which contained the dead in the houses of the Chinese. On enquiry he found that they had been there for years; and that some one of the family (generally the eldest son) never failed, morning and night, besides presenting rice, wine, and tea, to invoke the dead to be propitious to them, imagining that while the body is uninterred the spirit will continue to hover over it. If the habitation be too confined to admit of their reception, it is no unusual occurrence for the relatives to build outside the city wall a room of brick, large enough to contain one or two coffins; here the nearest male relation sleeps, (generally on a board,) whose duty, besides presenting the offerings, it is to see that the sticks of incense, commonly called *jos-sticks*, i. e. sacred sticks, are always burning: the observance of this ceremony is termed *completing filial piety*. In addition to the rice, &c., already mentioned, persons in affluent circumstances make offerings of a peculiar kind of pastry, sweetmeats, fowls, large roasted pigs, and even goats: and not unfrequently wardrobes, to the value of many hundred dollars, are burnt for the purpose of transmitting them, as is supposed, into another state for the use of the deceased. Anciently, ministers of state used to retire from office for three years on the death of a parent; but this custom has ceased. Persons in more humble circumstances will erect a shed of a kind of matting, where some one person will remain for months, sometimes years, disregarding the seasons, before the dead are interred. As the coffins are generally made of very hard wood, three or four inches thick, well dove-tailed, and cemented with chunam, they do not emit the least smell.

On the death of any one, the wife or nearest of kin, attended by some of his or her relations, repair to a stream of water outside the city wall, into which they throw a little salt, and then take home a portion of the water, with which the corpse is washed all over; the body being shaved, a little rice is put into the mouth and a coin in each hand, and the coffin is then fastened down. The whole of this ceremony is attended to with a great deal of weeping and lamentation. If the deceased had attained a great age, or been the mother of a large family, persons of different grades make large presents, and, without being invited, attend the funeral. In such cases, a long inscription, extending sometimes more than six feet in length, written in golden characters on crimson silk, is borne like a banner before the coffin, recording the numerous virtues of the deceased. Should the descendants of the deceased become reduced, the dead are often taken up and re-interred in a spot that is considered to be more propitious to the fortunes of the family. At such times, should there be but little remaining of the body, it is collected together and put into an earthen vessel, which is also interred, and before it is placed some unboiled rice, with wine and tea. All the priests of the Buddha sect in China, shortly after death, are burnt in an iron vessel in the open air, after which the ashes are collected and put into jars closely sealed, and either buried in their sacred enclosures or sent to some new temple to be there deposited.

The Ethiopians, according to Herodotus,* desiccate the bodies of their dead and after some process, the precise nature of which he does not describe, cover them all over with plaster and paint them, imitating as nearly as possible the life; they then are placed within columns of glass made hollow.† Deposited within these, the dead bodies appear through, emitting no unpleasant smell, nor exhibiting any thing whatever unsightly, and the whole case is visible, as well as the corpse itself. These columns were kept by the nearest relations of the deceased during the space of one year in their houses, presenting them with the firstlings of all, and honouring them with sacrifices, after which they were carried away, and set up without the town.

It may not be uninteresting here to notice the pious expression of regard shown by the people of the East to their dead at the present time. Sonnini‡ has told us that the traces of the precautions taken by the ancient Egyp-

* Thalia, Lib. iii. § 24. † De Pauw (Philosophical Dissertations on the Egyptians and Chinese, vol. I. p. 197,) conjectures these to have been composed of a resinous matter, something like yellow amber (which would most assuredly preserve bodies could means be devised of rendering it ductile or liquid), or of some transparent gum which is abundant in Ethiopia. But we learn from Ludolf (Hist. Æthiop. lib. i. cap. 7) that in some parts of Ethiopia a great quantity of fossil salt is found, which is transparent, and hardens by exposure to the air. M. Larcher (tom. III. lib. iii. § 24,) conceives that it was this salt which was taken for glass.

‡ II. 20.

tians in burying their dead are still to be found in their modern successors. Although unacquainted with the art of embalming, they, nevertheless, endeavour to preserve the body by the use of perfumes. As soon as a person is dead, the Egyptians hasten to press the different parts of the corpse, to free it from all impurities; wash it several times; shave it; pull out all the hair; stop up every aperture closely with cotton; and pour over it odoriferous waters, so that all its pores are penetrated with the perfumes of Arabia. After the body is committed to the earth, a little pillar of stone, terminated by a turban, is erected over the spot where the deceased reposes, and to this spot the friends repair every Friday to repeat their melancholy adieus.

From Wood * we learn that the uncommon magnificence of the monuments of the dead in ancient Palmyra seems to have been borrowed from Egypt, to which country they, of all people, come nearest in that sort of expense. Zenobia was originally of Egypt; she spoke their language perfectly well, and affected much to imitate in many things her ancestor, Cleopatra. But that they borrowed some of their customs from Egypt before her time seems plain, from a discovery of mummies in their sepulchral monuments. "We had been in Egypt a few months before," says this author, "and by comparing the linen, the manner of swathing, the balsam, and other parts of the mummies of that country with those of Palmyra, we found their methods of embalming exactly the same. The Arabs had seen vast numbers of these mummies in all the sepulchres; but they had broken them up, in hopes of finding treasures. We offered them rewards to find an entire one, but in vain; which disappointed our hopes of seeing something curious in the sarcophagus, or, perhaps, of meeting with hieroglyphics." I am happy to be able to add the testimony of Captain Mangles in favour of this account by Mr. Wood. This intelligent traveller has assured me that he saw many fragments of embalmed bodies wrapped up in similar swathings, and having quite the same appearance as those he had so frequently seen in Egypt.

* Ruins of Palmyra and Balbec, fol. Lond. 1827, p. 22.

CHAPTER IV.

ON EGYPTIAN TOMBS.

Practice of entombment by different nations—The tombs of Egypt—various articles found within them—Earliest known Tombs—The Pyramids—The Catacombs—Character of Egyptian architecture and sculpture—Opinions of Goguet—Denon—Hamilton—Legh—Light—Wilkinson—Champollion—Strabo—Woodward—Character of the ancient Egyptians—their high sense of virtuous conduct—the wisdom of some of their Laws—Examination into the Characters of the dead—confirmation of this by Diodorus Siculus—attested by Champollion—Description of the funeral ceremonies of the Egyptians by Diodorus Siculus—Description of the sacred barge—The catacombs—Correction of a statement made by De Pauw—Private tombs—Plain of mummies—Mr. Salt's opinion as to the antiquity of the catacombs—Evidence in favour of the casing of the pyramids—Mr. Davison's survey of the catacombs of Alexandria—Catacombs of Thebes—Royal tombs—Private tombs—Belzoni's account of Gournou—Mummy pits—position of the mummies.

An ingenious writer* has remarked that the people of polished nations accumulated riches in their temples, whilst those of barbarous ages deposited theirs in the tombs. Solomon honoured his father by burying near him all the riches he could obtain. Warlike nations have generally entombed the martial weapons of the deceased with the body. The ancient Gauls burnt their dead and interred their arms with their ashes. The tombs in Egypt have been found to contain all kinds of articles bearing reference to the habits and profession of the deceased. I have seen corn, barley, vetches, bread, fruits, artists' palettes, brushes, paints, various implements, &c. Instruments of war have been rarely found, although the Egyptians were so warlike a nation. Belzoni could only find one arrow, which was two feet long. At one extremity it had a copper point well fixed in it, and at the other a notch, as usual, to receive the string of the bow; it had evidently been split by the string and glued together again.† The armour of Alexander

---

* Roquefort (M. de) des Sépultures Nationales, 8vo. Paris, 1824.   † Travels, p.172.

is said to have been placed within his tomb, and Dion Cassius* relates that Caligula wore the breast-plate of Alexander, which he had taken from his tomb.

Perhaps the earliest known tombs for the reception of the dead are those alluded to by the late Dr. Clarke in his "Dissertation on the Sarcophagus brought from Alexandria." They consist of immense mounds of earth, and are to be found in almost every part of the habitable globe. Dr. Clarke states that he has seen these sepulchral heaps in Europe, in Asia, from the Icy Sea to Mount Caucasus, over all the south of Russia, Kuban Tartary, Asia Minor, Syria, Palestine, Egypt, and part of Africa.† A superstitious custom in the northern nations of casting a stone at them, he adds, prevents any appearance of their diminution; and this practice, according to Shaw,‡ prevails in Barbary, in the Holy Land, and in Arabia. They appear to present the most ancient mode of burial, and to be anterior to the pyramids, as having a less artificial form: and perhaps some proof of this may be derived from the appearance of one of the pyramids of *Saccara* in Upper Egypt, the stones of which, being further advanced in decomposition than those of *Djiza*, prove that they were erected at an earlier period, as they are exposed to the same atmosphere and at no great distance from the latter. This pyramid preserves almost the simplicity of the primæval conic mound, and shows only an approach to the more artificial structure of others.§

Next in point of antiquity are the pyramids and the catacombs. The former must always be classed among the most extraordinary works of the ancient Egyptians, but historians and antiquarians have failed in pointing out either the period of their erection, or the authors of such gigantic undertakings. The learned Goguet‖ infers that as Homer, who lived 900 years before Christ, sings of Thebes and her hundred gates, and makes no mention of the pyramids, they must have been built posterior to his time. In this respect Goguet is in agreement with the authority of Diodorus Siculus.¶ Hieroglyphical researches have hitherto thrown no light towards

* Lib. lix. cap. 17.   † P. 46, Note.   ‡ Travels, Pref. p. 10.   § Clarke, p. 47, Note.
‖ De l'Origine des Lois, des Arts et des Sciences, tom. III. p. 56. Paris, 1820.
¶ Lib. i. p. 72.

dispelling the mystery in which the erection of the pyramids is involved. We are in perfect ignorance as to their use or their builders. Abd'Allatif says that he saw a prodigious number of hieroglyphical inscriptions on the two great pyramids, as many as, if copied, would fill perhaps 10,000 volumes. No inscription is now to be found. It would be out of place here to attempt any description of these buildings, as it is to be obtained in the works of various travellers;* but I cannot omit noticing here that the Egyptians appear to have excelled in the gigantic style in all their specimens of sculpture and architecture. They display a fine and bold outline, but are deficient in the expression of passions and the representation of grace: due proportions and elegance of form are rarely to be met with. Immense masses astonish the eyes every where; indeed, so numerous and so stupendous are all the remains of the ancient monuments of Egypt, that Denon was tempted to say, " On est fatigué décrire, on est fatigué de lire, on est épouvanté de la pensée d'une telle conception ; on ne peut croire, même après l'avoir vu, à la réalité de l'existence de tant de constructions réunies sur un même point, à leur dimension, à la constance obstinée qu'a exigée leur fabrication, aux dépenses incalculables de tant de sumptuosité." Mr. Hamilton† has well expressed himself in allusion to the magnitude of that colossal fragment of antiquity called by the French Memnonuim. " Among other dimensions of this colossus," says he, " I found that it measured six feet ten inches over the foot, and sixty-two or sixty-three feet round the shoulders. This enormous statue has been broken off at the waist, and the upper part is now laid prostrate on the back. The face is entirely obliterated: and next to the wonder excited at the boldness of the sculptor who made it, and the extraordinary powers of those who erected it, the labour and exertions that must have been used for its destruction are most astonishing. It could only have been brought about with the help of military engines, and must then have been the work of a length of time. Its fall has carried along with it the whole wall of the temple, which stood within its reach. It was not without great difficulty and danger that we could climb on its shoulder and neck; and, in going from thence upon its chest,

* See Dr. Richardson's Travels along the Mediterranean, Greaves' Pyramidographia, &c.
† Remarks on several parts of Turkey. Part I. Ægyptiaca. 4to. Lond. 1809, p. 167.

E

I was assisted by my Arab servant, who walked by my side, in the hiero-glyphical characters engraven on the arm."

Mr. Legh* says that "from the appearance and present state of the temples (at Philæ) it appears clear that the system of building amongst the ancient Egyptians was first to construct great masses, and afterwards to labour for ages in finishing the details of the decorations, beginning with the sculpture of the hieroglyphics, and then passing to the stucco and painting. In Philæ, as at Thebes and Dendera, nothing is finished but what is of the highest antiquity."

Mr. Wilkinson has represented, in the 4th Plate of Part II., of his most valuable and interesting "Materia Hieroglyphica," the proportions of an Egyptian figure taken from the sculptures of the tombs at Thebes. He tells us, that "when the Egyptians intended to sculpture, or paint figures on a wall, they began by smoothing the surface, and drawing a number of parallel lines at equal distances; at right angles to which were traced other lines, forming a series of squares. The size of these squares depended upon the size of the figures to be introduced; but, whatever was their size, nineteen parts or spaces were always allowed for the height of the human figure; if smaller figures were to be introduced, intermedial lines were then ruled, which formed smaller squares, and consequently a figure of smaller pro-portion. The figures of the earlier times are of more lengthened proportions, because what is taken from the breadth of the limbs gives the appearance of greater height; but the total length of the figure is still divided into nineteen parts in their sculptures and fresco-paintings."†

Captain Light gives the following description of his visit to Kárnak, the ancient Diospolis:—" It was impossible to look on such an extent of build-ing without being lost in admiration; no description will be able to give an adequate idea of the enormous masses still defying the ravages of time. Enclosure within enclosure, propylæa in front of propylæa; to these, avenues of sphinxes, each of fourteen or fifteen feet in length, lead from

---

* Narrative of a Journey in Egypt and the Country beyond the Cataracts, by Thomas Legh, Esq. 4to. Lond. 1816, p. 51.

† P. 113. See also Appendix III. for Observations on the Sculpture and Drawing of the ancient Egyptians.

a distance of several hundred yards. The common Egyptian sphinx is found in the avenues to the south; but, to the west, the crio sphinx, with the ram's head, from one or two that have been uncovered, seems to have composed its corresponding avenue. Those of the south and east are still buried. Headless statues of grey and white granite, of gigantic size, lay prostrate in different parts of the ruins. In the western court, in front of the great portico, and at the entrance to this portico, is an upright headless statue of one block of granite, whose size may be imagined from finding that a man of six feet just reaches to the patella of the knee.

" The entrance to the great portico is through a mass of masonry, partly in ruins, through which the eye rests on an avenue of fourteen columns, whose diameter is more than eleven feet and whose height is upwards of sixty. On each side of this are seven rows, of seven columns in each, whose diameter is eight feet, and about forty feet high, of an architecture which wants the elegance of Grecian models, yet suits the immense majesty of the Egyptian temple.

" Though it does not enter into my plan to continue a description which has been so ably done by others before me, yet, when I say that the whole extent of this temple cannot be less than a mile and a half in circumference, and that the smallest blocks of masonry are five feet by four in depth and breadth, that there are obelisks of eighty feet high on a base of eighteen feet, of one block of granite, it can be easily imagined that Thebes was the vast city history describes it to be."*

Champollion calls Kárnak the Palace, or rather the City of Monuments. " Là m'apparut," says he, " toute la magnificence pharaonique, tout ce que les hommes ont imaginé et executé de plus grand. Tout ce que j'avais admiré avec enthousiasme sur la rive gauche, me parut misérable en comparaison des conceptions gigantesques dont j'étais entouré. Je me garderai bien de vouloir rien décrire ; car, ou mes expressions ne vaudraient que la millième partie de ce qu'on doit dire en parlant de tels objets, ou bien si j'en traçais une faible esquisse, même fort décolorée, on me prendrait pour un enthousiaste, peut-être même pour un fou. Il suffira d'ajouter qu'aucun peuple ancien ni moderne n'a conçu l'art de l'architecture sur une échelle aussi sublime, aussi large, aussi grandiose, que le firent les

* pp. 105—107.

vieux Egyptiens ; ils conçevaient en hommes des 100 pieds de haut, et l'imagination qui, en Europe, s'élance bien au-dessus de nos portiques, s'arrête et tombe impuissante au pied des 140 colonnes de la salle hypostyle de Karnak."*

The finest specimen of Egyptian sculpture hitherto discovered is unquestionably that of the "Young Memnon," as it is called, found at Thebes, whence it was removed by the intrepid and indefatigable Belzoni, and now placed in the British Museum. Mr. Hamilton was struck with its extraordinary delicacy, the very uncommon expression visible in its features, and the marked character that well entitled it to the admiration of Damies.†

M. Caviglia exhumed a magnificent colossal figure at Memphis. It is represented by M. Champollion to be a portrait of Sesostris, and he is confirmed in this opinion by the hieroglyphics on the breast and on the arms of the figure.‡

But M. Denon's description of the sphinx ought not to be overlooked : " L'expression de la tête," says he, " est douce, grâcieuse, est tranquille, le caractère en est Africain ; mais la bouche, dont les lèvres sont épaisses, a une mollesse dans le mouvement et une finesse d'exécution vraiment admirables ; c'est de la chair et de la vie." An earlier author (Abd' Allatif) seems to have felt the same sensations upon viewing this extraordinary specimen of Egyptian sculpture : " Un homme d'esprit," says he, " m'ayant demandé quel etoit, de tout ce que j'avois vu en Egypte, l'objet qui avoit le plus excité mon admiration, je lui dis que·c'étoit la justesse des proportions dans la tête du Sphinx." And he adds, " Or, il est bien étonnant que, dans une figure aussi colossale, le sculpteur ait su conserver la juste proportion de toutes les parties, tandis que la nature ne présentoit aucun modèle d'un semblable colosse, ni rien qui pût lui être comparé."§

The Egyptian sphinxes, we have the authority of Mr. Wilkinson for saying, are always representative of the male not female sex. They are either andro or crio-sphinxes, that is, having either the union of the lion and man, or the lion's body with the ram's head.‖

* Lettres écrites d'Egypte et de Nubie, p. 98.   † See Ægyptiaca.
‡ See Plate III. in Lettres écrites d'Egypte, &c., p. 66.   § p. 180. ' ‖ Mat. Hierog. p. 94.

The monotony of the Egyptian buildings is most striking; they are enormous masses, distinguished by a "calm and solemn grandeur of conception," but defective in spirit; all colossal, stupendous works of infinite labour, but deficient in taste. Strabo, speaking of the edifices of the ancient Egyptians, says they have neither design, genius, nor elegance.* Singularity and superstition form the peculiar character of the ancient Egyptian. I am, however, far from agreeing with a learned author,† who, in a "Discourse on the Wisdom of the Ancient Egyptians," affects to find them abounding in all that is bad, and deficient in all that is good. The first principles of the laws, the arts, and the sciences, have been derived from these people, from whom they have been transmitted to us through the Greeks and the Romans.‡ According to Herodotus, Diodorus Siculus, and other historians, the ancient Egyptians were a people holding truth and virtuous conduct in the highest estimation. Their penal laws applying to cases of homicide, parricide, perjury, adultery, &c., mark the high sense of justice entertained by them, and this is even carried to the verge of the tomb; for we learn from Diodorus Siculus§ that, upon the death of any one, the relations of the deceased were obliged to announce to the judges (forty, or forty-two, in number) the time at which it was intended to perform the ceremony of burial. This consisted in the first place of the passage of the deceased across the lake or canal of the department, or nome,‖ as it was called, to which the deceased had belonged. The day

---

* Lib. xvii. p. 1159. † Dr. Woodward.

‡ As the arts and sciences took their origin in Egypt, the Greeks began to visit it with a view to commerce, instruction, and curiosity, and it has been ingeniously and with great probability suggested that the Greeks must have looked upon Egypt with nearly the same feelings as we do on Greece and Rome. "Plan and Objects of the History of Herodotus," by P. E. Laurent.

§ Lib. i. § 92.

‖ Sesostris, who ruled 1659 years, A.C., divided ancient Egypt into thirty-six provinces. The name of nomes was given to them by the Greeks upon becoming the masters of Egypt under Alexander. The Romans afterwards under Augustus called them prefectures. Sesostris was perhaps the greatest sovereign of Egypt. He divided the people into seven classes, and obliged the children to take to the profession of their fathers. In his reign the celebrated temple of Vulcan was built. He is said to have been instructed by Mercury in politics and in the art of reigning. He ruled over Egypt thirty-three years, and the learned

being named, the judges* assembled, and the court of inquiry was open to all, so that any accusation might be urged against the defunct. Should his life have been bad, the right of sepulture was denied to him, which was considered as one of the greatest calamities that could occur. If, on the contrary, the life of the deceased had been well conducted and blameless, and that no reproach could attach to his memory, a eulogium was [pronounced upon him, and he was permitted to be entombed with all due honour. Diodorus Siculus informs us that in these eulogies no mention was ever made of the race or family of the defunct, all Egyptians being considered equally noble. No one was exempt from this ordeal—kings as well as the ordinary people were subjected to the same inquiry—those who during life no one dared to reproach, or whose actions no one dared to question, when dead, were submitted to a rigorous examination. A public audience was given to hear all accusations against the deceased monarch. The priests commenced by making his eulogy, and recounting his good actions. If the general opinion of the people as to the government and conduct of the monarch corresponded with that of the priests, the multitude poured forth their acclamations; but, if the contrary, murmuring succeeded; and Diodorus Siculus says there have not been wanting instances of the denial of burial to a deceased sovereign in accordance with the decision of the people. M. Champollion saw in Biban-el-Molouk the tomb of a king, in which the sculpture had been defaced from one end to the other, except in those parts where were sculptured the images of the queen his mother, and of his wife, which have been most religiously respected, as well as the hieroglyphical legends relating to them. M. Champollion conceives this to have been the tomb of a king condemned by the judgment after his death, and denied the rite of burial.†

Goguet gives to him the merit of having been the first to erect an obelisk; but Pliny assigns this distinction to Mestrès. The obelisk of Rameses, near the palace of Heliopolis, is the greatest.

* In some of the Papyri representations of these judges (forty-two in number) are to be seen. A good example may be found in the Catalago de' Papiri Egiziani della Biblioteca Vaticana, fol. Rom. 1825. This work is by the celebrated Angelo Mai.

† Lettres écrites d'Egypte et de Nubie, p. 96. M. Champollion has also seen the tomb of another king of Thebes of a most ancient period, from which it would appear that the tomb

This rigorous examination into the characters of the dead, either royal or plebeian, and the inquiry into their course of life, are surely entitled to praise, and shows in what estimation this people held good and virtuous conduct. The audience was public; the people pronounced sentence. The following is the account of this ceremonial as detailed by Diodorus Siculus:

" Τοῦ δὲ μέλλοντος θάπτεσθαι σώματος οἱ συγγενεῖς προλέγουσι τὴν ἡμέραν τῆς ταφῆς τοῖς τε δικασταῖς καὶ τοῖς συγγενέσιν, ἔτι δὲ φίλοις τοῦ τετελευτηκότος· καὶ διαβεβαιοῦνται, λέγοντες ὅτι διαβαίνειν μέλλει τὴν λίμνην τοῦ νομοῦ τοῦ τετελευτηκότος. ἔπειτα παραγενομένων δικαστῶν πλείω τῶν τετταράκοντα, καὶ καθισάντων ἐπί τινος ἡμικυκλίου, κατεσκευασμένου πέραν τῆς λίμνης, ἡ μὲν βάρις καθέλκεται κατεσκευασμένη πρότερον ὑπὸ τῶν ταύτην ἐχόντων τὴν ἐπιμέλειαν. ἐφέστηκε δὲ ταύτῃ πρωρεύς, ὃν Αἰγύπτιοι κατὰ τὴν ἰδίων διάλεκτον ὀνομάζουσι Χάρωνα. διὸ καὶ φασὶν Ὀρφέα τὸ παλαιὸν εἰς Αἴγυπτον παραβαλόντα καὶ θεασάμενον τοῦτο τὸ νόμιμον, μυθοποιῆσαι τὰ καθ' ᾅδου, τὰ μὲν μιμησάμενον, τὰ δ' αὐτὸν ἰδίᾳ πλασάμενον. περὶ οὗ τὰ κατὰ μέρος μικρὸν ὕστερον ἀναγράψομεν. οὐ μὴν ἀλλὰ τῆς βάρεως εἰς τὴν λίμνην καθελκυσθείσης, πρὶν ἢ τὴν λάρνακα τὴν τὸν νεκρὸν ἔχουσαν εἰς αὐτὴν τίθεσθαι, τῷ βουλομένῳ κατηγορεῖν ὁ νόμος ἐξουσίαν δίδωσιν. ἐὰν μὲν οὖν τις παρελθὼν ἐγκαλέσῃ καὶ δείξῃ βεβιωκότα κακῶς, οἱ μὲν κριταὶ γνώμας ἀποφαίνονται, τὸ δὲ σῶμα εἴργεται τῆς εἰθισμένης ταφῆς· ἐὰν δὲ ὁ ἐγκαλέσας δόξῃ μὴ δικαίως ἐγκαλεῖν, μεγάλοις περιπίπτει προστίμοις, ὅταν δὲ μηδεὶς ὑπακούσῃ κατήγορος, ἢ παρελθὼν γνωσθῇ συκοφάντης ὑπάρχειν, οἱ μὲν συγγενεῖς ἀποθέμενοι τὸ πένθος, ἐγκωμιάζουσι τὸν τετελευτηκότα, καὶ περὶ μὲν τοῦ γένους οὐδὲν λέγουσιν, ὥσπερ παρὰ τοῖς Ἕλλησιν, ὑπολαμβάνοντες ἅπαντας ὁμοίως εὐγενεῖς εἶναι τοὺς κατ' Αἴγυπτον· τὴν δ' ἐκ παιδὸς ἀγωγὴν καὶ παιδείαν διελθόντες, πάλιν ἀνδρὸς γεγενότος τὴν εὐσέβειαν καὶ δικαιοσύνην, ἔτι δὲ τὴν ἐγκράτειαν καὶ τὰς ἄλλας ἀρετὰς αὐτοῦ διεξέρχονται, καὶ παρακαλοῦσι τοὺς κάτω θεοὺς σύνοικον δέξασθαι τοῖς εὐσεβέσι. τὸ δὲ πλῆθος ἐπευφημεῖ, καὶ συναποσεμνύνει τὴν δόξαν τοῦ τετελευτηκότος, ὡς τὸν αἰῶνα διατρίβειν μέλλοντος καθ' ᾅδου μετὰ τῶν εὐσεβῶν. τὸ δὲ σῶμα τιθέασιν, οἱ μὲν ἰδίους ἔχοντες τάφους, ἐν ταῖς ἀποδεδειγμέναις θήκαις. οἷς δ' οὐχ ὑπάρχουσι τάφων κτήσεις, καινὸν οἴκημα ποιοῦσι κατὰ τὴν ἰδίαν οἰκίαν, καὶ πρὸς τὸν ἀσφαλέστατον τῶν τοίχων ὀρθὴν ἱστᾶσι τὴν

had been usurped by one of his successors of the nineteenth dynasty, and who has covered over with plaster all the old cartouches, and substituted for them his own, and also the bas-reliefs and inscriptions of his predecessor. The usurper had, however, cut a second tomb in which his sarcophagus was to be placed, so that that of his ancestor was not to be removed. It would seem that every king caused his tomb to be cut out of the rock during his life-time; for those who have reigned the longest period are found to have the largest tombs and the most elaborate sepulchres.

λάρνακα· καὶ τοὺς κωλνομένους δὲ διὰ τὰς κατηγορίας, ἢ πρὸς δανείων ὑποθήκας, θάπτεσθαι, τιθέασι κατὰ τὴν ἰδίαν ὀικίαν. οὓς ὕστερον ἐνίοτε παίδων παῖδες ἐνπορήσαντες, καὶ τῶν τε συμβολαίων καὶ τῶν ἐγκλημάτων ἀπολύσαντες, μεγαλοπρεποῦς ταφῆς ἀξιοῦσι."

Diodori Siculi Biblioth. Histor. lib. i. § 92.

" The relations of the dead person fix the day of his obsequies, that the judges and all the friends of the deceased may assemble ; and they appoint it by declaring that he will pass the lake of his nome. The judges, more than forty in number, then repair to the spot, and form a semicircle on the further side of the lake. A boat containing those who are to officiate in the ceremony then approaches, under the direction of a navigator, whom the Egyptians, in their language, call ' Charon.' It is said that Orpheus, having in his travels to Egypt witnessed this ceremony, took from it his fable of the passage into the infernal regions, imitating a part of the cere-monies, and inventing the remainder. Before the coffin containing the corpse is placed within the boat, the law permits any person to accuse him ; if it is proved that he has led a bad life, the judges condemn him, and he is excluded from the place of burial. If it appears that he has been un-justly accused, the law inflicts a severe punishment on the accuser. If no one undertakes to accuse him, or if the accuser is convicted of calumny, the relations take off the badges of mourning, and pronounce the panegyric of the deceased, without speaking of his birth, as is done in Greece ; for they think that all Egyptians are equally noble. They expatiate upon the manner in which he has been brought up and instructed from his in-fancy, upon his piety, his justice, his temperance, and his other virtues, since he attainèd the age of manhood, and they pray the gods of the in-fernal regions to admit him into the abode of the pious. The people applaud and congratulate the defunct, who is about to pass a blissful eternity in the residence of the blessed.* If any one has a tomb destined

---

* " According to the theology of the Egyptians, the philosophers, and those who had practised the most rigid virtue, were the only people whose souls went directly to dwell with God, without passing through purgatory, or ever being subject to resurrection. In the Egyptian ceremonies a public confession was made in the name of some dead persons, declaring that they had constantly honoured their parents ; that they adhered invariably to the religion of the state ; that their hearts were never sullied with a crime, nor their hands tinged with human

for his sepulture, his body is placed in it; if not, a chamber is constructed in his house, and his bier is placed close against the most solid part of the wall. They place in their houses those to whom sepulture has been denied, whether on account of the crimes of which they have been accused, or of debts which they have contracted; and it sometimes occurs that they afterwards receive honourable burial, because their descendants, having become rich, pay their debts, or purchase absolution."

In the family sepulchral chamber discovered in 1823 by Mons. Passalacqua, in the Necropolis of Thebes, he found two models of boats, one for the ordinary purposes of navigation on the Nile, the other for conveying the mummy of a deceased person across the lake of his nome. Of the latter, as closely connected with the subject of this work, I have, by the kindness of M. Passalacqua, obtained a drawing from the original now in the collection at Berlin. (See Plate III.) The boat or bark is cut out of sycamore wood, and measures two feet eight inches and six lines, French measure. The boat is furnished with a large projecting portion of wood at the prow and at the poup. In the centre is a male mummy extended on a sofa or table, of which the legs are formed of the limbs of a lion. This is surmounted by a canopy, on which are inscribed various hieroglyphical characters, and is supported by six pillars painted successively in red, black, white, and green. At the head and feet of the mummy are two female figures; the former is in an attitude of great grief and desolation, represented by the hair of her head falling upon the mummy, whilst her arms are employed in embracing the deceased. The hands of the latter are placed upon the feet of the mummy. Four priests are seated upon the deck of the vessel, one at each corner of the table or bier, whilst another in front is observed to be holding out a MS. unrolled before him, and appears

blood in the midst of peace; that they had preserved and religiously discharged every trust confided to them; and, finally, that during their whole lives they had never given reason to any person to complain of an injury. All these conditions were evidently indispensable for those who hoped to escape the *amenthes* or purgatory; and to me it appears obvious that this doctrine on the duties of the man and of the citizen is an extract from what was read in the lesser mysteries, where it was probably displayed on two tables of stone."—De Pauw, Phil. Diss. vol. ii. p. 247.

F

to be delivering a funeral oration. Another, a sacrificer, is, with knife in hand, prepared to immolate an ox which lies bound at his feet. The first figure on the prow has his right arm extended, and appears to be watching the course of the vessel. The pilot, whom from his long white tunic we must suppose to be a priest, is seated at the poup between the two oars, the mechanism for moving which is well worthy of observation. The oars and the pillars on which they move are crowned with the head of a hawk. The body of the vessel is of a green colour, the extremities of the same colour, but of a deeper tinge. Paints and frames, to serve in the representation of religious ceremonies, are lying on the vessel, and at the sides of the fore part are emblematical representations of the sacred eye, the Eye of Osiris, which is also represented on the flat part of the oars surrounded by leaves of the lotus. The plank to descend from the vessel, and the pegs to fasten it, together with the club to drive them into the earth, are also on the deck. The male figures in the vessel have a red tinge of countenance, the women a yellow one, which corresponds with what is commonly seen in the ancient Egyptian paintings. It is to be observed that the priests as well as the females have their heads well covered with hair, which was permitted to grow during the term assigned for the mourning for the dead. This has induced M. Passalacqua to conceive the funeral ceremony here represented to be that of a priest, and the hieroglyphical inscription on the MS. reads, according to M. Champollion, " Grand Prêtre." In the tomb, in which three coffins or cases enclosed one within another were found, these hiero-glyphical symbols were seen marked upon each, together with the names of different divinities, to the worship of which probably the deceased had been particularly devoted.

But, to return to the catacombs. Five series of these subterraneous caverns have been described by travellers in Egypt as being in various states of preservation. They are those of Alexandria, Saccara, Silsillis, Gournou (Qoorna), and the tombs of the kings of Thebes. These vary considerably in extent. Those at Thebes are the most extensive. Over these hypogæa were built the city of Memphis and other places. It must be admitted that in the selection of these places for depositing the dead,—places where the water of the Nile could not reach, and where the air could scarcely penetrate, in caverns hidden from the view of men, and hewn out of the solid rock, surmounted by the base of the pyramids,—the ancient Egyptians must have been deeply impressed with the necessity (agreeably to their religious opinions on the subject of the Metempsychosis), and thus made choice of, situations beyond all others calculated to receive and to preserve from decay and corruption the remains of their dead. According to M. De Pauw,* an Egyptian law† preserved by Plato declares that no person should be buried on any spot capable of producing a tree. The soil in the environs of the pyramids and around the sepulchres of Thebes would be in agreement with this regulation. But at Sais the tombs are erected upon mounds of earth ; it is not rocky here. So numerous are the masses in the catacombs that they are said to extend to the distance of some miles, even to the temple of Ammon and the oracle of Serapis. The city of Saccara is the nearest to the cave of the mummies, as it has been called, and the inhabitants of Saccara are said to have derived the means of subsistence by breaking open these caves and extracting from them the embalmed bodies‡ The

* II. 23.

† This is one from a large number of instances that might be adduced of the carelessness in the mode of citation adopted by this author. The law here referred to is not an Egyptian law, but one by Plato himself, and inserted in the 12th book of his Laws. It runs thus :

θημας δ' ειναι, των χωριων οποσα μεν εργασιμα μηδαμου, μη τι μεγα μητε τι σμικρον μνημα. ἁ δε η χωρα προς τουτ' αυτο μονον φυσιν εχει, τα των τετελευτηκοτων σωματα μαλιστα αλυπητως τοις ζωσι δεχομενη κρυπτειν, ταυτα εκπληρουν. τοις δε ανθρωποις οσα τροφην μητηρ ουσα η γη προς ταυτα πεφυκε βουλεσθαι φερειν, μητε ζων μητε τις αποθανων στερειτο τον ζων θ' ημων.

i. e. " Let there be no sepulchres in cultivated places, neither large nor small. But that place alone receive the bodies of the dead which is useless for other purposes, and will in the smallest degree injure the living. For no one, either living or dying, should impede the fecundity of mother earth, and thus deprive some living person of aliment."—Plat. de Legibus, lib. xii.

‡ M. Champollion is the latest traveller from whom we have an account of the plain of Saccara, the ancient cemetery of Memphis, which he describes as " parsemé de pyramides et de tombeaux violés." "This spot," says he, " thanks to the barbarous rapacity of the dealers in antiquities, is absolutely barren for the student. The highly sculptured and ornamented tombs are destroyed and lie in ruins. The place is frightful, being formed only of mountains of sand strewed with human bones, the remains of former generations."—Lettres de Champollion, p. 68.

Mahommed Ali accompanied Mons. Cailliaud to visit the tombs at Gournou, and he was

excavations are formed in calcareous substances where no humidity can remain. The labour in their execution could not have been so great as may at first be imagined, as the layer of stone is soft; its consistence is hardened by exposure to the air. About half a league from Siut or Siout, one of the largest cities of Upper Egypt, on the site of the ancient Lycopolis, there are a great many tombs or excavations more or less magnificent. M. Denon has figured the largest. They are so numerous that the whole rock resounds under your feet.

Mr. Salt considers the catacombs to have been built as a place of sepulchre for the ancient kings of Egypt anterior to the construction of the pyramids, and connected with the city of Heliopolis before the seat of empire had been transferred to Memphis. But an able writer in the Quarterly Review* thinks differently, and conjectures that many of these edifices have been constructed from the dilapidated casing of the pyramids. From Herodotus we learn that they were originally so cased, and M. Belzoni has told us that the second pyramid retains a portion of its casing at the present time. The opinion hazarded by the writer in the Quarterly Review is strengthened by a statement of Mr. Salt, who says that one of the stones, bearing an inscription of hieroglyphics and figures, is built into the walls upside down, which certainly goes to prove that it had originally belonged to some other building: and the writer I have alluded to conceives the walls of these sepulchral edifices to have been constructed of the fragments of the casing of the pyramids. The tumuli, mentioned by Dr. Clarke, this writer regards merely as similar buildings of higher antiquity, mouldered away to their present shape; or that they were originally composed of more perishable materials.

Mr. Davison examined and surveyed the catacombs at Alexandria. He found some Greek inscriptions in them, from which one would be led

___

shocked at the spectacle presented by the fragments of human remains that every where were scattered about. Venting reproaches against the consuls and others who had permitted and encouraged such devastation, he exclaimed, "Quoi! ces cadavres n'etaient ils pas autrefois des hommes comme nous? On ne pense qu'à acquérir de brillantes collections; et ces chairs, ces ossemens, sont jetés çà et là sans respect; ces restes humains deviennent tous les jours la proie des plus vils animaux, et l'on y fait à peine attention." He then commanded the Turks to cover the remains with sand. Cailliaud, Voyage à Meroé, tom. I. p. 294.   * No. 38.

to conclude that these sepulchral receptacles had been made about or a little after the time when Alexandria was built. Mr. Davison remarks[*] that the paintings in the catacombs appeared to him to be of ordinary execution. Mr. Walpole[†] considers them to belong to the period when the arts were declining, and thinks that they might have been the works of the pagan inhabitants of the city in the sixth century; for at that time paganism was not altogether abolished, as we learn from a curious passage in Cyril.[‡] These paintings were seen only by the light of torches and lamps, when visits to the tombs of the dead were paid by their relatives, and the colour of them must necessarily have been such as admitted of a strong contrast.

Almost every city had its necropolis or cemetery at a distance from the town. Here the mass of people belonging to the city were interred; but there were many private tombs, and, according to Herodotus and Diodorus Siculus, in some instances the mummies, after being placed in their sarcophagi, were deposited in recesses in the habitations of their relatives or successors. Here, it is said, they were placed in niches *upright against the walls.*[§] This may probably have been the case with mummies kept in houses; but in the tombs, both public and private, all travellers agree in saying that they were always found lying down. The public cemeteries were always formed in a situation so as to be above the level of the water in the highest known inundations. They are principally excavated in the side of the great Libyan chain of hills which forms the western boundary of Egypt.[‖]

The catacombs of Thebes are the most extraordinary and magnificent. The Necropolis, or City of the Dead, of this place, a spot described as "devoted by nature to silence and death," is situated on the west bank of the Nile, and formed the burial place of the people as well as of the kings. Diodorus Siculus mentions[¶] that, according to history, there were

---

* p. 382.   † Id. 382.   ‡ In Esaiæ, cap. 18. Opp. tom. xi.

§ Belzoni says (p. 170) the wooden case is first covered with a layer or two of cement not unlike plaster of Paris, and on this are sometimes cast figures in *basso relievo,* for which they make niches cut in stone.

" ‖ Hypogées qui criblent la montagne Libyque."—*Champollion.*

¶ Lib. i.

forty-seven royal tombs at Thebes,* of which only seventeen remained at the time of Ptolemy Lagus. In the time of Diodorus Siculus most of them were destroyed. Strabo† says there were forty royal sepulchres cut out of the rock, and that they had obelisks and inscriptions setting forth the riches, power, and empire of the several kings.

The sepulchral monuments of the private inhabitants of Thebes, Mr. Hamilton states to be equally interesting with those of the kings. The painted sculptures on the walls represent the economical pursuits of those interred within them, and show to what degree of excellence the arts of design were cultivated in the earlier periods of the Theban monarchy. The reader will be amply compensated for his labour by referring to the work of Mr. Hamilton‡ for an account of the paintings which adorn the walls and ceilings of these catacombs, representing feasts, funeral processions, agricultural scenes, fishing, fowling, &c. The plan of these sepulchres is uniform and regular, and formed out of a kind of limestone; the roofs are in general flat, but some are arched, and in one instance Mr. H. observed a shelving or oblique roof in that form which seems to have been very general among the Egyptians for their chests and arbours, but more particularly destined for funeral purposes and other religious ceremonies.

Belzoni has given an interesting account of Gournou,§ the burial place of the renowned city of Thebes. It is a tract of rocks, about two miles in length, at the foot of the Lybian mountains, on the west of Thebes. Every part of this immense tract is cut out into large or small chambers, each having its separate entrance, and there is seldom a communication from one to the other. According to this traveller there are no sepulchres in the world like them, no excavations or mines that can be compared to

---

* Biban-el-Molouk, the place of the tombs, or rather "the Gates of the Kings," is, according to the learned De Sacy, a corruption of the ancient Egyptian name, Biban-Ourôon. This royal Necropolis is situated in an arid valley enclosed by very high rocks. No one tomb communicates with another; they are all isolated. M. Champollion was convinced that they contained the bodies of the kings of the eighteenth, nineteenth, and twentieth dynasties. He perceived the most ancient of all, that of Aménophis-Memnon, in the isolated valley at the west.—See Lettres, p. 221.

† Lib. xvii.   ‡ Pp. 161-167.   See also the work of M. Cailliaud.

§ Narrative of the Operations and Recent Discoveries within the Pyramids, Temples, Tombs, and Excavations in Egypt and Nubia, 4to. Lond. 1821, p. 156.

them, and no exact description can be given of their interior, owing to the difficulty of visiting these recesses, not to mention that the inconveniency of entering them is such that few would be able to support the exertion. I cannot do better than give the account of Belzoni's visit to those caverns in his own words, and it is too interesting to be abridged. " A traveller," he observes, " is generally satisfied when he has seen the large hall, the gallery, the staircase, and as far as he can conveniently go : besides, he is taken up with the strange works he observes cut in various places, and painted on each side of the walls ; so that when he comes to a narrow and difficult passage, or to have to descend to the bottom of a well or cavity, he declines taking such trouble, naturally supposing that he cannot see in those classes any thing so magnificent as what he sees above, and consequently deeming it useless to proceed any farther. Of some of these tombs many persons could not withstand the suffocating air, which often causes fainting. A vast quantity of dust rises, so fine that it enters the throat and nostrils, and chokes the nose and mouth to such a degree that it requires great power of lungs to resist it, and the strong effluvia of the mummies. This is not all ; the entry, or passage where the bodies are, is roughly cut in the rocks, and the falling of the sand from the upper part or ceiling of the passage causes it to be nearly filled up. In some places there is not more than a vacancy of a foot left, which you must contrive to pass through in a creeping posture like a snail, on pointed and keen stones, that cut like glass. After getting through those passages, some of them two or three hundred yards long, you generally find a more commodious place, perhaps high enough to sit. But what a place of rest! surrounded by bodies, by heaps of mummies in all directions, which, previous to my being accustomed to the sight, impressed me with horror. The blackness of the wall, the faint light given by the candles or torches for want of air, the different objects that surrounded me, seeming to converse with each other, and the Arabs with the candles or torches in their hands, naked and covered with dust, themselves resembling living mummies, absolutely formed a scene that cannot be described. In such a situation I found myself several times, and often returned exhausted and fainting, till at last I became inured to it, and indifferent to what I suffered, except from the dust, which never failed to choke my throat and nose; and though, fortunately, I am destitute of the sense of smelling, I could taste that the mummies were rather unpleasant to swallow. After the exertion of entering into such a place, through a passage of fifty, a hundred, three hundred, or, perhaps, six hundred yards, nearly overcome, I sought a resting place, found one, and contrived to sit; but, when my weight bore on the body of an Egyptian, it crushed it like a band-box. I naturally had recourse to my hands to sustain my weight, but they found no better support; so that I sunk altogether among the broken mummies, with a crash of bones, rags, and wooden cases, which raised such a dust as kept me motionless for a quarter of an hour, waiting till it subsided again. I could not remove from the place, however, without increasing it, and every step I took I crushed a mummy in some part or other. Once I was conducted from such a place to another resembling it, through a passage of about twenty feet in length, and no wider than that a body could be forced through. It was choked with mummies, and I could not pass without putting my face in contact with that of some decayed Egyptian; but as the passage inclined downwards, my own weight helped me on; however, I could not avoid being covered with bones, legs, arms, and heads rolling from above. Thus I proceeded from one cave to another, all full of mummies piled up in various ways, some standing, some lying, and some on their heads."*

Captain Light crept into one of the mummy pits or caverns, which were the common burial places of the ancient Thebans. As it happened to be newly discovered, he found thousands of dead bodies, placed in horizontal layers side by side; these he conceives to be the mummies of the lower order of people, as they were covered only with simple teguments, and smeared over with a composition that preserved the muscles from corruption. " The suffocating smell," he says, " and the natural horror excited by being left alone unarmed with the wild villagers in this charnel house, made me content myself with visiting two or three chambers, and quickly return to the open air."†

Herodotus mentions the mummies as being placed erect. Belzoni says‡ that, although he had opened a great number of pits, he had never seen a

* pp. 156, 7.   † Quarterly Rev. No. 37.   ‡ P. 167.

single mummy standing.* On the contrary, he found them lying regularly in horizontal rows, and some were sunk into a cement, which must have been nearly fluid when the cases were placed on it. The lower classes were not buried in cases; they were dried up, as it appears, after the regular preparation of the seventy days. Mummies of this sort, Belzoni calculates, were in the proportion of about ten to one of the better class. M. Passalacqua met with only one instance in which the mummy was placed in an upright posture: this was before the door of a sepulchral chamber in which were found two Greek mummies.

* I do not know how to reconcile this with what he says respecting the caves at Gournou, p. 157.

CHAPTER V.

ON EMBALMING.

Embalming—definition—Ethiopian, Persian, and Scythian methods of preserving their dead —also of the Greeks and Romans—Egyptian method the most perfect—unknown at this day—accounts of by Herodotus and Diodorus Siculus—difficulty of assigning with precision the antiquity of a mummy—points to be attended to in this enquiry—Count de Caylus's opinion—the testimony of St. Athanasius and of St. Augustine—embalming of strangers— examination of the ancient accounts of this process—embalmers probably an inferior kind of priesthood—honours paid to the embalmers or swathers—three methods described by Herodotus—these admit of many subdivisions—price of embalming—First method: Extraction of the brain—insects found in the head of a Græco-Egyptian mummy—extraction not practised in all cases—Dr. Lee's mummy—head filled with bituminous matter and other substances—Dr. Perry's mummy—Dr. Mead's mummy—Mr. Davidson's mummy—ventral incision—the scribe—representations of this part of the process in papyri—the dissector —Æthiopic stone—prayer uttered by the embalmers—record of it by Porphyry—evisceration of the body—canopi or vases for the intestines—palm wine—aromatics—replacing of the viscera—discovery of the heart in the author's Græco-Egyptian mummy—restoration of different parts to a natural state—extraction of the viscera not always practised in the most expensive mode—use of spices—resinous matters—natrum—period for which the body was to lie in a solution of this substance—removal of the cuticle—great care taken to preserve the nails—body anointed with oil of cedar, &c.—probable application of heat—gilding of mummies—testimony of Abd'Allatif, Hertzog, Denon, Jomard, Rouyer, Passalacqua, Madden, &c., to the application of gold on different parts of the body—probability of the whole body having been gilt in the author's Græco-Egyptian mummy—the body of Alexander adorned with a chase work of gold—practice of wrapping the dead in sheets of gold, observed in the sepulchres on the banks of the Volga, the Tobol, the Irtish, and the Ob—staining of the nails and hands with henna—amulets found on the surface of the body—position of mummies—wonderful preservation of the hair—Second method: Non-extraction of the brain— no ventral incision—no resinous or aromatic substances—oil of cedar—natrum—probability of the injection of a caustic alkaline solution—Third method: Washing the body with surmaia—natrum—impossibility of classing all the embalmed under the three divisions— Rouyer's method of classing the mummies—rarity of the mummies of children—mummy of a fœtus in the author's collection—case of a similar kind in Dr. Lee's museum—also in the Earl of Munster's possession—Denon and Cailliaud's notices of these cases—Captain Henvey's fœtal mummy.

BY embalming we are to understand an artificial operation, in which, by the aid of various medicaments, a dead body may be rendered capable of resisting the process of putrefaction. The ancient Egyptians are the only people who have practised this art with any thing like method or success, and by these people, the Persians, and the Arabians, the bodies so prepared have been, according to the Arabic language, denominated mummies. The process has been variously termed and described as BALSAMATIO—MUMISATIO—CAROMOMIA—EMBERUMA—HONESTA ANATOMIA—UNCTURA FERALIS—CADAVER MEDICATUM—FUNUS MEDICATUM—CADAVER CONDITUM.

The Ethiopians employed a diaphanous resin to preserve their dead bodies; the Persians enveloped theirs in wax; the Scythians folded their dead in skins; and the Greeks and Romans employed perfumes and unctions with the same intent. The unctions were performed by ordinary servants, whilst the perfumes were made and applied by the medical attendants.

The art of embalming among the Egyptians of the present day is entirely unknown; we are, therefore, compelled to have recourse to ancient authorities in order to learn the particulars of the modes of embalming adopted by the Egyptians. Herodotus, who lived 484 years B.C., is the most ancient author from whom we can derive any information upon the subject. This is particularly contained in the second Book of his History, the "Euterpe," which gives the history of the kings of Egypt, and goes down to the invasion of that country by Cambyses, and from which the following extract is taken:—

"Εἰσὶ δὲ οἳ ἐπ' αὐτῷ τούτῳ κατέαται, καὶ τέχνην ἔχουσι ταύτην. οὗτοι ἐπεάν˙ σφικομισθῇ νεκρὸς, δεικνύασι τοῖσι κομίσασι παραδείγματα νεκρῶν ξύλινα, τῇ γραφῇ μεμιμημένα. καὶ τὴν μὲν σπουδαιοτάτην αὐτέων φασὶ εἶναι, τοῦ οὐκ ὅσιον ποιεῦμαι τὸ οὔνομα ἐπὶ τοιούτῳ πρήρματι ὀνομάζειν. τὴν δὲ δευτέρην δεικνύασι ὑποδεεστέρην τε ταύτης καὶ εὐτελεστέρην˙ τὴν δὲ τρίτην, εὐτελεστάτην. φράσαντες δὲ, πυνθάνονται παρ' αὐτέων κατὰ ἥν τινα βούλονταί σφισκευασθῆναι τὸν νεκρόν, οἱ μὲν δὴ ἐκποδὼν, μισθῷ ὁμολογήσαντες, ἀπαλλάσσονται˙ οἱ δὲ ὑπολειπόμενοι ἐν οἰκήμασι, ὧδε τὰ σπουδαιότατα ταριχεύουσι. πρῶτα μὲν σκολιῷ σιδήρῳ διὰ τῶν μυξωτήρων ἐξάγουσι τὸν ἐγκέφαλον, τα μὲν αὐτοῦ οὕτω ἐξάγοντες, τὰ δὲ ἐγχέοντες φαρμακα. μετὰ δὲ, λίθῳ Αἰθιοπικῷ ὀξέι· παρασχίσαντες παρὰ τὴν λαπάρην, ἐξ ὧν εἷλο τὴν κοιλιὴν πᾶσαν· ἐκκαθήραντες δὲ αὐτὴν καὶ διηθήσαντες οἴνῳ φοινικηΐῳ, αὖτις διηθέουσι θυμιήμασι τετριμμένοισι. ἔπειτα τὴν νηδὺν σμύρνης ἀκηράτου τετριμμένης, καὶ κασίης, καὶ τῶν ἄλλων θυωμάτων, πλὴν λιβανωτοῦ, πλήσαντες, συρράπτουσι ὀπίσω. ταῦτα δὲ ποιήσαντες, ταριχεύουσι λίτρῳ, κρύψαντες ἡμέρας ἑβδομήκοντα· πλεῦνας δὲ τουτέων οὐκ ἔξεστι ταριχεύειν. ἐπεὰν δὲ παρέλθωσι αἱ ἑβδομήκοντα, λούσαντες τὸν νεκρὸν, κατειλίσσουσι πᾶν αὐτοῦ το σῶμα σινδόνος βυσσίνης τελαμῶσι κατατετμημένοισι, ὑποχρίοντες τῷ κόμμι τῷ δὴ ἀντὶ κόλλης τὰ πολλὰ χρέωνται Αἰγύπτιοι. ἐνθεῦτεν δὲ παραδεξάμενο μιν οἱ προσήκοντες, ποιεῦνται ξύλινον τύπον ἀνθρωποειδέα· ποιησάμενοι δὲ, ἐσεργνῦσι τὸν νεκρόν. καὶ κατακληΐσαντες οὕτω, θησαυρίζουσι ἐν οἰκήματι θηκαίῳ, ἱστάντες ὀρθὸν πρὸς τοῖκον. οὕτω μὲν τοὺς τὰ πολυτελεστατα σκευάζουσι νεκρούς. Τοὺς δὲ τὰ μέσα βουλομένους, τὴν δὲ πολυτελητην φεύγοντας, σκευάζουσι ὧδε. ἐπεὰν τοὺς κλυστῆρας πλήσωνται τοῦ ἀπὸ κέδρου ἀλείφατος γινομένου, ἐν ὧν ἔπλησαν τοῦ νεκροῦ τὴν κοιλίην, οὔτε ἀναταμόντες αὐτὸν, οὔτε ἐξελόντες τὴν νηδὺν, κατὰ δὲ τὴν ἕδρην ἐσηθήσαντες· καὶ ἐπιλαβόντες τὸ κλύσμα τῆς ὀπίσω ὀδοῦ, ταριχεύουσι τὰς προκειμένας ἡμέρας· τῇ δὲ τελευταίῃ ἐξιεῖσι εκ τῆς κοιλίης τὴν κεδρίην, τὴν ἐσῆκαν πρότερον· ἡ δὲ ἔχει τοσαύτην δύναμιν, ὥστε ἅμα ἑωυτῇ τὴν νηδὺν καὶ τὰ σπλάγχνα κατατετηκότα ἐξάγει. τὰς δὲ σάρκας τὸ λίτρον κατατήκει· καὶ δὴ λείπεται τοῦ νεκροῦ τὸ δέρμα μοῦνον, καὶ τὰ ὀστέα. επεὰν δὲ ταῦτα ποιήσωσι, ἀπ' ὧν ἔδωκαν οὕτω τὸν νεκρὸν, οὐδὲν ἔτι πρηγματευθέντες. Ἡ δὲ τρίτη ταρίχευσίς ἐστι ἥδε, ἣ τοὺς χρήμασι ἀσθηνεστέρους σκευάζει. συρμαίῃ διηθήσαντες τὴν κοιλίην, ταριχεύουσι τας ἑβδομήκοντα ἡμέρας, καὶ ἔπειτα ἀπ' ὧν ἔδωκαν ἀποφέρεσθαι. Τὰς δὲ γυναῖκας τῶν ἐπιφανέων ἀνδρῶν, ἐπεὰν τελευτήσωσι, οὐ παραυτίκα διδοῦσι ταριχεύειν, οὐδὲ ὅσαι ἂν ωσι. εὐειδέες κάρτα καὶ λόγου πλεῦνος γυναῖκες· ἀλλ' ἐπεὰν τριταῖαι ἢ τεταρταῖαι γένωνται, οὕτω παραδιδοῦσι τοῖσι ταριχεύουσι. τοῦτο δὲ ποιέουσι οὕτω τοῦδε ἕινεκεν, ἵνα μή σφι οἱ ταριχευταὶ μίσγωνται τῇσι γυναιξί. λαμφθῆναι γάρ τινά φασι μισγόμενον νεκρῷ προσφάτῳ γυναικός· κατεῖπαι δὲ τὸν ὁμότεκνον."

Herodoti Historiarum, lib. ix. *ed. Schweighaeuseri*, 8vo. Lond. 1817, lib. ii. § 86-9.

"There are certain individuals appointed for that purpose (the embalming), and who profess that art; these persons, when any body is brought to them, show the bearers some wooden models of corpses, painted to represent the originals; the most perfect they assert to be the representation of him whose name I take it to be impious to mention in this matter; they show a second, which is inferior to the first, and cheaper; and a third, which is the cheapest of all. They then ask of them according to which of the models they will have the deceased prepared: having settled upon the price, the relations immediately depart, and the embalmers, remaining at home, thus proceed to perform the embalming in the most costly manner. In the first place, with a crooked piece of iron, they pull out the brain by the nostrils; a part of it they extract in this manner, the rest by means of pouring in certain drugs: in the next place, after making an incision in the flank with a sharp Egyptian stone, they empty the whole of the inside; and after cleansing the cavity, and rincing it with palm-wine, scour it out again with pounded aromatics: then having filled the belly with pure myrrh pounded, and cinnamon, and all other perfumes, frankincense excepted, they sew it up again; having so done, they steep the body in natrum, keeping it covered for seventy days, for it is not lawful to leave the body any longer in the brine. When the seventy days are gone by, they first wash the corpse, and then wrap up the whole of the body in bandages cut out of cotton cloth, which they smear with gum, a substance the Egyptians generally use instead of paste. The relations, having then received back the body, get a wooden case, in the shape of a man, to be made; and, when completed, place the body in the inside; and then, shutting it up, keep it in a sepulchral repository, where they stick it upright against the wall. The above is the most costly manner in which they prepare the dead. For such as choose the middle mode, from a desire of avoiding expense, they prepare the body thus:—They first fill syringes with cedar oil, which they inject into the belly of the deceased, without making any incision, or emptying the inside, but sending it in by the seat; they then close the aperture, to hinder the injection from flowing backwards, and lay the body in brine for the specified number of days, on the last of which they take out the cedar oil which they had previously injected, and such is the strength it possesses that it brings away with it the bowels and inside in a state of dissolution: on the other hand, the natrum dissolves the flesh, so that, in fact, there remains nothing but the skin and the bones. When they have so done they give back the body without performing any farther operation upon it. The third mode of embalming, which is used for such as have but scanty means, is as follows:—After washing the inside with syrmaea, they salt the body for the seventy days, and return it to be taken back. The wives of men of quality are not given to be embalmed immediately after their death, neither are those that may have been extremely beautiful, or much celebrated; but they deliver them to the embalmers after they have been three or four days deceased: this they do for the following reason, that the workmen may not be able to abuse the bodies of those females; for it is reported by them that one of those artificers was discovered in the very fact on the newly-deceased body of a woman, and was impeached by his fellow workman."

Laurent's Translation.

The next authority is that of Diodorus Siculus, who lived 440 years after Herodotus. He has detailed several particulars not mentioned by the preceding historian, and entered more at large upon the funeral ceremonies of the Egyptians.

"Ὅταν γάρ τις ἀποθάνῃ παρ' αὐτοῖς, οἱ μὲν συγγενεῖς καὶ φίλοι πάντες καταπασάμενοι πηλῷ τὰς κεφαλὰς, περιέρχονται τὴν πόλιν θρηνοῦντες, ἕως ἂν ταφῆς τύχῃ τὸ σῶμα, οὐ μὴν οὔτε λουτρῶν, οὔτε οἴνου, οὔτε τῆς ἄλλης τροφῆς ἀξιολόγου μεταλαμβάνουσιν, οὔτε ἐσθῆτας λαμπρὰς περιβάλλονται. τῶν δὲ ταφῶν τρεῖς ὑπάρχουσι τάξεις, ἥτε πολυτελεστάτη καὶ μέση καὶ ταπεινοτάτη. κατὰ μὲν οὖν τὴν πρώτην ἀναλίσκεσθαι φασὶν ἀργυρίου ταλαντον, κατὰ δὲ τὴν δευτέραν μνᾶς εἴκοσι, κατὰ δὲ τὴν ἐσχάτην παντελῶς ὀλίγον τι δαπάνημα γινεσθαι λέγουσιν. οἱ μὲν οὖν τὰ σώματα θεραπεύοντες, εἰσὶ τεχνῖται τὴν ἐπιστήμην ταύτην ἐκ γένους παρειληφόντες. οὗτοι δὲ γραφὴν ἑκάστου τῶν εἰς τὰς ταφὰς δαπανωμένων τοῖς οἰκείοις τῶν τελευτησάντων προσενέγκαντες, ἐπερωτῶσι τίνα τρόπον βούλονται τὴν θεραπείαν γενέσθαι τοῦ σώματος. διομολογησάμενοι δὲ περὶ πάντων, καὶ τὸν νεκρὸν παραλαβόντες, τοῖς τεταγμένοις ἐπὶ τὴν κατειθισμένην ἐπιμέλειαν τὸ σῶμα παραδιδόασι. καὶ πρῶτος μὲν ὁ γραμματεὺς λεγόμενος, τεθέντος χαμαὶ τοῦ σώματος, ἐπὶ τὴν λαγόνα περιγράφει τὴν εὐώνυμον ὅσον δεῖ τεμεῖν. ἔπειθ' ὁ λεγόμενος παρασχίστης, λίθον ἔχων Αἰθιοπικὸν, καὶ διατεμὼν ὅσα νόμος κελεύει τὴν σάρκα, παραχρῆμα φεύγει δρόμῳ, διωκόντων τῶν συμπαρόντων καὶ λίθοις βαλλόντων, ἔτι δὲ καταρωμένων, καὶ καθαπερεὶ τὸ μῦσος εἰς ἐκεῖνον τρεπόντων. ὑπολαμβάνουσι γὰρ μισητὸν εἶναι πάντα τὸν ὁμοφύλῳ σώματι βίαν προσφέροντα, καὶ τραύματα ποιοῦντα, καὶ καθόλου τι κακὸν ἀπεργαζόμενον. οἱ ταριχευταὶ δὲ καλούμενοι πάσης μὲν τιμῆς καὶ πολυωρίας ἀξιοῦνται, τοῖς τε ἱερεῦσι συνόντες καὶ τὰς εἰς ἱερὸν εἰσόδους ἀκωλύτως ὡς ἱεροὶ ποιοῦνται. πρὸς δὲ τὴν θεραπείαν τοῦ παρεσχισμένου σώματος ἀθροισθέντων αὐτῶν, εἷς καθίησι τὴν χεῖρα διὰ τῆς τοῦ νεκροῦ τομῆς εἰς τὸν θώρακα, καὶ πάντα ἐξαίρει, χωρὶς νεφρῶν καὶ καρδίας. ἕτερος δὲ καθαίρει τῶν ἐγκοιλίων ἕκαστον, ἐγκλύζων οἴνῳ φοινικείῳ καὶ θυμιάμασι.

καθόλου δὲ πᾶν τὸ σῶμα τὸ μὲν πρῶτον κεδρίᾳ καὶ τισιν ἄλλοις ἐπιμελείας ἀξιοῦσιν·.ἐφ' ἡμέρας πλείους τῶν τριάκοντα, ἔπειτα σμύρνῃ καὶ κιναμώμῳ, καὶ τοῖς δυναμένοις μὴ μόνον πολυχρόνιον τήρησιν, ἀλλὰ καὶ τὴν εὐωδίαν παρέχεσθαι, θεραπεύσαντες, παραδιδόασι τοῖς συγγενέσι τοῦ τετελευτηκότος ὄντως ἕκαστον τῶν τοῦ σώματος μελῶν ἀκέραιον τετηρημένον ὥστε καὶ τὰς ἐπὶ τοῖς βλεφάροις καὶ ταῖς ὀφρύσι τρίχας διαμένειν, καὶ τὴν ὅλην πρόσοψιν τοῦ σώματος ἀπαράλλακτον εἶναι, καὶ τὸν τῆς μορφῆς τύπον γνωρίζεσθαι. διὸ καὶ πολλοὶ τῶν Αἰγυπτίων ἐν οἰκήμασι πολυτελέσι φυλάττοντες τὰ σώματα τῶν προγόνων, κατ' ὄψιν ὁρῶσι τοὺς γενεαῖς πολλαῖς τῆς ἑαυτῶν γενέσεως προτετελευτηκότας· στε ἑκάστων τά τε μεγέθη καὶ τὰς περιοχὰς τῶν σωμάτων, ἔτι δ' τοὺς τῆς ὄψεως χαρα κτῆρας ὁρωμένους, παράδοξον ψυχαγωγίαν παρέχεσθαι, καθάπερ συμβεβιωκότας τοῖς θεωρουμένοις."

Diodori Siculi Bibliothecæ Histor. lib. i. § 91.

" When any one among the Egyptians dies, all his relations and friends, putting dirt upon their heads, go lamenting about the city, till such time as the body shall be buried. In the mean time they abstain from baths and wine, and all kinds of delicate meats, neither do they during that time wear any costly apparel. The manner of their burials is three-fold; one very costly, a second sort less chargeable, and a third very mean. In the first, they say, there is spent a talent of silver, in the second twenty minæ, but in the last there is very little expense. Those who have the care of ordering the body are such as have been taught that art by their ancestors. These, showing to the kindred of the deceased a bill of expenses of each kind of burial, ask them after what manner they will have the body prepared; when they have agreed upon the matter, they deliver the body to such as are usually appointed for this office. First, he who has the name of scribe, laying it upon the ground, marks about the flank on the left side how much is to be cut away. Then he who is called the cutter, or dissector, with an Æthiopic stone cuts away as much of the flesh as the law commands, and presently runs away as fast as he can : those who are present, pursuing him, cast stones at him, and curse him, hereby turning all the execrations which they imagine due to his office, upon him. For, whosoever offers violence, wounds, or does any kind of injury to a body of the same nature with himself, they think him worthy of hatred; but those who are called the embalmers they esteem worthy of honour and respect; for they are familiar with their priests, and go into the temples as holy men, without any prohibition. So soon as they come to embalm the dissected body, one of them thrusts his hand through the wound into the abdomen, and draws forth all the bowels but the heart and kidneys, which another washes and cleanses with wine made of palms and aromatic odours. Lastly, having washed the body, they anoint it with oil of cedar and other things for above thirty days, and afterwards with myrrh, cinnamon, and other such like matters, which have not only a power to preserve it for a long time, but also give it a sweet smell; after which they deliver it to the kindred, in such manner that every member remains whole and entire, and no part of it changed, but the beauty and shape of the face seems just as it was before, and may be known, even the hairs of the eye-lids and eye-brows remaining as they were at first. By this means many of the Egyptians, keeping the dead bodies of their ancestors in magnificent houses, so perfectly see the true visage and countenance of those that died many ages before they themselves were born, that in viewing the proportions of every one of them, and the lineaments of their faces, they take as much delight as if they were still living among them."

These are the two principal accounts of the processes of embalming adopted by the ancient Egyptians, and the statement of these will prepare the way for a more detailed account upon the subject, previously to which, however, I shall make a few general observations.

It would, I fear, be a task of no little difficulty to assign the period and give any thing like the precise age of a mummy; but much may be done by a careful comparison of the observations of Herodotus, Diodorus Siculus, and other historians, and an attentive examination into the physical forms of the individuals thus converted into mummies. Professor Blumenbach felt the difficulty of the investigation when he proposed, in order to obtain this object, the two following *Pia Desideria*, as he terms them, to be first accomplished:—

" 1. A more accurate determination of the *various*, so strikingly *different*, and yet as strikingly *characteristic* national configurations in the monuments of the Egyptian arts, together with a determination of the periods in which

H

these monuments were produced, and the causes of their remarkable differences.

" 2. A very careful technical examination of the characteristic forms of the several *skulls* of mummies we have hitherto met with, together with an accurate comparison of those skulls with the monuments above mentioned."*

Count Caylus is of opinion that no mummies have been made since the conquest of Egypt by the Romans. The Christians in Egypt, St. Athanasius tells us, in his Life of St. Anthony, were in the habit of keeping in their houses the embalmed bodies not only of their martyrs, but also of all who died among them. St. Anthony opposed this custom, and, fearing that his body might be so disposed of, he withdrew with two of his monks into the desert, and directed that they should, after his death, bury him in secret and not let the place of his entombment be known.† And St. Augustine bears testimony‡ to mummies having been made in his time (the beginning of the fifth century). As in relation to the religious opinions of the ancient Egyptians, as we have already seen,§ it was essential the bodies of all classes should be preserved, it may naturally be asked what was the practice adopted with the poorest or lowest order of society? Were they also embalmed ? Not according to the methods mentioned by Herodotus and Diodorus Siculus most assuredly. The ordinary mode of sepulture among the Egyptians effected a kind of natural embalming: they were laid upon beds of charcoal, ‖ according to Maillet, and wrapped round only with a few swaddling clothes, covered with a mat, upon which was heaped a quantity of sand seven or eight feet in thickness. This material served as a bed to absorb all moisture from the body, and it thus became shrivelled and dried up.

Herodotus gives some curious information upon the embalming of strangers, or those destroyed by crocodiles or drowned in the Nile, though

---

* Philos. Trans. 1794, p. 189.   † Montfauçon Antiquité Expliqué, tom. V., Part II., p. 176.
‡ Serm. 361, oper. tom. V., p. 981.   § Chap. III.
‖ Does it not then appear that the Egyptians were acquainted with the antiseptic properties of this substance ?

it is to be regretted that his detail relative to the sacred repository is not more particular.

"Ὃς δ' ἂν ᾖ αὐτῶν Αἰγυπτίων, ἢ ξείνων ὁμοίως, ὑπὸ κροκοδείλου ἁρπαχθεὶς ἢ ὑπ' αὐτοῦ τοῦ ποταμοῦ φαίνηται τεθνηὼς, κατ' ἣν ἂν πόλιν ἐξενειχθῇ, τούτους πᾶσα ἀνάγκη ἐστὶ ταριχεύσαντας αὐτὸν, καὶ περιστείλαντας ὡς κάλλιστα, θάψαι ἐν ἰρῇσι θήκῃσι. οὐδὲ ψαῦσαι ἔξεστι αὐτοῦ ἄλλον οὐδένα, οὔτε τῶν προσηκόντων, οὔτε τῶν φίλων· ἀλλά μιν οἱ ἱρέες αὐτοὶ, οἱ τοῦ Νείλου, ἅτε πλέον τι ἢ ἀνθρώπου νεκρὸν, χειραττάζοντες θάπτουσι."

Herod. Hist. lib. ii. § 90.

" If any one, no matter whether one of the Egyptians themselves or a foreigner, is found having been carried off by a crocodile, or merely drowned in the river, whatever be the city near which he is cast up, the inhabitants must necessarily embalm and dress his body in the most sumptuous manner, and inter him in the sacred repository: no one must touch him, whether relation or friend; the priests of the Nile alone handle the body and bury it, as though it were the corpse of something more than a man."

Laurent's Translation.

This practice was doubtless a wise one, and the effect of it was to induce vigilance on the part of the authorities of the different cities, and prevent accidents, in order to avert the very expensive process of embalming.

The account of Herodotus, as we have seen, commences with stating that the persons employed in embalming, the κατέαται, were individuals specially appointed for the purpose; but he does not inform us of their quality. The term used to denote the persons performing this office applies generally to those following any *sedentary arts.* It is not unlikely that the embalmers were an inferior kind of priesthood; for Diodorus Siculus informs us that they were esteemed " worthy of honour and respect," that they were " familiar with their priests," and that " *they went into the temples as holy men without any prohibition;*" whereas the *Paraschistes*, the cutter or dissector, who was employed in making the incision into the left flank of the body for the extraction of the bowels, was held in abhorrence, and obliged to fly away for safety after the performance of his task. M. Peyron supposes the honours mentioned by Diodorus Siculus as given to the *Taricheutæ*, or embalmers, were really paid only to the *Chol-chytæ* or swathers.   From papyri, not long since discovered, M. Peyron states we derive the knowledge that the latter part of the embalming process was performed by a peculiar class of priests, of the lowest order, yet possessed of great privileges, and much respected by their countrymen.*

To the embalmers the relatives of the dead made application for the purpose of preserving the body, and selecting the mode by which it should be effected.   Herodotus mentions three modes; but, from the examination of mummies of various kinds, it is clear that others may be added, and these probably admit of subdivisions.†   The price attending each mode is stated by Diodorus Siculus.‡   The first method cost a talent of silver,§ which is equal to £225 of English money; the second 20 minæ, or £75; and the third a much smaller sum, which is not mentioned.

The FIRST and the most costly mode of embalming described by Herodotus is that which commenced by the operation of the extraction of the brain through the nostrils, which was effected by the aid of iron (bronze) crotchets.   I, at first, was tempted to conceive that it was not possible to empty the skull of its contents by these means, and at least it seemed to me to be an operation of exceeding difficulty.   But the examination of more than one specimen has convinced me of the practicability of it.‖ Not only has the brain been entirely removed from the head of the mummy I opened, and which I have called the " Græco-Egyptian Mummy," but also the whole of the membranes have been dragged through the nostrils without in any way defacing them, disturbing the *septum* of the nose, or disfiguring this organ in any manner whatever, as will be seen by a reference to

* Peyron, Papyri Egypt. pp. 84—89.

† The observation of Belzoni is, doubtless, correct, when he states, in relation to the three several modes of embalming, that he " will venture to assert that the high, middling, and poorer classes all admit of farther distinction."

‡ Lib. i. § 91.

§ The Babylonian talent, according to Taylor (Translation of the History of Herodotus), is worth about £226; the talent of Eubœa is believed to be nearly the same as the Attic, and is valued at £193. 15s. English money.   See also Browne's Travels, p. 8.

‖ Greenhill, in his " Art of Embalming," p. 249, speaks of the extraction of the brain through the nostrils as an amusing story of a thing " impracticable and ridiculous."

Plates I. and II. It would appear that the crotchets (*Fig.* 9, 10, Plate IV.) had been introduced up the nostrils, made to perforate the ethmoid bone at the upper part of the nostrils, and then by a circular rotatory movement to break down the cribriform plate of that bone, together with the adjacent portions of the frontal bone, of sufficient size to admit a crown-piece, and through which opening the brain and membranes could be extracted and any fluid injected into the skull that might be thought necessary to cleanse that cavity.* In the instance to which I have alluded the skull was quite empty—the only contents, if such they can be called, consisted of some insects and the pupæ of others.† I observed a similar opening in Mr.

* In a remarkably fine specimen of mummy, supposed to have been brought from Egypt by M. Passalacqua, and opened in 1828 at the Leeds' Philosophical and Literary Society, the brain was found to have been extracted through the right nostril. The opening into the skull was made through the sphenoidal sinuses and not through the cribriform plate. The membranes were preserved entire. In Mons. Cailliaud's Græco-Egyptian Mummy the nose was disfigured and broken by the operation.

Dr. Granville observed small crystals of what appeared to be an animal substance resembling steatine, studded on the inner surface of the skull of his mummy. I found similar crystals on the surface of the body of my Græco-Egyptian Mummy, and I transmitted them to Dr. Faraday, the highly-talented professor of chemistry at the Royal Institution, for his examination. The following account is worthy of notice :—" The small needle-like crystals are very curious, but too minute in quantity, and too vague as to their origin, to allow of much being made out relative to them. The crystallization is very perfect and acicular, and, from the appearance, one might suppose them the result of sublimation; but when the substance is heated it does not prove to be volatile. It fuzes, and upon cooling concretes again, crystallizing the whole like spermaceti. It burns with a bright flame, and evidently abounds in carbon and hydrogen. It is not soluble in water, and has the odour, when heated, of a fatty matter; but then alkali acts very feebly upon it, and dissolves only a very small portion. On the contrary, it is very soluble in alcohol, the solution being precipitated by water. The substance may probably be a result of slow action upon organic (perchance animal) matter, and has, perhaps, been assisted in its formation by *heat*." Extract of a letter from Dr. Faraday, May 23, 1823. On the body of the Mummy opened at Leeds, upon exposure of any part to the operation of the atmosphere, small white crystals were found to be produced; they consisted of natrum, which had been employed in the process of embalming.

† I submitted these to the examination of my friend the Rev. F. W. Hope, whose minute acquaintance with entomological science eminently qualifies him to detect all the peculiarities of the beings composing this curious division of animated nature. He has kindly favoured me with the following description :

Saunders's mummy, and Mr. Brodie acquaints me that he found the same in

1. NECROBIA MUMIARUM. *Long. lin.* 3. *Lat. lin.* 1¼. *Purpurascens hirta, antennis pedibusque flavo-rubris. Antennæ rubræ, totum corpus fere supra violaceum punctatum marginibus elytrorum rufescentibus lineato-punctatis. Corpus infra nigrum hirtum, pedibus flavo-rubris.* As this species of Necrobia appears distinct from any previously described, Mr. Hope has named it *N. Mumiarum. N. Rufipes Fab.*, an African species, seems closely allied to it; it differs, however, in the colour of the antennæ, *rufipes* having black antennæ with the basal joint red, the Fabrician species is also a broader insect and differs from *mumiarum* in its sculpture and hirsuties. Mr. Hope thinks it probable that these insects, when alive, were of a violet or deep purple colour, the medicaments used in the process of embalming having partly discharged the colouring matter. Some of them also exhibit the appearance of immaturity.

2. DERMESTES VULPINUS? In the Appendix to the 14th vol. of the Linnæan Transactions, there is a notice of this insect being found, together with *Corynetes violaceus*, in a mummy at Thebes. The only *dermestes* Mr. Hope could find in the collection from the head of my Græco-Egyptian mummy appears however quite distinct. Several species of true *Dermestes* are found in Egypt, and at the Cape of Good Hope. It is almost absolutely necessary to describe the species of this genus as soon as they are captured, as they are liable to become greasy, and the colour and appearance of them so changed that it is difficult to name them accurately.

3. PUPÆ OF DIPTEROUS INSECTS. In the head of the mummy was found a considerable quantity of the *pupæ* of dipterous insects, apparently of two distinct species, and from their appearance Mr. Hope was led to remark, that the process of embalming could not possibly be a rapid one. Some of the pupæ cases were empty, and the major part of them contained the dried-up insects almost in a state of perfection.

Mr. Hope has been so kind as to examine a number of insects obtained from the head of a mummy brought for me from Thebes by Mr. Wilkinson. The account of these will, I trust, be truly acceptable to entomologists, as opportunities of examining insects under such circumstances are unquestionably of rare occurrence.

DERMESTES POLLINCTUS. *Long. lin.* 4. *Lat. lin.* 2.

Totum corpus supra castaneum, subtomentosum, pedibus concoloribus, abdomineq. infra albido. Caput fusco-rubrum¦ oculis nigris, antennis rubro-castaneis. Thorax castaneus, punctatus medio nigricanti, marginibusq. lateralibus albo-tomentosis. Scutellum hirsutum, seu pilis albis obsitum. Elytra castanea, subtomentosa. Corpus infra albido-pilosum segmentis abdominis castaneo-maculatis, trigonoq. concolori, in medio singulorum posito. Pedes castanei.

This Dermestes appears to Mr. Hope to differ from any species hitherto described. In form it resembles D. domesticus Steven. from Siberia. Its light colour is remarkable, arising probably from the exclusion of light, and not in this case, he imagines, from the effects of the drugs used in embalming. The thorax in many of the specimens is nearly black: in two of them the elytra are of a dark chesnut colour, almost approaching to black. From one skull

three mummies belonging to Lord Mountnorris. M. Lancret says* that
he had found the nose preserved entire, notwithstanding the extraction of
the brain through the nostrils. M. Rouyer† has made the same remark,
but observes that several had the nose broken or destroyed. In Dr.

more than 270 tolerably perfect specimens were taken; and, from the remaining fragments of
others, probably double that number lived, propagated their species, and died without ever seeing
the light. The perfect pupæ are not abundant; the remnants of the empty cases, however,
would lead one to believe that the greater part of them arrived at the imago state some time
after the process of embalming was completed, when as mummies, they were deposited in
their respective mausolea.

DERMESTES ROEI.—*Long. lin.* 3. *Lat. lin.* 2½.

Totum corþus supra nigrum, subtus albopilosum. Antennæ capitulo nigro cæteris articulis
rubris. Thorax ater lateribus thoracis cinereo-villosis. Corpus infra albopilosum lateribus abdominis antice maculâ magnâ ovatâ notatis, posticeque segmentis utrinq. minoribus maculis
variegatis.

The above species agrees very well with several specimens of Dermestes which were brought
to Mr. Hope from the shores of the Red Sea by Lieutenant Roe, in honour of whom he named
the insect. There is a third species also from the same mummy differing from all others of the
genus by its elongate oblong form. It is, however, in too mutilated a state to describe, as the
antennæ and legs are wanting. Among the broken fragments of insects taken from the mummies, there are remnants of some large species of Pimelia, probably Pimelia spinulosa, Klug,
not uncommon in Egypt. There are also immense numbers of Pupæ of some dipterous insects,
certainly of three different species, if not more. The recorded mummied insects, including
those described at present, are the following :—

1. *Corynetes* violaceus Fab. vid. Linn. Tran. Vol. XIV. Appendix.

2. *Necrobia* Mumiarum, Hope.

3. *Dermestes* vulpinus, Fab. vid. Linn. Tran. Vol. XIV. Append.

4. ———— pollinctus, ⎫
5. ———— Roei,   ⎬Hope.
6. ———— elongatus, ⎭

7. *Pimelia* spinulosa, Klug?

8. Copris Sabæus? found by Passalacqua, embalmed, and so named on the testimony of
Latreille.

9. —— Midas, Fab.

10. —— Pithecius, Fab.

11. A species of Cantharis in the collection of Passalacqua from Thebes (No. 442.)

* Jomard Description des Hypogées de la Ville de Thèbes, in the Description de l'Egypte.

† Notice sur les Embaumemens des Anciens Egyptiens in the Description de l'Egypte, par
M. Rouyer, tom. I. p. 207.

Granville's mummy the brain and part of the membranes were extracted through the nostrils.* In many cases, however, the brain was not removed at all, and yet the body very carefully and perfectly preserved. This was the case in Dr. Lee's mummy, the brain of which is in my possession. It has sunk down into a cake-like mass, bearing the impress of the crucial ridge in the internal part of the back of the skull, and shows that the body had been placed in a horizontal posture after being embalmed. I have another head from Thebes, showing the same fact. In this specimen the nostrils are plugged with cotton cloth. M. Rouelle states† that in the head of the mummy sent to the Count de Caylus he perceived a hole in the cranium, made at the extremity of the nostrils, and that the end of the orbit on the right side was actually open. Through these apertures doubtless the brain had been extracted, and the cavity was, as in many other instances, filled up with bituminous and resinous matter.‡ In the mummy, which formerly belonged to Dr. Perry, and which is now in my collection, I found the head filled with these substances. Dr. Mead's mummy, the remains of which are in the Museum of the Royal College of Physicians, was in the same state. Mr. Davidson's mummy also contained this matter, and it is remarkable that in this instance the apertures of the nostrils, with part of the cavity of the skull, was plugged up and filled with twisted portions of cloth introduced through the nostrils, which Mr. Davidson " drew out to the extent of nine yards. It was of very fine texture, and about three inches in width."§ Mr. Madden mentions that he saw heads of mummies crammed with fine linen, which must have been introduced through the nose.‖ The head of the mummy opened at Leeds was found to be rather more than half filled with spices in a state of coarse powder, amongst which were a few lumps of resinous matter, particularly about the base of the skull. The right nostril was also filled with a resinous substance. Dr. Granville's mummy had a lump of rags dipped in pitch and placed in the mouth.

The head being thus deprived of that matter which most readily runs

---

* Philos. Trans. 1825.   † Mem. de l'Acad. Roy. des Sciences, 1750.
‡ The nature of the substances will be treated of in the Chapter on Medicaments.
§ Address on Embalming, 8vo. Lond. 1833, p. 20.
‖ Travels in Turkey, Egypt, Nubia, and Palestine, ii. 88.

into putrefaction, the next step in the process of embalming was the making of the incision into the flank for the evisceration of the body. Diodorus Siculus, describing this part of the embalming, says, " He who has the name of Scribe (ὁ γραμματεὺς), laying the body upon the ground, marks about the flank on the left side,"·&c. Now, all the representations of this process, and they are very numerous, both upon the cases of mummies and on the papyri which have been found within them, represent the body as lying extended upon a table furnished with a lion's head.* I am at a loss to account for this emblem, which is constant in MSS., on cases, tablets, &c. Count Caylus has figured in his *Recueil d'Antiquités Egyptiennes* (tom. IV., Pl. XIV., *fig.* 4) an Egyptian engraving on a hæmatite of a female mummy, stretched on the back of a lion, and Anubis standing by its side, with his arms extended as in the act of invoking protection for the body. Be that as it may, a line is marked out by the scribe, and the dissector (ὁ παρασχιστης) makes his incision according to this direction, and with an Ethiopic stone,† which is of exceeding hardness, and capable of bearing a very keen cutting edge. The man who makes this incision, it is most singularly said, is obliged to fly with all speed even from the assistants in the embalming, who throw stones after him, and load him with curses, it being considered as odious to do any act of violence to a body of the same nature as their own.

Herodotus and Diodorus Siculus leave us in ignorance as to what is done with the intestines after they are extracted from the body by the embalmers, through the incision made in the left flank by the cutter; but Porphyry‡ here affords us some curious and important information. This author has handed down to us the prayer said to have been uttered by the embalmers in the name of the deceased, " entreating the divine powers to receive his soul into the region of the gods." It is as follows:—" When those who have the care of the dead proceed to embalm the body of any

---

* The embalmers are figured with the head of a jackal, and are painted black, &c.

† Egyptian pebbles of pyromachous silex, according to M. Brogniart. *Fig.* 6, 7, 8, Plate IV., are representations of what is supposed to be the knife for making the incision. They are taken from M. Passalacqua's Collection at Berlin.

‡ De Abstinentia, lib. iv. cap. 10.

person of respectable rank, they first take out the contents of the belly, and place them in a separate vessel. After the other rites for the dead have been performed, one of the embalmers, laying his hand on the vessel, addressing the sun, utters on behalf of the deceased the following prayer, which Euphantus has translated from the original language into Greek:— " O thou Sun, our lord, and all ye gods who are the givers of life to men, accept me, and receive me into the mansions of the eternal gods; for I have worshipped piously, while I have lived in this world, those divinities whom my parents taught me to adore. I have ever honoured those parents who gave origin to my body; and of other men I have neither killed any, nor robbed them of their treasure, nor inflicted upon them any grievous evil; but if I have done any thing injurious to my own soul, either by eating or drinking any thing unlawfully, this offence has not been committed by me, but by what is contained in this chest,—meaning the intestines in the vessel, which is then thrown into the river. The body is afterwards regarded as pure, this apology having been made for its offences, and the embalmer prepares it according to the appointed rites." Plutarch confirms the authenticity of this account:—" The belly being opened," he says, " the bowels were cast into the river Nile and the body exposed to the sun. The cavities of the chest and the belly were then filled with unguents and odorous substances."

In the representations of embalming to which I have alluded, four vases will be constantly seen placed beneath the embalming table.* Each of these vases is furnished with a cover, having on it either the head of a human being, a cynocephalus, a jackal, or a hawk. These are the four genii of the Amenti or Amun-ti, which, in Coptic, exactly corresponds with αϑης in Greek. It signifies the *receiver and giver*. Mr. Wilkinson says it was, therefore, a temporary abode. This agrees with the idea of the Egyptians returning again to the earth, after a stated period. The names of the genii are:

1. NETSONOF, or KEBHNSNOF, with the hawk's head.

---

* In Dr. Middleton's miscellaneous works, vol. IV., p. 166, there is a representation of the embalming of a body, the principal operator, and two assistants. There are four vases (Canopi) beneath the table. It occurs in the description of the case, paintings, &c., of an Egyptian mummy given to the University of Cambridge by Captain George Townshend. See Tab. 22 and 23.

2. SMOF, or SMAUTF, with the jackal's head.

3. HAPEE, with the head of the cynocephalus.

4. AMSET, with the human head. (See Plate III., *fig.* 1, 2, 3, 4.*)

The vases containing the embalmed intestines are made either of baked clay or of alabaster: the latter are so rare that Belzoni had only met with fragments of this kind. I have seen one perfect and most beautiful set, and some others imperfect. Lord King has a very fine set measuring 16¾ inches in height. They have most commonly hieroglyphics upon them. In size they vary from about nine inches to a foot and a half.

To return to the process :

The intestines and other viscera being removed through the incision just mentioned, and which is usually about five inches in length, Herodotus tells us they were cleansed and steeped in palm wine. In several instances they were neither placed in vases nor thrown into the river; for, in Dr. Lee's mummy, I found the intestines had been taken out from the opening (5¼ inches in length) in the left flank, and washed I presume in the palm wine ; they had been sprinkled with aromatics, which were also thrown into the cavity of the belly, and then replaced in one mass into that cavity. These are now in my possession. Belzoni remarks that the entrails of mummies are often bound up in linen and asphaltum.† In Mr. Davidson's mummy the arrangement was somewhat different; for, after their removal, they were rolled up in four distinct portions, enclosed in cotton bandages, and then returned into the body. The cut surfaces of this incision were, in all the instances I have seen, merely brought together, not sewed, as stated by Herodotus. M. Rouyer's experience coincides with mine. In the Leeds mummy the edges of the incision were also brought together, but not by any sewing—a simple apposition of surfaces. The contents of the chest and abdomen in this case were removed, with the exception of the liver, the kidneys, and the heart, which had been embalmed, wrapped up in fine cloth, and returned into the cavity. In my " Græco-Egyptian Mummy" the cavity was quite empty. I could not find even the kidneys, which are especially mentioned by Diodorus Siculus as parts that were not to be

* These are taken from four carved figures in my possession. They are of great rarity.

† Travels, p. 170.

removed. So, also, he says of the heart, and this substance I found placed between the thighs of the mummy, without any bandaging or protection of any kind. I have had this figured in Plate IV., *fig.* 3, and the reader will easily observe, by a reference to Plate XXIII. in the Phil. Trans. for 1825, its striking resemblance to the form of the heart belonging to Dr. Granville's mummy. I was for a long time at a loss to ascertain what it really was. I succeeded, however, by macerating it in spirit, and I found the mass to consist of the muscular or fleshy part of the heart. Upon examination of the chest, or thoracic cavity, I was enabled to obtain some portions of membrane (the pleuræ), a portion of the windpipe, and some of the larger blood-vessels coming from, and going to, the heart. This division of the heart from the vessels has evidently been effected by a cutting instrument, and the surfaces receiving this violence are clearly apparent; for, having macerated the portions in warm water, I completely soaked out the mummifying matter, and have since preserved the specimens in spirit; for, the drugs of preservation being removed, the parts began immediately to putrefy, after the lapse of a period of probably three thousand years! Dr. Lee's and Mr. Davidson's mummies had the kidneys as well as the other viscera.

The extraction of the intestines by means of an incision does not appear to have been exclusively practised in the mummies prepared according to the most expensive process, detailed by Herodotus as the first mode; for many have been found, as we learn from Passalacqua* and other competent authorities, with this incision, that had not been enclosed in a sarcophagus. The amount of the expense of the process would rather depend upon the nature and quantity of the spices used, and the profusion of idols with which the mummy should be decorated. Mummies very richly furnished, and prepared in the most costly manner, have been found without the ventral incision.† Passalacqua remarks‡ that the mummies in which the intestines had been removed through the incision had always the place supplied by asphaltum; but I have seen the cavity merely filled with dust of cedar, cassia, &c., and an earthy matter. And Passalacqua himself had

* Catalog. No. 1547.   † Ib. No. 1552.   ‡ Ib. p. 179.

the mummy of a child,* the abdomen of which had been emptied of its contents, and no substance was found to replace them. In Dr. Granville's mummy no ventral incision had been practised, nor had the greatest part of the viscera been displaced; for, upon removing the integuments of the belly, the stomach was found adhering to the diaphragm, the spleen much reduced and flattened, the kidney, gall-bladder, &c. The contents of the chest were entire, and those of the pelvis were found *in situ;* and Dr. Granville has detailed some appearances which he conceives to be indicative of a diseased state of some of those organs, previously to the death of the individual.†

The great cavities of the body being cleansed and prepared, they are, according to Herodotus, filled with aromatic substances, stated to be myrrh and cinnamon or cassia. The use of frankincense was forbidden. Resinous matters were also thrown into the body,‡ which is now to be steeped § in a solution of natrum, a composition of carbonate, sulphate, and muriate of soda, and in this liquid it was to remain for seventy days and no longer. This would appear to be precisely the time necessary for the operation of the alkali on the animal fibre. Having remained in this solution for the time specified, the body was withdrawn and washed. At this stage of the process I suspect the cuticle was removed; for, in all the instances I have been able to meet with, this appears to have been an operation to which much attention has been paid.‖ Great care has been observed in the removal of it, not to disturb any of the nails. My " Græco-Egyptian mummy " has two of the nails fastened on by means of thread, they having been loosened by the detachment of the cuticle.

* No. 1549.

† For the particulars, the reader is referred to the Philosophical Transactions for 1825.

‡ Dr. Granville found several lumps of brittle resin and two or three small pieces of myrrh in their natural state, mixed up with a compound of a bituminous and resinous matter and argillaceous earth. These Dr. G. supposes were placed to fill up the vacancies created by the removal of portions of the intestines. Dr. Verneuil says, he has been able to recognize myrrh among the balsamic substances employed in embalming. The abdomen of the Leeds mummy was filled with aromatic powder.

§ Herodotus is most likely incorrect here as to the order of proceeding, for the placing the body in this saline liquid would, of necessity, precede the application of the aromatics.

‖ In the Leeds mummy, it is said, the cuticle had not been removed.

Dr. Granville has noticed the appearance of minute saline crystals, both on the exterior and interior surfaces of his mummy and upon collecting them together a sufficient quantity was obtained to be submitted to various analyses, and they were found to consist of nitrate of potash, carbonate, sulphate, and muriate of soda, and traces of lime. There is no difficulty in accounting for the presence of all these substances, from the body having been subjected to the operation of the natrum, excepting that of the lime, and the existence of this substance Dr. Granville supposes is owing to an operation preliminary to embalming, namely, the removal of the cuticle by the agency of this caustic matter.

The cuticle removed, the body would more readily receive the benefit of the ablution with palm wine, which would act as an astringent, and in a manner tan the true skin.

The body now, according to Herodotus, is fitted for bandaging; but Diodorus Siculus (who makes no mention of the natrum) says that the body was "anointed with oil of cedar and other things for thirty days, and afterwards with myrrh, cinnamon, and other such like matters;" and I suspect also, from the examinations I have made, that in this process the body must have been subjected to a very considerable degree of heat; for the resinous and aromatic substances have penetrated even into the innermost structure of the bones, an effect which could not have been produced without the aid of a high temperature, and which was absolutely necessary for the entire preservation of the body. The heat would essentially destroy all insects, and remove all fatty matter, so powerful in promoting putrefaction. M. Rouyer, I find, also conceives that the bodies must have been put into stoves, or kept at a certain temperature in convenient vessels, to incorporate most intimately the resinous substances with the animal matter. His words are, " Cette opération, dont aucun historien n'a parlé, étoit sans doute la principale et la plus importante de l'embaumement."*

The mummy opened at Leeds presented an appearance different from any I have either seen or read of. On the surface of the body there was a coating of the dust of woods and barks, nowhere less than one inch in thickness; and this extended all over the body, even to the extremities of

*Description de l'Egypte, p. 212.

the fingers and toes. It had the smell of cinnamon or cassia. The body contained within it also a quantity of a similar powder, which, upon being mixed with alcohol and water and exposed to the action of heat, emitted an odour resembling that of myrrh.

The body being embalmed, the additions of gilding and otherwise orna-menting, in some instances, must be presumed to precede the enveloping it in its proper bandages. The gilding of mummies has been most fre-quently observed on the nails of the fingers and toes,* but it has also been seen on the eye-lids, on the lips, the face, on the sexual organs,† and on the hands and feet. Abd'Allatif states ‡ that leaves of gold have been found on the forehead, eyes, and nose of the bodies—also on the sexual parts of the women, and some bodies entirely covered with this precious metal. He also mentions that it was customary to lay a small leaf of gold on the body, and in some instances a lingot of gold was placed in the mouth. A cadi of Bousir reported to Abd'Allatif that he had removed three of these lingots, and that they weighed together nine mithkals.§ Mr. Wilkinson has fa-voured me with a drawing of a plate of gold beaten very thin, and found upon the tongue of a mummy. From the hieroglyphics upon it, it appears to be of the time of Ramses the Great. See Plate VI., *fig.* 1.

Dr. Lee has a beautiful specimen of the hand of a female mummy, in which the nails of the fingers are gilt. The mummy described by Hertzog, the apothecary of Gotha, had the nails of the fingers and toes gilt.‖ In my " Græco-Egyptian mummy" the gilding has been over the whole of the body, and appears, as Plates I. and II. will show, in the form of square patches, which, it has been conjectured, have remained most apparent in consequence of their having been applied to fill up spaces where the gilding has originally been defective, similar to the process now in use among the picture-frame gilders of the present day. M. Cailliaud's mummy was gilt in the same manner. A few years since I saw an unwrapped mummy that

* Denon Voyage dans l'Egypte, tom. II. p. 33.

† Jomard, p. 42, and Rouyer, p. 216.

‡ P. 200.

§ A mithkal is 1½ drachm Arab. or 90 grs., and a grain Arab. is ⅔ English.

‖ Hertzog (Christ.) Essai de Mumiographie, 12mo. Gothe 1718, p. 55. The head of this mummy was wanting.

was exhibited in the Haymarket, said to have been brought from Thebes by Captain Jefferson, and upon this there were here and there small portions of gold leaf apparent. Mr. Madden saw some mummies in which the fingers, toes, lips, and eyes were gilt.* M. Rouyer thinks that these gilded mummies are too numerous to produce assent to the opinion that they only are bodies of persons of the highest rank and importance. He says that mummies not having the ventral incision are never gilt. My specimen contradicts this assertion. Passalacqua regards all the mummies that are found gilt *on the flesh* as Greek mummies—the mummies of those Greeks who either in the time of the Pharaohs or Lagides were living in Egypt. Many have been found with Greek inscriptions or characters impressed on the bandages or cases.† Very thin plates of gold, or silver gilt, are sometimes found in mummies without any Greek inscription. Mons. Cailliaud's mummy had a plate of gold over each orbit representing an eye, with the eye-lashes, &c., and another plate of gold in the shape of a tongue over the mouth, which was effectually closed. According to Mons. Letronne all the Egyptian mummies have the mouth open,‡ which is not the case in the Græco-Egyptian mummies. " Lorsqu'une personne venait d'expirer, ses parens et ses amis avaient le soin de lui fermer la bouche. Nous voyons le disciple de Socrate, Criton, s'empresser de rendre à son maître ce pieux devoir, aussitôt qu'il eut rendu l'âme ;§ c'est ce qu'on appellait συλλαμβάνειν τὸ στόμα. On allait même plus loin : en ornant le corps pour l'exposition, on serrait ses mâchoires avec des bandelettes de laine, rattachées par dessus la tête." " Par Tisiphone (dit Lucien, en faisant parler un mort de ses parens), en vous voyant dire et faire tant de sottises à mes funérailles, j'aurais éclaté de rire, si les bandelettes de laine dont vous m'avez si bien serré les mâchoires ne m'en eussent empêché." " Rien ne me paroit plus propre (continue M. Letronne) à expliquer cette circonstance. C'est vraisemblablement par une sorte d'expression symbolique

* Travels, vol. II. p. 90.

† Passalacqua, Catalog. Nos. 1543, 1588. Augusteum; ou Description des Monumens Antiques qui se trouvent à Dresde, par G. G. Becker, Leip. 1804, folio.

‡ This was not the case in Dr. Lee's Egyptian mummy.

§ Plat. Phædon. § 66. fin. ubi, vide Wyttenb.

de ce dernier devoir rendu aux morts, qu'on avait placé sur les lèvres de la momie une lame d'or qui a la forme d'une langue, et dont l'objet semble avoir été de sceller la bouche."* M. Cailliaud's mummy had an artificial crown of olive in copper gilt placed round the head. This appears to be somewhat in conformity with a custom of the Greeks, who were in the habit of exhibiting their renowned dead with a crown of gold until the time of their burial, when it was either placed on the tomb or in a funeral urn.

The mummy I opened, and which from the character of its skull I am disposed to conceive to be that of a Greek, had no inscription whatever on its bandages. There may probably have been one on some outer bandage or case that did not reach this country. It cannot be a matter of surprise that the Greeks, who adopted so much of the mythology of the Egyptians, should also have adopted their manners in the treatment of their dead. The body of Alexander was preserved, not only free from corruption by the process of embalming, but from external injury by being cased in the most precious of metals, and the one of all others the least liable to alteration. Diodorus Siculus has given † an account of this splendid preparation. The covering of gold was a sort of chase-work, and of such a nature that it could be applied so closely to the skin as to preserve not only the form of the body, but also to give the expression of the features of the countenance. The practice of wrapping the dead in sheets of gold, Dr. Clarke has remarked,‡ is strictly oriental. The Rev. Mr. Tooke § has also made us acquainted with the fact that among the sepulchres discovered on the banks of the Volga, the Tobol, the Irtish, and the Ob, bodies are found wrapped in thin plates of gold. Sheets of the purest gold have been found extending from the head to the feet, and so great a quantity has been seen in these eastern tumuli, that the borderers upon the Siberian and Tartarian deserts have, for years, been in the habit of digging for the treasures contained within them. It is stated that in one sepulchre alone in Siberia, opened by the order of the Russian government, two sheets of gold covering two bodies were found amounting to no less than forty pounds' weight of fine gold. ‖ Mr. Forster supposes the prince and princess thus buried to have been Mun-

* Voyage à Meroé, Tom. IV. p. 13.   † Lib. xviij. c, 26.   ‡ P. 51.
§ Archæologia, VII. 224.   ‖ Forster in Archæologia, II. p. 233.

golians, of the family of Genghiz-Khan, and to have lived between the years 1295 and 1370.   Similar plates of gold, or this metal in the form of vessels, bracelets, or other ornaments, have been found in the country near the Tanais, and in the territory near the Mœotis;* and this it is that Dr. Clarke supposes has given rise to the erroneous notion of the body of Alexander having been deposited in a golden coffin. The chase-work upon the body of this hero was protected by a further golden veil or garment, which was placed immediately over it, then a splendid purple vest variegated with gold, and to this succeeded his armour, that he "might appear as he had lived, and the whole be accordant with his past actions."   In later times a covering of glass was substituted for that of gold by one of the Ptolemies, and the body placed in a sarcophagus, which, it is said, "bids defiance to the arts, at any other period than that of Ptolemy and in any other country than that of Egypt.†

Passalacqua says that the position of the bodies of Greek mummies varies somewhat from that of the Egyptians, that the arms were always extended along the sides, and that the fingers were invariably extended, and the limbs separately bandaged.   This was certainly not the case in my specimen.

The nails of the fingers and toes of some mummies have been observed to be stained, as if with henna. (*Lawsonia inermis*, Forskal Flor. Egypt). Whether this be really the case is not at all clear; the colour may probably be produced by the medicaments employed in the process of embalming.

M. Rouyer notices the staining of the nails, and also the palms of the hands and the soles of the feet, and attributes it to the henna.   Mr. David-son's mummy presented this stained appearance on the nails.   Mr. Madden also says that the hands of many were dyed with the juice of the henna, as is the custom of the Arabs.‡   The henna is the gopher of Scripture and the cyprus of the Greeks.   The shrub is called the Tamar-hhenné, and is common in Sharkiyyeh and Kelyúb.   In the month of April, suckers pro-perly prepared are planted vertically, three feet apart, in land twice ploughed, and irrigated abundantly.   In a year's time the plants have ac-quired a considerable size, and the leaves are then fit for gathering.   These

---

* See Rennell's Geographical system of Herodotus, p. 107.   † Clarke, p. 75.
‡ Travels II. 90.

are dried and powdered, and formed into a paste, which is very commonly used throughout Asia to stain the nails of the hands and feet, and the palms of the hands and soles of the feet. The colour is a kind of scarlet. Sonnini has figured it in his *Travels*, Plate III. The flowers are extremely fragrant.

Scarabæi or other amulets or ornaments are but rarely found in contact with the body of a mummy, but in Mr. Davidson's specimen there was a collar adherent to the neck of the mummy, from the centre of which hung a scarabæus an inch and a half in length and an inch in breadth, having the remains of some written (not carved) hieroglyphical characters, impressed on it.* In the mummy of Horseisi, an incense-bearing priest of the temple of Ammon, unrolled by me at the Royal College of Surgeons, I found also a necklace and a scarabæus. The necklace appears to have been composed of seven separate portions, which, by the pressure of the bandages, have been forced down upon the upper part of the breast. At the pit of the stomach there was a scarabæus in the usual light green stone, an inch in length, and proportionably broad; no inscription was upon this amulet.

It is not a little remarkable that the scarabæus is more frequently found upon the naked flesh than any other divinity or amulet.

As to the position of the bodies of mummies, the only difference is to be found in the mode of disposing of the arms; the body is always extended and the head erect. The legs are invariably placed at their full length, and brought close together. The arms are found either lying along the sides of the body, the palms of the hands in contact with the thighs, or placed upon the groins,† or brought forward in contact with each other, or they are placed across the breast, or, as in some rare instances, one arm extended along the side of the body, whilst the other is carried across the chest. I believe these postures to have been indiscriminately employed; for they are to be found in males, females, and children. Passalacqua says that the greater number of instances in which the arms are crossed are those of females, though my limited experience does not serve to support this opinion,

* Mr. D. has represented it in his Address on Embalming.
† This was the position of the mummy of Horseisi.

and M. Jomard,* who enjoyed abundant opportunities, states the reverse to be the case. Dr. Granville's female mummy had the arms crossed. This was also the case in the female mummies described by Gryphius and Hertzog.

In Dr. Perry's, Dr. Lee's, Mr Davidson's, and in the mummy opened at the Mechanics' Institution, they were extended. Mons. Villoteau, one of the members of the French Commission in Egypt, and who has communicated to Mons. de Sacy an account of the observations he made during his stay in that country, a detail of which will be found in M. de Sacy's interesting edition of Abd'Allatif's History of Egypt, states, among other things, that in a female mummy, remarkably well preserved, and in which he observed the hair was of great length, and flowing in tresses which must have hung down the back extending even to the waist; the arms were extended along the sides—whereas in a male mummy they were crossed; and he adds that he had observed this to be constantly the case in male and female mummies. Passalacqua had the mummy of a boy† with the arms crossed. Denon had the mummy of a female, in which one hand was inclined towards the sexual organ, whilst the other was carried to the throat in the position of the Venus di Medicis, and Passalacqua had one‡ in the same attitude. M. de Verneuil has suggested that women of a certain age had the arms crossed; but that virgins and younger females had them extended.§ The arms were extended in M. Cailliaud's male mummy.

Passalacqua has remarked that the Egyptians had the fingers of the right hand extended, and those of the left clenched, a remark I am not able to confirm. The fingers of the left hand of Dr. Granville's mummy were bent inwardly, but the thumb was extended.

The body being thus prepared, the bandages‖ are applied, and the whole is placed in its proper case or coffin.¶

The SECOND mode described by Herodotus differs from the preceding in the non-extraction of the brain, in having no ventral incision, and in the absence of the resinous and aromatic substances. The intestines were

---

* P. 42.   † No. 1547.   ‡ No. 1546.   § Catal. de M. Passalacqua, p. 284.

‖ For particulars as to the nature of these, and the mode of application, see chap. VII.

¶ See chap. IX.

filled with oil of cedar, after which the body was placed in a solution of natrum for the specified number of days,* at which time it is said the oil is withdrawn, and along with it the bowels.   M. Rouelle† has doubted the possibility of this injection into the body without the aid of incisions, and my specimen of Græco-Egyptian mummy goes to confirm this opinion; for there have evidently been incisions made in the neighbourhood of the rectum.   It has been doubted whether the oil of cedar has the power of destroying the viscera.‡   A mummy opened at the Mechanics' Institute, in 1832, presented the appearances described by Herodotus: the skin and bones alone remained, the flesh was entirely destroyed by the natrum. Abd'Allatif says that he saw human bones in so decayed a state that they resembled the white fibres which surround the base of the leaves of the palm-tree.

The THIRD mode simply consisted in washing the inside (but in what manner is not stated) with syrmæa, or surmaia (a purgative liquor, supposed to have been composed of an infusion of senna and cassia, both of which plants are natives of Egypt,) and then salting the body for seventy days.   Upon comparing the accounts given by modern travellers with those of the ancient authorities, it will be seen that it is impossible to class the whole of the mummies that have been discovered under one or other of the three modes above detailed.   The observations I have made, *en passant*, are sufficient to show that in no one case have they been strictly true, and yet nothing has been described by Herodotus that has not in some instance or other been detected: M. Rouyer, whom I have had occasion frequently to refer to, and whose " Notice sur les Embaumemens des Anciens Egyptiens," in the large and splendid work published in France, the result of the labours of the celebrated Commission, furnishes us with many curious and interesting particulars, has endeavoured to class the mummies he saw in Egypt under two principal divisions, and these he subdivides into others. The principal divisions are :—

---

* Seventy days, the precise period of mourning for the dead. Joseph was mourned for during this time.   See Genesis, chap. l. ver. 3.

† Mem. de l'Acad. des Sciences, 1750, p. 139.

‡ See Chap. VI. on Medicaments.

I. Those having an incision in the left flank for the eviscerating of the body.

II. Those without any incision.

I. Of the mummies with the ventral incision, they are those preserved

1. By balsamic matter.

2. By natron.

Those dried by balsamic and astringent substances are filled with a mixture of resin and aromatics, and the others with asphaltum or pure bitumen. Those filled with resinous matter are of an olive colour, the skin dry, flexible, and like a tanned skin, retracted and adherent to the bones. The features are preserved, and appear as during life. The belly and chest are filled with resins, partly soluble in spirit of wine. These substances have no particular odour by which they can be recognized; but, thrown upon hot coals, a thick smoke is produced, giving out a strong aromatic smell. These mummies are dry, light, and easily broken; the teeth, hair of the head, and eye-brows preserved. Some of these are gilt on the surface of the body, others only on the face, or the sexual parts, or on the hands and feet. The mummies filled with bitumen are black, the skin hard and shining, and as if coloured with varnish. The features perfect, the belly, chest, and head filled with resin, black and hard, and having little odour; and, upon being examined, are found to yield the same results as the Jews' pitch met with in commerce. These mummies are dry and heavy. They have no smell, and are difficult to develope or break. They have been prepared with great care, and are very little susceptible of decomposition from exposure to the air.*

The mummies with ventral incisions, and prepared by natron, are also filled with resinous substances, and also asphaltum. The skin is hard and elastic. It resembles parchment, and does not adhere to the bones. The resins and the bitumen injected into these mummies are little friable, and give out no odour. The countenance of the body is little altered, and

---

* When the asphaltum incorporates with the body, it becomes brown and greasy, and easily crumbles into powder; when it does not incorporate with the flesh it retains its shining black colour.

the hair is badly preserved: what remains usually falls off upon being touched. These mummies are very numerous, and if exposed to the air they become covered with an efflorescence of sulphate of soda. They readily absorb humidity from the atmosphere.

II. Those without the ventral incision.

These are also of two kinds:—1. Salted and filled with bituminous matter less pure than the others, and called pissasphaltum.—2. Simply salted. The mummies preserved with pissasphaltum are not recognizable; all the cavities are filled, and the surface of the body is covered with this mineral pitch. It penetrates the body, and forms with it one undistinguishable mass. These mummies, M. Rouyer conceives, were submersed in vessels containing the pitch in a liquid state. They are the most numerous of all kinds, black, dry, heavy, and of a disagreeable odour, and very difficult to break. Neither the eye-brows nor hair is preserved, and there is no gilding upon them. The bituminous matter is fatty to the touch, less black and brittle than the asphaltum, and yields a very strong odour. It dissolves imperfectly in alcohol, and when thrown upon hot coals emits a thick smoke and disagreeable smell. When distilled, it gives an abundant oil, fat and of a brown colour and fœtid odour. Exposed to the air, these mummies soon change, attract humidity, and become covered with an efflorescence of saline substances.

2. The mummies simply salted and dried are generally worse preserved than those filled with resins and bitumen. The skin is dry, white, elastic, light, yielding no odour, and is easily broken. The skin is blanched and supple, and masses of adipocere are frequently found in them. The features are destroyed, the hair is entirely removed, the bones are detached from their connexions with the slightest effort, and they are white like those of a skeleton. The cloth enveloping them falls to pieces upon being touched. These mummies are generally found in particular caves, which contain great quantities of saline matters, principally the sulphate of soda.

The state of preservation in which the hair has frequently been found has excited astonishment. M. Belzoni brought away from Gournou some hair from a well embalmed mummy that was plaited and measured eighteen inches in length. M. Villoteau, I have already stated, saw hair of great length and flowing in tresses, which must have reached to the waist, and my friend Dr. Sayer has a very fine specimen of the head of a female mummy, in which the hair hangs in elegant tresses. This head was taken from the tombs at Kárnak. I have the head of a female mummy from Thebes, in which the hair is of considerable length, and what is more singular there are three plaited portions turned up from behind over the skull, precisely in the way the Egyptians of the present day wear their hair, and as it is commonly done in this country. De Breves, who was French Ambassador at the Porte for twenty-two years, mentions having seen the preservation of the hair and the nails in mummies. Count de Caylus only displayed his own want of knowledge when he called in question the veracity of this traveller. "M. de Breves," says he, "étoit sans doute un bon ministre, mais un mauvais observateur. Cette conservation est physiquement impossible; et il aura été trompé par les Arabes qui font métier d'en imposer aux Francs. Ils lui auront présenté quelques corps embaumés selon les usages qui se pratiquent aujourd'hui."*

M. Rouyer, M. Passalacqua, M. Champollion, and many other travellers have expressed their surprise at the very small number of the mummies of children in the tombs. Maillet states that separate caverns were appropriated to males, females, and children; but this observation has not been confirmed by any traveller. M. Rouyer remarks† that the bodies of the females differ from the males in the manner of their embalming, in the nature of the substances employed in the operation, and in the arrangement of the bandages in which they are enveloped. He has not, however, favoured us with any relation of these peculiarities, nor have I been able to distinguish any, either by my own personal inspection of mummies or by my enquiries among those of my friends who have enjoyed extensive opportunities of examining the caves and tombs in Egypt, and who have favoured me with their opinions on this subject.

The smallest mummy in Passalacqua's collection measures fifteen inches. Denon had a mummy twenty-five inches and another thirty inches. At a late sale of Egyptian antiquities, I purchased, perhaps, the smallest known mummy in the world. It measures only three inches and a quarter, and was enclosed in a wooden case upon which was rather rudely carved a repre-

* Mem. de l'Acad. des Belles Letters, xxiii. 135.   † P. 215.

sentation of the god Osiris seated. The eyes are in enamel. The figure has originally been gilt; but traces only of that operation are now visible. I have figured this (Plate IV. *fig.* 1) and the mummy as enclosed in its bandages (Plate IV. *fig.* 2). Dr. Lee has the case of a similar one rather larger than mine, but varying very little from it. The opening in his is from the back part; in mine it is from the bottom. There is no inscription on either. In Dr. Lee's specimen the mummy is wanting. The Earl of Munster has kindly shown me a case of the same description, but rather smaller than my specimen. It measures barely four inches; the back part and sides are wanting. It has also been gilt. In the Catalogue of the Antiquities of the late Baron Denon two cases of this description are noticed. They are numbered 107 and 108. The former was four inches and a half high, and represented Osiris seated on a throne furnished with his ordinary attributes. Behind the figure was a cavity like Dr. Lee's, with a little board to open and shut at pleasure: the cavity contained a mass of bitumen. The figure had been gilt. The second-specimen was also an image of the same deity, in the same attitude, and of the same size; it had been gilt and had contained an embalmed object, which, I presume, is alluded to in the same catalogue (No. 236), as " un fœtus humain, enveloppé de langes, et formant une petite momie." In the tombs of Thebes M. Cailliaud saw some human fœtuses enclosed in small wooden cases, " accolés à des figures assises et dorées."* Captain Henvey, R. N., favoured me with the sight of a portion of a mummy case, the lower part of which was unfortunately wanting. It had been obtained, I believe, from Thebes. The case was formed of cloth plastered over, and then covered with hieroglyphics. The face had been gilt. When entire it probably measured five inches. A mass of waxy substance filled the inside of this curious specimen.

* Voyage à Meroé, tom. I. p. 264.

L

POSTSCRIPT TO CHAPTER V.

———

SINCE writing the preceding chapter I have made a more minute examination of the mummy of Horseisi at the Museum of the Royal College of Surgeons. From the appearance of the outer table of the skull, Mr. Clift, the intelligent Conservator of the Museum, suspected that there had been a fracture, and upon removing a portion of the skull this was found to have been the case. The occipital bone had been broken, and on the inner surface an exudation, or rather deposition, of bone, extending upwards of one inch in length, was found to have taken place, thereby marking the process of nature in repairing an injury of the frame. The skull was half filled with three bandages of cotton cloth, one of which measured ten feet three inches, the others eleven feet six inches each. These had been introduced through the right nostril, by which it appears the whole of the brain and its investing membranes had been extracted. The inner surface of the skull was entirely denuded and perfectly clean. Not an insect was contained within it. In the abdomen the viscera were found rolled up in three distinctly-bandaged portions. One of these is easily recognized as the liver and gall-bladder; a second consists of the intestines; and the third probably the spleen, stomach, &c. The cavity of the belly was filled with earthy matter and asphaltum. Specimens of all these may be seen at the Museum.

CHAPTER VI.

ON THE MEDICAMENTS EMPLOYED IN EMBALMING.

Imperfection of the present state of chemical knowledge—unable to detect the precise nature of vegetable substances—bituminous matter in the head of a mummy—Rouelle's examination of the embalming materials of six different mummies—asphaltum or Jews' pitch—description of it by Dioscorides—Dr. Verneuil's examination of M. Passalacqua's balm—Mr. Davidson's analysis—particular kind of balsam found by Mr. Madden in the head of a mummy— aromatics mentioned by Diodorus Siculus—myrrh, cassia, cedar—pissasphaltum—balm— different species—of Judea—of Syria—of Egypt—of Mecca—powdered aromatics—colocynth—aloes—examination of the contents of canopi—natrum—its nature and effects—erroneous opinion of Rouelle pointed out—Blumenbach's analysis of mummies—crystals of natrum obtained—Bahr-bélà-mà natron lakes—pure nitre in the heart of a mummy— cedria—description of it by Pliny and Dioscorides—embalming materials not mentioned by Herodotus—honey—wax—bitumen—resin—preservative powers of honey noticed by Alexander ab Alexandro, Columella, Lucrètius, Josephus, Abd'Allatif—anecdote from this author of a child found in a vessel of honey—body of Alexander the Great embalmed by honey— Statius's allusion to it—wax—Dr. Granville's demonstration of it in mummies—body of Agesilaus enveloped in wax.

In entering upon the subject of the medicaments employed in the process of embalming, one cannot but express regret that the present state of chemical knowledge is not sufficiently advanced to be capable of detecting the precise nature of the substances, chiefly of a vegetable kind, that have been used in this ancient operation. A variety have been named merely upon conjecture, and observations lightly made have been regarded as authorities of weight and consequence. In treating of these substances I shall endeavour to preserve the same order as that pursued in the previous chapter on embalming, taking the accounts of Herodotus and Diodorus Siculus, as the most ancient, for a kind of text upon which comments can be conveniently made. According to these authorities, and particularly the former one, after the extraction of the brain the cavity of the skull was filled with " certain drugs."

In the head of a well-embalmed mummy which Mr. Greaves caused to be opened, there were found in the cavity of the skull two pounds of bituminous matter, which by the heat of the sun had become soft. He conjectures that this could have been injected into the head only through the nostrils, according to the method described by Herodotus. The tongue of this mummy weighed only seven grains English, " so light was that member which St. James* calls a ' world of iniquity.'"

M. Rouelle† has examined the embalming materials of six different mummies. These resinous and bituminous substances he has carefully analysed. In the head of a mummy sent to him by the Count De Caylus, the substance taken was soft, as in Mr. Greaves's specimen. By distillation in a retort, the heat being applied gradually, it gave at first a little insipid water, which, as the distillation proceeded, became more and more acid; then a limpid oil, slightly coloured, of an odour resembling that of amber. A further distillation produced a thicker oil, which, when congealed, also retained a similar odour to that of the first drawn oil. He tried whether it were possible to make the acid liquor crystallize in the same manner as the liquor of amber does. He washed the oils in boiling water in order to separate the acid and the liquor; being filtrated, he evaporated it; it diffused a smell of amber and all was dissipated—there was too little matter to furnish crystals.

From the head of another mummy, which belonged to M. de Jussieu, he drew a clearer and more abundant oil, an acid more concentrated, and an oil which did not congeal as the oil in the former instance had done. The

---

* Chap. III. v. 6.

† The memoir of M. Rouelle, inserted in the Mémoires de l'Academie Royale des Sciences for 1750, contains the best analysis of the materials employed in the process of embalming by the Egyptians. The Memoir is styled the first, but it was not succeeded by a second, which was intended to have embraced an account of the experiments Mons. Rouelle had made to imitate the Egyptian embalmings, and some methods founded on the same principles for making anatomical preparations. The published Memoir is not confined merely to a chemical analysis of the medicaments used in the making of mummies, but extends to a history of the subject, beginning with the account given by Herodotus.

products were much the same with respect to the taste and smell of the acid and oils, and resembled the products of the distillation of amber. The matter remaining in the retorts was rarefied like bituminous substances, more so in the latter than in the former experiment. In appearance the two substances very much resembled each other; the first was rather blacker and more shining than the second, which had precisely the characters described by Dioscorides * as belonging to the Jews' pitch. By bruising it, it became of a dirty red and like bullocks' blood dried. M. Rouelle compared this with a small specimen of true Jews' pitch, and found them to resemble each other. From these experiments M. Rouelle infers that the mummy to which the second specimen belonged had been embalmed with Jews' pitch, but that there was something mixed with it, though so inconsiderable in quantity that it was almost impossible to detect it without comparing, because the matter differs only in being a little more black, less reddish when crumbled, and in yielding by distillation an oil that congealed.

Dr. Verneuil analysed the balm extracted from the head of a mummy in the collection of M. Passalacqua,† and found it to consist of a quantity of silicious sand mixed with argillaceous matter and asphaltum. Mr. Madden ‡ found in the head of a mummy of a superior kind a quantity of balsam different from any hitherto described. In colour and transparency, he says, it was not to be distinguished from pink topaz; it burned with a beautiful clear flame, without leaving any residue, and emitted a very fragrant odour, in which the smell of cinnamon predominated. Mr. Davidson found four ounces and a half of soft matter in the head of his mummy; it burned with a dark red flame, leaving a considerable residue of carbon; it was but slightly acted upon by water, or spirit of wine, the latter dissolving a minute portion.§

* Ex Dioscoride, cap. 100, et cap. 102. "Bitumen omne aliud antecedit Judaicum. Probatur quod purpuræ modo splendet, ponderosumque et firmo odore est. Damnatur contrà quod nigro colore sordet. Adulteratur enim admista pice. Nascitur in Phænice, Sidone, Babylone, et Zacyntho. Gignitur et in Sicilia Agrigentinorum agro liquidum, fontibus supernatans, quo ad lucernarum lumina vice olei incolæ utuntur, Siculum oleum falso appellantes: siquidem liquidi Bituminis, genus est. Vocatur et quoddam bitumen naphtha, quæ Babylonii bituminis destillatio est, colore candidum, invenitur et nigrum."

† No. 1556.   ‡ Travels, II. 88.   § Address on Embalming, p. 20.

Abd'Allatif* says that the balsam extracted from the heads and bodies of mummies is black like bitumen. When exposed to heat, it adheres to all around it ; and if thrown on a fire it exhales an odour resembling that of white pitch and myrrh, which, he says, are supposed to constitute its composition. The brain being extracted, and the " certain drugs" injected into the skull, the next step, according to Herodotus, was to wash the body with palm wine, and Diodorus Siculus adds, with "aromatic odours." The intestines removed, " pounded aromatics, pure myrrh, pounded cassia,† and all other perfumes except frankincense, which was forbidden, were employed. Diodorus Siculus bears his testimony to the employment of myrrh and cassia, and also that the body was anointed with oil of cedar. In a specimen of mummy which belonged to M. de Jussieu, of which there was only a part of the thigh and the leg, black and very shining, and scarcely affording any red colour when bruised, M. Rouelle, by distilling it in the same manner as in the former instances, obtained first an acid liquor and a small quantity of lightly-coloured fluid oil, but in much less proportion than in the previous experiments. The acid and oil he describes as having a resinous odour, and as very quick and penetrating. At the end of the distillation a thick oil was obtained, having the smell of amber, but in a much weaker degree than in the experiments upon the masses taken from the skulls of mummies. M. Rouelle also examined specimens of a similar nature to that of M. de Jussieu, from the mummy of the Celestins and the mummy of St. Geneviève. That of the former was of the same colour and the same consistence as the specimen of Jussieu, and by distillation the same products were obtained. The latter specimen yielded the same products, varying only in having the odour of the bitumen Judaicum a little less distinct, arising perhaps from the nature of the specimen, for it was taken from the skull and contained several portions of bandages so closely connected together that there was scarcely any thickness of bituminous matter between them.

The sixth and last examination made by M. Rouelle was of the balsamic matter found in a vessel preserved in the chambers of the mummies. It was of a black colour, brilliant, soft, and flexible. Upon handling it an

---

* P. 201, De Sacy's edition.

† Probably the *laurus cassia* or bastard cinnamon.

agreeable odour was diffused. Its nature was purely resinous, uniform in its substance, not bitter like aloes to the taste, and perfectly soluble in spirit of wine. By distillation, a small quantity of water, slightly aromatic, was obtained, to which, upon an increase of the heat, some drops of an acid, and a light oil, scarcely coloured, but quick and penetrating in its nature, such as that of the most essential oils, and retaining the smell of the balsamic matter, were produced. The quantity of the oil thus obtained amounted to almost one-fourth of the weight of the balsamic matter. This oil was followed by another more thick, which had the smell of the Jews' pitch, and the acid accompanying this oil possessed the same odour. Thus it appeared that there entered into the composition of this substance some matter of an aromatic and resinous nature, abounding with an essential oil —the basis of the balsam is Jews' pitch.

The Jews' pitch, or *bitumen Judaicum*, called also asphaltum, from the name of the lake whence it has been obtained, is a solid friable substance of a brownish-black colour, brilliant in its fracture, and giving out a bituminous odour. It has been named *funeral gum*, and *gum of mummies*, from its use in the preparation of mummies. Chemical analysis demonstrates the composition to be a compound of oily matter and mineral acids. *Pissasphaltum* is a compound of asphaltum and common black pitch. It is known also by the name of *mineral pitch, pitch of the mountain,* &c.* M. Rouelle distilled different mixtures of resins and pitch, with the bitumen Judaicum, and he found the odours produced in no manner to resemble those of the mummies. As the resinous matter mixed with the Jews'-pitch was aromatic and very penetrating, he conjectured that it might be the liquor of the cedar. The matter of these mummies may be regarded as the pissasphaltum. Pursuing this subject with ardour, M. Rouelle obtained another specimen from a mummy in the custody of the *Augustins déchaussés*, and by distillation, as before, he obtained a light aromatic oil; then a thicker oil, more penetrating in its odour; then one more thick, and having the smell of the Jews' pitch. The results vary in a very trifling degree from the previous experiments. It results from the whole of these analyses that

* See chap. I.

M. Rouelle has detected three modes of embalming, differing in the materials used :—1. With the asphaltum or Jews' pitch. 2. With the mixture of asphaltum with the liquor of cedar or the cedria. 3. With this mixture, to which were added some resinous and aromatic ingredients. The matter contained in the vessel found in the chamber of the mummies probably furnishes another method more balsamic, and perhaps more precious.

Penicher* enumerates four species of balm, supposed to have been used in embalming. 1. That of Judæa. 2. Of Syria. 3. Of Egypt. 4. Of Mecca. The trees yielding these were formerly trained with as much care in the countries where they were cultivated as the vine ; they are now so rare as scarcely to be met with except in the gardens of the Grand Seignior. The mode of obtaining the balm is by making an incision through the bark of the plant during the dog-days, avoiding the use of any instrument having an iron point. The liquor produced by this incision is described as yielding a very fine and agreeable odour, aromatic, and abounding in volatile oils. The colour is white, approaching to a yellowish tint, similar to that of citron. The taste is slightly astringent and sharp. Its odour and fluidity are lost by being kept any length of time, but its qualities are said to remain. Abd'Allatif gives a very detailed account of the tree yielding the balm, and of the mode of collecting and preparing it.†

No pounded aromatics have been found mixed with the bituminous matter ; they would have destroyed the uniformity of the mass, and served rather to attract humidity, and thus promote putrefaction than resist it. These vegetable substances were sprinkled into the cavities of the body. Resinous matters would afford the best protection against moisture, and such were evidently employed, forming a kind of varnish on the surface of the body.

Mr. Madden's account of the penetrating nature of the particles of mummy dust agrees in every respect with that of Belzoni. His throat was

---

* Traité des Embaumemens, p. 2.

† See also Prosper Alpinus de Balsamo dialogus. Observations de P. Bellon ; Linné Amœnitat. Acad. tom. VII., and various other authors, from whom M. De Sacy has cited the most important passages in his valuable notes appended to his edition of Abd'Allatif's History of Egypt.

frequently excoriated by it, and this, he says, tended to make him acquainted with the component parts of the balsam employed in the preparation of mummies, which he conceives essentially consists of powdered *colocynth*, commonly called bitter apple. By analysis, he says, he has found this substance to form a very large proportion of the balsam. The resin being insoluble in water, he thought he might get an infusion of colocynth, if it existed in it, by pouring a quantity of water on four ounces of the coarse powdered balsam. He then made an infusion of colocynth and found the taste of the two mixtures to be the same. Colocynth, in the form of powder, he found was largely employed in Upper Egypt for destroying vermin in clothes'-presses and store-rooms ; and the ostrich feathers which are sent to Lower Egypt are sprinkled with this substance as they are packed.*

The mention of aloes in the embalmings frequently occurs, but there is no positive authority for its use as relating to the Egyptian embalmings. I have already noticed that it is recorded by St. John that Nicodemus brought about 100 lbs. weight of a mixture of myrrh and aloes to preserve the body of Christ (John xix. 39) ; and aloes is mentioned as a perfume in other parts of scripture: "I have prepared my bed with myrrh, aloes, and cinnamon" (Prov. vii. 17). "Spikenard and saffron; calamus and cinnamon, with all trees of frankincense; myrrh and aloes, with all the chief spices" (Solomon's Song, iv. 14).

Dr. Verneuil examined a compound found in two of the vases called canopi, containing the intestines, in M. Passalacqua's collection,† and he found it to consist of the same materials as those of the substance taken from the head of a mummy.‡ Other vases contained the intestines simply enveloped with asphaltum, and in some§ Dr. Verneuil found cloth impregnated with blood and filled with cedar dust and natrum. He also found the abdominal cavity of a mummy‖ filled with the dust of sandal wood. The embalming matter in vases for the ibis and cynocephalus consisted of the balm of Mecca, altogether different from that employed for human mummies.

---

* Travels II. 86 † Nos. 1422 and 1423. ‡ No. 1556. § Nos. 771, 1553.
‖ No. 1554.

M

M. Julia Fontenelle examined the contents of one of Passalacqua's vases,* consisting of a liquid matter, and, from various experiments, concludes that it was not a balsam, but the asphaltum or bitumen of Judæa.

The next part of the process to be remarked upon is that of salting the body, or immersing it in a solution of natrum. M. Rouelle condemns the idea entertained by many ancient writers, that the body being first salted was then embalmed in such a manner that the balsamic, resinous, and bituminous matters united with the flesh, the fat, and the different fluids, so as to form a uniform mass, as is observed in mummies: the inspection alone of the dryness and aridity of a mummy he conceives is sufficient to dispel this opinion. "Tous ces corps," says he, "sont dans un tel état de sécheresse et d'aridité qu'il est impossible de pouvoir imaginer qu'une si grande quantité de differentes liqueurs telles que celles de certains corps, morts de maladies inflammatoires, qui sont, pour ainsi dire, dissouts par des pourritures et des corruptions subites, puissent être absorbées par les matières résineuses et balsamiques, qu'on sait d'ailleurs ne faire aucune union avec l'eau: ainsi cette grande quantité d'humidité auroit été, par la suite, une cause de destruction du corps. Si les momies avoit été préparées suivant cette méthode, on devroit en trouver qui eussent conservé quelque trace de cette humidité; mais on trouve le contraire: tous ces corps sont très-secs, et n'ont aucune humidité."† Now it is quite clear from this statement that all the mummies seen and experimented upon by M. Rouelle have not been those in which the art has been carried to its highest degree of perfection; for had he seen Dr. Granville's mummy, or Dr. Lee's mummy, or Mr. Davidson's mummy, or my Græco-Egyptian mummy, he would have found that they were all so well embalmed that the whole substance of the body and its embalming materials had so coalesced as to form one uniform mass, and of a substance so soft and ductile that it could easily be divided by the knife; nay, further, that by proper management, as in Dr. Granville's specimen, and also in mine, the embalming material could be so completely subtracted from the body as to display clearly the original texture of which it was composed, and then to run to decay, unless placed in

---

* No. 708.   † Mem. de l'Acad. des Sciences, 1750, p. 125.

spirit or some other material capable of resisting the process of decomposition.

Professor Blumenbach obtained from John Hawkins, Esq., F.R.S., some pieces of mummy which he had bought of a druggist at Constantinople, one of which was covered and impregnated with a saline matter. Being dissolved in water, the solution filtered, and evaporated, a true soda, or mineral alkali (*natrum*), was obtained, exhibited in very neat and regular crystals. They are figured in the Philosophical Transactions for 1794. Tab. XVI., *fig.* 4.

The natron, natrum, or nitrum of the ancient Egyptians was used for the purpose of cleansing, scouring, and bleaching the stuffs and linen, and it was also employed in the manufactory of glass. It must, therefore, have been a fixed alkali, and not a neutral salt like the nitre or saltpetre of the present day. Common nitre we know will act as an antiseptic and preserve the animal matter; but it will do this, retaining all the animal juices. This is certainly not the case in the mummies; and the presence of these fluids would necessarily, after a certain period, tend rather to promote putrefaction. The fixed alkali, on the contrary, dries up the fibre, and without destroying it. The length of time in which the bodies are said to have been immersed in a solution of natron would be sufficient to incorporate the salt with the fatty matter, and thus form a kind of soap.

Dr. Ure has been so kind as to make an analysis of a quantity of this salt, which I collected from within the body of my Græco-Egyptian Mummy, and he found it to consist of common culinary salt, chloride of sodium, mixed, as usually happens in nature, with minute portions of sulphate of soda and muriate of lime, and imbued with much animal matter, derived from the human body. When the crystalline matter was ignited in a platina capsule, it emitted a copious flame by the combustion of that animal impregnation, and lost about one-sixth part of its weight. No nitre or corbonate of soda was present; the antiseptic function of the salts is therefore traceable entirely to the muriate of soda.

The order of the process of embalming, as detailed by Herodotus, has been justly considered obscure, and every one must admit that to fill the body with aromatic and balsamic substances, prior to placing it in the saline solution, would be not only unnecessarily to waste a considerable quantity of the materials of the most expensive kind used, but also, by the union which would be produced between these and the alkaline salt, a soapy matter very soluble in its nature would be created, and thus the preserving effect of the aromatic substances prevented. The perfuming of the body we must therefore believe to have been a process posterior, not antecedent to the salting.

My friend Mr. Davidson feels satisfied in his opinion as to the nature of the saline substance employed in this part of the process, from finding that the Bahr-bélàmà (waterless sea), natron lakes, and saline incrustation of soil are confined to the Lybian side of the Nile, on which side the great necropolis of Thebes, of Memphis, and of Abydus are situated. The Faioom to this day, and the natron lakes to the north, he tells me, continue to furnish abundant quantities of this salt; and, about the period of and previous to the visit of Herodotus, persons of consequence were buried on the borders and islands of Lake Mœris, situate in the Faioom, whereas the nitre beds, combined with the muriate of soda, said to be a recent discovery, are situated on the Asiatic side, and where very few if any sepulchral ruins are to be found. Sonnini* says that it is uncommon to meet with natron perfectly pure, that earthy matter is almost always mixed with it, and that it is not entirely a free alkali, being usually combined with marine salt, Glauber's salt, and in a small degree vitriolic tartar.†

Mr. Madden‡ states that he found in the heart of a mummy about three drachms of pure nitre, which must have been injected through the bloodvessels, for the heart was entire. That the substance was nitre, he says he proved by the crackling noise it made on throwing it into the fire, and by the peculiarity of its taste.

The oil of cedar, mentioned by Herodotus as injected into the body in the second mode of embalming is also noticed by Diodorus Siculus as employed in anointing the body. The liquor from the cedar has been

* Vol. I. p. 320.

† For an account of the natron lakes the reader is referred to the Appendix, No. VII., in Denon's Voyages, by General Andréossi.　　　　‡ Travels II. 88.

called *cedria*, and this, we learn from Pliny, was obtained by burning the wood, cut into small pieces, in a sort of kiln. The liquor is not caustic, and could not therefore produce the effect ascribed to it by Herodotus, namely, that of destroying the entrails.* Nor could it be injected in sufficient quantity *per anum* to fill the cavity of the belly. It is clear, therefore, that an incision must necessarily have been made, either through the lower bowel or on the side of it, to permit the free injection into the body. My Græco-Egyptian Mummy bears evidence of violence of this kind having been committed. Dr. Granville's also had similar appearances. The effect of an injection of cedria would, I conceive, serve to destroy all insects, and to dry up the animal fibre, by which the most powerful agent in putrefaction would be overcome. The cedria is, doubtless, insufficient for the destruction of the bowels, and M. Rouyer has, therefore, conjectured that injections were used composed of a solution of natron rendered caustic prior to the use of the cedria. That such an injection was used my Græco-Egyptian Mummy serves to confirm; for I have removed from within the body a very considerable quantity of this salt.

Herodotus makes no mention either of honey, wax, bitumen, or resin. But another authority expressly names these substances along with others as used in embalmings, and other writers strengthen the statement made. "Condiebant, enim cadavera myrrha, aloë, cedro, *melle*, sale, *cerâ*, *bitumine*, et *resinâ* odoribus et unguentis delibuta."† Columella speaks of the property of honey in preserving bodies for several years.‡

Lucretius also refers to the preservative power of honey:

> " Nam si in morte malum est, malis morsuque ferarum
> Tractari; non invenio quî non sit acerbum
> Ignibus impositum calidis, torrescere flammis ;

---

* Pliny and Dioscorides describe the cedria as being so *lively* that it injures living bodies, but that its quality is to preserve dead bodies; hence it has been called the *death of the living and the life of the dead.* "Defuncta corpora incorrupta ævis servat, viventia corrumpit : mira differentia, cum vitam auferat spirantibus, defunctisque, pro vita sit." Plin. lib. xxiv. cap. 5.

† Alexand. ab Alex., Dier. genial. lib. iii. cap. 2.   ‡ Lib. iii. cap. 45.

"Aut in *melle* situm suffocari, atque rigere
Frigore, cùm in summo gelidi cubat æquore saxi." *

Josephus records that the Jewish king Aristobulus, whom Pompey's partisans destroyed by poison, lay buried in honey till Antony sent him to the royal cemetery in Judæa.† The Assyrians placed the bodies of their dead in honey to preserve them from corruption. The Romans also used honey for the same purpose.‡ Abd'Allatif relates§ an anecdote of a man who had found a sealed cruise, and, having opened it, he discovered it to contain honey, which he began to eat, until one of his companions observed a hair upon his finger, when the vessel was more closely examined, and a little child, all perfect, was withdrawn from it. The body was well preserved, and furnished with rich jewels and ornaments.

The body of Alexander the Great was rubbed with and embalmed by honey. Thus Statius:‖

"Duc et Aemathios manes, ubi belliger urbis
Conditor *Hyblæo* perfusus *nectare* durat."

Dr. Clarke has remarked that the like application of *nectar* to *fluid honey* was common both in Latin and Greek. Thus Virgil:¶

"Qualis apes æstate novâ per florea rura
Exercet sub sole labor; cùm gentis adultos
Educunt flores, aut cùm liquentia mella
Stipant et dulci distendunt Nectare cellas."

* "Grant the corse torn by ravening fangs a curse,
Is hence no ill in funeral flames to burn;
Or, pent in cold obstruction, stiffening lie
Immers'd in *honey*, while entomb'd in stone."

† Antiquitat. lib. xiv. c. 7.
‡ Montfaucon Antiquité Expliquée, tom. V. part ii., pp. 185, 186.   § p. 199.
‖ Lib. iii. carm. 2., v. 117.   ¶ Æneid. lib. i. 433.

And Euripides,*

'Ρεῖ δὲ γάλακτι πέδον
'Ρεῖ δ' οἶνῳ, ῥεῖ δὲ μελισσᾶν
ΝΕΚΤΑΡΙ, Συρίας δ' ὡς λιβάνου καπνός.

Compare also Exodus, chap. xxxiii., ver. 1—3; and Numbers, chap. xiii., ver. 26, 27.

Wax is also mentioned as an article used in embalming, but I believe Dr. Granville to be the first person who has demonstrated its existence in a mummy. He observed a resino-bituminous substance between some of the folds of the peritonæum, and, upon examination, he ascertained it to consist of bitumen, with wax, in a proportion sufficient to render it plastic. Dr. Granville succeeded in separating the wax from the soft parts, leaving the muscular fibres perfectly distinct and apparent.

According to the quantity of this material used in the preparation would, of course, depend the softness of the mummy, and there can be no doubt but that the body was perfectly soft at the time of the application of the bandages, since the folds and wrinkles occasioned by the cloth is, in all well-prepared mummies, most distinctly visible.

The body of king Agesilaus was enveloped in wax and thus conveyed to Lacedæmon.† This is confirmed by Cornelius Nepos, and also by Plutarch, who ascribe the adoption of wax to the want of honey for this purpose. Cicero reports the use of it by the Persians.‡ " Persæ jam *cera* circumlitos condiunt, ut quam maximè permaneant diuturna corpora."

* Bacch. v. 142. † Æmilius Probus. ‡ Tuscul. I.

CHAPTER VII.

ON THE BANDAGES.

*Bandages not applied to all mummies—quantity of bandages—the use of woollen garments for-
bidden—bandages generally supposed to be of cotton, not linen—coarsest applied nearest the
body—fringed bandage—various kinds—different textures—colour of the bandages—to
what attributable—hieroglyphical characters on the bandages—in the mummy of Horseisi—
in Greek mummies—application of the bandages—compresses—applied wet—leathern amulet
placed over the heart—limbs sometimes separately bandaged—condensed bandages by the
application of bituminous matter—varieties in the mode of bandaging—in the priests are of
different colours—artificial eyes in mummies—masks for the hands and feet—varnished
bandages—ancient portrait attached to a mummy in the British Museum—branch of rosemary found in a mummy—bulbous root at the soles of the feet.*

THE body of the mummy being washed, according to Herodotus, after its
immersion in the solution of natron, and thus all superfluous salt likely to
attract moisture removed, the bandages are to be applied. All mummies,
however, were not bandaged. Many had only the covering of a mat which
surrounded them. Denon states that he saw bodies without bandages in
the Necropolis of Thebes, and Belzoni saw the bodies of two females lying
on the ground in a corner of a chamber in one of the tombs in the valley
of Biban el Molouk without any bandages; they were well preserved, their
hair long, and flowing in tresses. The quantity of bandages on some mummies have been computed to consist of not less than 1000 ells.* Abd'Allatif
says that in some mummies more than 1000 yards have been used, and that
the Bedouins were in the habit of taking it away to make vestments, or to
sell for the manufacture of paper for the grocers. The bandages on Mr.
Davidson's mummy weighed twenty-nine pounds and a half. The mummy

---

* Greaves' Pyramidographia, p. 69.

N

of Horseisi thirty-five pounds and a half. Herodotus states that it was profane for the Egyptians either to be buried in woollen garments or to use them in their temples. " Les Prêtres ne pouvoient porter ni des habits de laine, ni des souliers de cuir; parceque la laine engendre la vermine, et que le cuir vient d'une bête morte."*

The bandages generally employed in the enveloping of the mummies have been supposed to be of cotton. Jomard says that in the catacombs at Philæ linen was clearly to be detected; it was of a coarse description, and he conceives answered for the poorer class of people. Rouyer also noticed a difference in the texture of the bandages. Jomard has gone more particularly into the manufacture of it.†

I have invariably found the coarsest kind of bandage the nearest to the body, both in the human species and in animals. The bandages have sometimes a border of a blue colour; this was the case in Dr. Lee's mummy. Jomard has represented some portions of bandage of this kind and others furnished with a kind of fringe and terminating in knots.‡ I have also seen this in bandages from a mummy.

Mons. Cailliaud found in his mummy a kind of cravat tied with a flat knot round the neck. He also found four Egyptian chemises without sleeves, three feet eight inches in length, and well made. One had been very neatly repaired, and they were marked in characters in ink. Between the bituminous coverings were several napkins, and in such a state of preservation that M. Cailliaud had one of them washed in lye, and he states that it underwent this process eight times before it showed any sensible marks of deterioration. " C'est," says he, " avec une sort de vénération, je l'avoue, que chaque jour je déployais ce linge si perissable, qui cependant avait été tissu depuis plus de dix-sept cents ans."§ On a scarf of the same mummy he also observed the two initials of the Greek name of the defunct, A. M., embroidered "au crochet." The mummy opened at Leeds had also a chemise without sleeves; the aperture answering to the collar was cut out and hemmed round. The holes for the arms were also hemmed like the collar. Round the bottom was a fringe an inch and a

* Martin. Religion des Egyptiens, p. 168.　　† See Memoir sur les Hypogées, p. 36.
‡ Plate 48. Description de l'Egypte.　　§ Voyage à Meroé, tom. IV. p. 11.

half in breadth.   Several portions had been mended.   In one of the bands was an arm-hole, the hem of which had been sewed round with remarkable neatness, proving that garments which had been worn were used by the embalmers.

The bandages vary very much in length, and are sometimes even a yard or more in breadth; they do not, however, generally exceed seven or eight inches, and many are much less.   They appear to have been indiscriminately used.   Belzoni saw bandages as fine as muslin, and of a very strong and uniform texture.   I have various specimens of these kinds.   Count de Caylus and M. Rouelle state that they found all the bandages to be of cotton or byssus, and the latter enquires whether the cotton might not have been consecrated by religion for the service of embalming.   " Le lin des Egyptiens étoit-il le coton? ou le coton étoit-il consacré par la religion pour les embaumemens ?" *

Larcher is of this opinion, and conceives the custom to have originated in the circumstance of Isis having folded up in cotton the scattered members of Osiris, killed by Typhon (see Diodorus Siculus, lib. i. § 85). Larcher regards cotton and the byssus as the same, and he quotes the following from Julius Pollux in support of his opinion :—" The byssus," says he, " is amongst the Indians a kind of linen.   In Egypt, on a certain shrub is found a species of wool, of which cloth is made, which considerably resembles linen cloth, but that the texture is more substantial.   On this shrub grows a fruit much like a nut; this fruit has three divisions; when it is ripe it separates; they then draw from it a substance resembling wool.†   And Arrian says,‡ " The Indians make use of linen garments, as Nearchus says; I mean that kind of linen which is gathered from trees, and of which I have before spoken." §

* Mem. de l'Acad. des Sciences, pour 1750, p. 150.

† Onomasticon, lib. vii. cap. 17. § 75.   ‡ Indic. cap. xvi. § 1.

§ Dr. Ure has been so good as to make known to me that which I conceive to be the most satisfactory test of the absolute nature of flax and cotton, and in the course of his microscopic researches on the structure of textile fibres he has succeeded in determining their distinctive characters.   From a most precise and accurate examination of these substances he has been able to draw the following statement :—" The filaments of flax have a glassy lustre when viewed by daylight in a good microscope, and a cylindrical form, which is very rarely flattened.   Their diameter is about the two-thousandth part of an inch.   They break

Greaves says that the habits of the Egyptian priests were made of linen,* and Plutarch tells us† that the priests of Isis used linen vestments, and were shaved. So also Suetonius,‡ " Sacra etiam Isidis sæpe linteâ religiosâque veste propalam celebrasse." The goddess Isis is called by Ovid " linigera :" §

> " Nec tu linigeram fieri quid possit ad Isim
> Quæsieris."

Mr. Hamilton gives his testimony in favour of all the bandages being of cotton. The cotton-plant was successfully cultivated by the ancient Egyptians ; and Apuleius, and Pliny the elder, tell us that the habits worn by the priests were of this substance.‖ Larcher thinks Greaves had not examined the bandages with sufficient care. He thinks also that Herodotus, Plutarch, and others are mistaken in asserting that the habits of the Egyptian priests were of linen. If they meant linen that grows on trees, he thinks they should have mentioned it, to obviate all doubt. According to Pliny garments of cotton were very agreeable to the Egyptian priests : " Vestes indè sacerdotibus Ægypti gratissimæ."¶ Apuleius says the initiated wore garments of cotton : " In ipso ædis sacræ meditullio, ante deœ simulacrum constitutum tribunal ligneum jussus superstiti, byssinâ quidem, sed floride depicta veste conspicuus."**

M. Rouyer says that he found a great number of mummies enveloped with bandages of linen, and that he observed this especially in the mummies

transversely with a smooth surface, like a tube of glass cut with a file. A line of light distinguishes their axis, with a deep shading on one side only, or on both sides, according to the direction in which the incident rays fall on the filaments.

" The filaments of cotton are almost never true cylinders, but are more or less flattened and tortuous ; so that when viewed under the microscope they appear in one part like a riband from the one-thousandth to the twelve-hundredth part of an inch broad, and in another like a sharp edge or narrow line. They have a pearly translucency in the middle space, with a dark narrow border at each side, like a hem. When broken across, the fracture is fibrous or pointed. Mummy-cloth tried by these criteria in the microscope appear to be composed both in its warp and woof-yarns of flax, and not of cotton. A great variety of the swathing fillets have been examined with an excellent achromatic microscope, and they have all evinced the absence of cotton filaments."

* Pyramidographia, p. 68.   † De Iside et Osiride.   ‡ In Othone, c. 12.
§ VII. Amor. Eleg.   ‖ See Egyptiaca, p. 320.   ¶ Hist. Nat. lib. xix cap. 1.
** Metamorph. lib. xi. lin. 9.

of birds, and particularly that of the ibis. All the cloths taken from mummies, and not imbued with resinous matter, examined by M. Rouelle, he says he found to be entirely of cotton. This was the case with the bandages surrounding birds, &c., as well as the bodies of the human species. Abd'Allatif saw many skeletons of dogs, bulls, and cats, all enveloped in bandages of hemp (chanvre), in the cemetaries of Bousir. In the Leeds mummy the remains of a covering of very fine white linen still adhered to the outermost of the folds.

The bandages are variously tinged; those nearest to the body are the only ones saturated with bituminous matter. Greenhill thinks the bandages have been dipped in the cedria. Abd'Allatif thinks the bandages were soaked in aloes and goudron. Dr. Granville made some experiments on portions of the bandages of his mummy, and found that they had been steeped in some vegetable solution, which, when treated with gelatine, exhibited the presence of tannin in considerable quantity. From this he infers that the Egyptians were acquainted with the antiseptic powers of astringent and vegetable infusions. What the precise nature of this vegetable was, whether the bark of the acacia, the bark of the oak from the coast of Syria, or the gum hinted at by Dr. Granville, does not appear; but certain it is that a gum similar to that known by chemists as kino, was found by Dr. Granville in the belly of his mummy, and exhibited by him to the Royal Society.

Mr. Davidson is of opinion that the colour of the bandages is derived from the gum of an acacia, which Strabo calls the thorn of the Thebais—called by the Arabs "Sount," and is very common all over Egypt and Arabia: it grows to a considerable size, and Theophrastus in his History of Plants states that beams twelve cubits in length were cut from it; and Pliny mentions that its seeds and bark were used instead of galls for tanning hides, &c. The several uses of the tree are well expressed by this author: "Spina celebratur in eadem gente, duntaxat nigra, quoniam incorrupta etiam iu aquis durat, ob id utilissima navium costis. Candida facilè putrescit. Aculeus spinarum et in foliis semen et in siliquis, quo coria perficiuntur gallæ vice. Flos et coronis jucundus et medicamentis utilis. Manat et gummi ex ea, &c."

The coarse bandages around the mummies of the poorer class M. Jomard found charged with natron, not bitumen. M. Rouyer says the bandages were impregnated with resin.

Sometimes the bandages are found marked with hieroglyphical characters or alphabetical letters. M. Jomard found on a mummy at Thebes a bandage negligently written on in hieroglyphical characters.* In the mummy of Horseisi I met with hieroglyphical characters on various parts of the bandages no less than five times—they all gave the name and profession of the deceased. These interesting specimens are preserved ·in the Museum of the Royal College of Surgeons. M. de Maillet caused a female mummy to be opened in the convent of the Capuchins at Memphis, and the fillets were imprudently cut with scissars. The bandages were very long and broad, and were covered with hieroglyphical figures, and also some unknown characters written from right to left, and forming a sort of verses. He observed the same termination to several succeeding lines, and he presumes this to have been an *éloge* on the person embalmed.† Some portions were sent into France and afterwards engraven ; but I have not been able to meet with the specimen.

The names of some of the Greek mummies have been found inscribed in Greek characters on the bandages enveloping the body. These mummies M. Passalacqua‡ regard. as the bodies of Greeks who have died in Egypt at a most distant period (the time of the Pharaohs), and he conceives that it is not at all surprising that these people should have adopted, for the preservation of the deceased, the same method of embalming as that of the Egyptians, seeing that it formed so remarkable a dogma of the religion of a people highly respected by the Greeks, and from whom they drew the origin of their laws and their mythology. The most ancient customs, particularly as it regarded the funeral obsequies, were preserved in Egypt in the time of the Ptolemy's, as we learn from Diodorus Siculus.§

Count de Caylus has given‖ a fac-simile of a MS. taken from a bandalette found upon a mummy. It is in the Enchorial character, is upon linen cloth, coloured apparently by asphalt, and measures twenty-one feet in length. He also describes¶ another from the Cabinet of St. Geneviève, two

---

* Plate XLVIII., *fig.* 4.   Description de l'Egypte.·   † Maillet, Letter VII., p. 278.

‡ Catal. p. 185.   § Lib. i. § 36.

‖ Recueil d'Antiquités Egyptiennes V., tab. xxvi—xxix.   ¶ Ibid. I. p. 65.

feet four inches six lines in length, and six inches seven lines in breadth. The bandage was terminated by a compartment, containing, besides some words, various figures painted in red. I recognise two of the deities of the Amenti among them. This bandage also covered a mummy and was stained with a brown colour.

The bandages then we have seen are principally composed of cotton, though occasionally of linen. They vary in texture, the coarsest being always nearest to the body; they vary also in length and breadth, and they are either endued with bitumen, resin, gum, or natron. They are also occasionally bordered with blue and sometimes fringed and knotted, and they have also been found impressed with characters both hieroglyphical and alphabetical. Our attention must next be directed to their mode of application. This part of the process is done with a neatness and precision that astonishes all who behold it.* Every method of bandaging is, perhaps, to be found in the Egyptian mummies, and to effect their immediate application to the body compresses are placed in various parts that no space or deficiency may be left. By this means the air is effectually excluded and decay prevented. The bandages vary very much in thickness in different mummies; sometimes they are found twenty or thirty times around the members and body. Mr. Hamilton examined several mummies from the pits opposite Philæ on the eastern shore, and in some instances he counted six-and-forty folds of cotton cloth, resembling exactly that which is now worn at this place by the common peasants, and is manufacted in Nubia, where it is called Zabouk; and at Es Souan, Gibbe.†

Dr. Granville says he has seen in the bandages of his mummy the *couvrechef*, the *scapularium*, the *eighteen-tailed bandage*, the *T bandage*, as well as the *linteum scissum* and *capistrum*. I cannot say that I have witnessed these in any of the mummies it has been my fortune to inspect. Throughout the whole the object has appeared to me to be close and effective binding by compresses and rollers, and all shapes and positions were adopted to effect this purpose, and I am perfectly satisfied that the

* Plate VI. *fig*. 2, represents a mummy in the outer bandages. This was drawn from Dr. Lee's specimen, and shows the position of the leathern finger (amulet). *Fig*. 3, represents the second layer of bandages, and marks the precision with which the rollers were applied.

† Egyptiaca, p. 55.

bandages were applied wet. There is, however, something like regularity in their mode of application; thus, upon the face we generally meet with square portions affixed by a long and broad envelope extending over the head, and reaching down to the feet in one continued piece. But exterior to this is an envelope like a sheet fastened at the back, and secured by fillets, and I must here allude to a curious circumstance I met with in the unfolding of Dr. Lee's mummy. Over the heart, and beneath one of these fillets, I found that which I conceive to be an amulet in the shape of the finger of a glove, composed of leather stained red.* At first I thought some characters had been impressed on it; but, upon closer inspection, it was found to be only the structure of the leather. Belzoni says the Egyptians knew how to stain leather like our Morocco, and occasionally embossed it. I am entirely ignorant of the meaning of this leathern finger— the manner in which it was placed forbids my attributing its presence to accident, and I am at a loss to conceive that which it might imply. I can only regard it as an amulet, and Dr. Richardson tells me has seen them not only of leather but also of painted cloth. In M. Passalacqua's Catalogue I observe the following notices:

"1589. Matières diverses. Six paires de doigts accouplés deux par deux et dont l'emploi nous est inconnu.—Memphis et Thebes.—Hauteur moyenne, quatre pouces." "Les six paires de doigts, placées sous le même 1589, dont on ne saurait assigner l'usage, furent découvertes en partie, dans le ventre d'autant de momies, et en partie sur leurs poitrines."†

I have obtained drawings of these,‡ and I regret to say that they throw no light upon my accidental discovery. The "six paires de doigts" are really so many specimens of that which is erroneously described by Hertzog as the Æthiopic stone, used in making the ventral incision. I look upon them as benedictions for the deceased. A leathern amulet was found upon the mummy opened at Leeds. A few folds of the bandages being removed from the head, a singular ornament presented itself. It is evidently an amulet, and consists of three straps of red leather sewed together by a single stitch. One of these portions was attached to the others by two leathern

---

* See Plate IV., *fig.* 4, and Plate VI., *fig.* 2.   † Pp. 109—210.

‡ One is represented in Plate IV., *fig.* 5.

thongs, and resembled in form the portion of leather I have mentioned, as upon the breast of Dr. Lee's mummy. Upon the crown of the head of the Leeds mummy was another piece of leather, but of a different form; it was probably a continuation of one of the other straps, turned over the head, and broken off by its brittleness. Upon these portions of leather hieroglyphics were impressed, evidently by the application of heated metal types.* The hieroglyphics inscribed denote the name of the monarch during whose reign the mummy was supposed to have been embalmed. Mr. Osborn has laboured with great assiduity to make out these characters, as well as those upon the sarcophagus which contained the body, and by reference to the works of Dr. Young and M. Champollion he may fairly be said to have ascertained the subject of his investigation to have been a priest† of the name of Natsif-Amon, and contemporary of Rameses V., who began to reign in the year 1493, A.C., and who continued to do so for nineteen years and six months. He was the last monarch of the eighteenth dynasty of the kings of Egypt.

To return to the bandaging :—Immediately beneath the envelope long and broad bandages are found to proceed somewhat in the figure of 8 from the head to the feet. Of these there are several folds, and then a more regular application of the roller is observable around the body and limbs in a spiral manner. Compresses at the sides of the body and limbs extend the length of two feet or more, to admit of the firm and steady application of the rollers, which now become of a finer texture, and some of which are continuous for four, five, or even six yards together. I have seen one piece measuring nine yards. After these succeeds a coarser kind, and the cloth increases in looseness of texture until the bandage comes in contact with the body. Compresses will now be found between the thighs and legs, where occasionally papyri and other substances are met with. In the mummy of Horseisi, at the Royal College of Surgeons, I found the remains of an Egyptian idol. It was in a state of decomposition, although the body

* They are represented in Plate II. of Mr. Osborn's Account of an Egyptian mummy, &c. Leeds, 1828.

† This opinion is strongly supported by the appearance of the mummy; the head, eye-brows, and beard were closely shaved, the arms were bent across, &c.

o

had undergone no change. It measured in length eight inches, and in breadth
three inches.   In some instances the limbs are found separately bandaged,
whilst in others they are included in the general bandaging.   When distinctly bound it is done with exceeding neatness, beginning with the
extremity of each finger or toe, and extending upwards.   Compresses are
placed in the palms of the hands and in the soles of the feet.   The bandages in contact with the body are frequently so condensed by the application of the bituminous matter that they cannot be separated ; this was the
case in my Græco-Egyptian mummy and in Mons. Cailliaud's mummy of
the same description, in both of which they were so consolidated together
that it was quite impossible to unravel them, and indeed a very considerable degree of force was necessary to separate them from the body.   M.
Cailliaud states that he was occupied during four days in endeavouring to
remove them, which at last he was obliged to do with the hammer and the
chisel.   Mummies of different classes it would appear are differently bandaged.

An able writer in the Encyclopædia Metropolitana* is disposed to con-
sider that as every thing in the religion of Egypt is symbolical,† so no
doubt was the mode in which the embalmed bodies were swathed.   " The
bandages of mummies," says he, " are sometimes crossed, at others laid
obliquely or straight."   These, and their various ornaments and appendages, he regards as symbolical of the embalmed body of Osiris, which
was carried about by Isis ;‡ and Damascius§ expressly calls these " the
bandages (περιβολαὶ) of Osiris."

Upon removing a few of the folds from the breast of the mummy examined at Leeds, a wreath or fillet was discovered, exactly resembling in
form the collars which are constantly represented round the necks of
Egyptian figures.   It consisted of two garlands ; the upper one was composed of nine strings, each of which was double.   A row of red berries
strung upon a straw or stalk was connected, at intervals of eight berries,
with another string, by little loops of the same material, and to this string
were sewed the petals of the lotus.   Each petal had been neatly folded,

* Art. Mummy.   † Peyron, Papyri Egypt. p. 82.   ‡ Plutarch. de Iside et Osiride.
§ Phot. Biblioth. Cod. ccxlii.

and being bent over the string was completely secured in its place by two very thin stalks, which passed on each side of it, and crossed each other like wicker-work. The strings were plaited together at the ends. The lower garland consisted also of nine strings, with petals of the lotus, and were likewise plaited; but on the two higher ones (or those which were next the throat, when it was worn round the neck) there was a small compound globular flower enclosed within each petal, and standing just above it. The execution of these intricate pieces of flower-work is described as being very neat and accurate. Upon examination Mr. Osborn found that the garland painted on the case was composed of strings and berries, and flowers arranged in exactly the same manner as that which was around the neck.*

Some of the mummies Belzoni observed to have garlands of flowers and leaves of the Acacia-tree over their heads and breasts. This tree is common on the banks of the Nile above Thebes, and particularly in Nubia. The flower is of a yellow colour, and so hard in substance that it appears artificial; the leaves are strong, and though turned brown by being dried still retain their firmness.†

The mummies of priests (respecting which, and those of kings, neither Herodotus nor Diodorus Siculus furnish us with any particulars) Belzoni conceives to be folded in a manner altogether different from that appropriated to other classes. Greater respect appears to have been paid to these personages, and the bandaging to have been performed with more care and attention. The bandages, according to Belzoni,‡ are strips of red and white linen intermixed, covering the whole body, and forming a curious effect from the two colours. The arms and legs are not enclosed in the same envelope with the body, but are bandaged separately, even the fingers and toes being preserved distinct. Sandals of painted leather are applied to the feet, and bracelets are fixed on the arms and wrists. The arms are always found folded across the breast. The body is enveloped in a vast quantity of linen, but the shape of the figure is most carefully preserved. The cases containing these choice specimens of mummy are also of much superior execution to the ordinary ones. Belzoni saw one with

---

* Account of an Egyptian mummy, &c. p. 3. † Travels, p. 170. ‡ P. 170.

the eyes and eye-brows of enamel, beautifully executed in imitation of nature. Mr. Madden was fortunate enough to procure the head of a mummy * in which enamelled glass eyes were substituted; but he has not given us any description of the mummy. He states the eye-balls to be invariably wanting. I have in my own possession three specimens which contradict this statement, and I know of several other instances. The mummy at the Royal College of Surgeons had artificial eyes; the sclerotic coat or white of the eye was represented by pieces of ivory, and the transparent cornea and dark part of the eye by portions of a black composition. The application of the bandages had disturbed the position of these, so that one eye is placed two-thirds of an inch lower than the other, giving by no means a prepossessing appearance to the mummy.

In addition to the bandages thus enumerated, M. Jomard tells us † that some mummies are furnished with masks for the hands and feet, as well as the face, and that these coverings have imprinted in relief the several fingers, toes, and even the nails. It would appear that they had been formed in a wooden mould.

In examining one of the cases transmitted to the British Museum several years since by Mr. Salt, I found in a highly-ornamented sarcophagus, covered with mythological emblems and hieroglyphical characters, the mummy of a male, in which the bandages presented an appearance quite new to me, and of which I can find no notice, nor have I yet met with any traveller who has witnessed the same circumstance. The mummy appeared to have been bandaged with great precision and neatness, and over the whole surface a coat of varnish of a dark leaden colour had been thickly spread. It is in amazingly fine preservation, very few, and those exceedingly small portions, being detached, and it gives to the body the appearance of a uniform coat of mail.

In another case sent to the British Museum by Mr. Salt, I found a portrait of exceeding interest placed upon the bandages, and secured at the edges by the outer envelope. This painting is upon a thin plate of cedar-wood, and presents probably the earliest portrait known. The trustees of

---

* Travels II. 90.   † P. 34.

the Museum have permitted me to have a copy of this interesting figure (see Plate VII.), and it will be clear that this must be a portrait of the deceased, for there is no mythological emblem whatever attached to it. The colours appear to have been fixed by a strong gluten, and the mode of reflecting light and marking shade exhibits more of the management of modern art than could have been expected. I presume the portrait to be that of a youth. Mr. Sams has a portion of a similar portrait, which in the style, management of colour, &c., bears a strong resemblance to that in the Museum.

After the first or outer series of bandages, it is not at all uncommon to meet with various idols, papyri, &c., which will be noticed hereafter. I shall only stop here to introduce the accounts of two substances, one of which was found in the chest of a mummy, the other in the bandages on the sole of the foot. The former instance is recorded by Prosper Alpinus. It shows the perfection of the art of embalming by the Egyptians, and how great a length of time putrefaction or decay may be resisted by artificial means. In the breast of a mummy was found, according to this author, some branches of rosemary, so well preserved that they appeared as though they had been but just gathered and dried. These are the words of Prosper Alpinus : "Nos intra quoddam medicatum cadaver invenimus scarabæum magnum ex lapide marmoreo efformatum, quod intra pectus cum libano-tidis coronarii ramis colligatum, fuerat repositum. Incredibile dictu, ramorum roris marini, qui unà cum idolo inventi fuerunt, folia usque adeo viridia et recentia visa fuerunt, ut eâ die à plantâ decerpti et positi apparuerint."* M. Rouelle, quoting this passage, suggests that the embalmer, in placing this plant in the mummy, might have had a mind to leave to posterity a proof of the excellence of his art. The other instance I have to notice is recorded by Dr. Hadley in the Philosophical Transactions for 1764.

In Dr. Grew's catalogue of the rarities belonging to the Royal Society, the first article mentioned is an Egyptian mummy, presented by Henry Duke of Norfolk. This mummy had been greatly injured, and the body

---

* Hist. Ægypt. Natural. pars. I., lib. i. cap. 7.

was in a very indifferent state. The feet had been broken off the legs, but they constituted the most interesting part of the whole. On cutting into the bandages of the sole of the left foot, they were found to enclose a bulbous root. The appearance of this was very fresh, and part of the thin shining skin came off with a flake of the dry brittle filleting with which it had been bound down; it seemed to have been in contact with the flesh : the base of the root lay towards the heel.* "The fillets were removed from this foot with great care; they were much impregnated with pitch, excepting about the toes, where the several folds united into one mass, being cut through, yielded to the knife like a very tough wax. The toes being carefully laid bare, the nails were found perfect upon them all, some of them retaining a reddish hue, as if they had been painted; the skin also, and even the fine spiral lines on it, were still very visible on the under part of the great toe, and of the three next adjoining toes. Where the skin of the toes was destroyed there appeared a pitchy mass, resembling in form the fleshy substance, though somewhat shrunk from its original bulk. The natural form of the flesh was preserved also on the under part of the foot near the bases of the toes. On the back of the toes appeared several of the *extensor* tendons. The root just mentioned was bound to the foot by the filleting that invested the metatarsal bones; no more of this filleting was cut away than was just sufficient to show, without removing it from its place, a substance which had been preserved in so extraordinary a manner. The right foot had also had a bulbous root placed under the sole, for the impression made by it was apparent, and some of the external shining skin still remained. It is not a little singular that the feet were the only portions of this mummy in any thing like a state of nature; all other parts were lost in a mass of pitch.

* P. 8, and Tab. I.

CHAPTER VIII.

ON THE EGYPTIAN IDOLS, AMULETS, ORNAMENTS, &c.

Hertzog's mummy—number of ornaments contained in it—description of them—necklaces—glass—manufactory of by the Egyptians—gold ornaments—shells—silver—precious stones—varnished clay—ear-rings—rings—bracelets—metallic mirror—quantity of gold and silver in Egypt—alabaster vases, &c.—Body of a soldier—poignard—hatchet—triangular stone on the breast—ivory bracelet—enamelled divinities and amulets—more frequent at Memphis and Hermopolis than at Thebes—scarabæi in various substances with and without hieroglyphics—breast-plates—singular mummy-case seen by Belzoni—the Amenti—statue of wood lying over the heart of a mummy—no money under the Pharaohs—medals found at Memphis and Lower Egypt struck under the Greeks, Romans, and Arabs—first current coin of Egypt struck by Aryandes—no medel found older than the reign of Alexander—brass coin of Ptolemy found in a mummy—leaden seals taken from a Greek mummy—emblems of different trades, &c., found in the tombs—objects of the toilet and jewels—various utensils.

BEFORE I proceed to treat of the cases in which the mummies are contained, I must draw the attention of the reader to the idols, amulets, &c., that have been found within the mummies themselves, or among the bandages with which they are surrounded. These ornaments are of various kinds, and are found chiefly between the first and second layers of bandages. The hieroglyphical and alphabetical characters impressed on the bandages, as well as the name of the embalmed, in the Greek mummies, have already been considered.

Christopher Hertzog, apothecary to the Duke of Saxe-Gotha, opened a mummy in 1715, and published an account of the same under the title of "Mumiographia." The head of this mummy was wanting; but the body contained probably more ornaments of its kind than any other on record. "Tous les ongles des doigts des mains et des pieds dorés, les bras entortillés de plusieurs petits rubans large et étroits, dorés par-ci par-là, et sans les bras, nous eumes le plaisir de voir soissante et quatorze figures differentes de jaspe, d'agathe, et d'autres pierres rares et curieuses, qui representoient toutes quelque chose particulière, comme on le voit dans la planche que nous avons," &c.* The stones were either lapis lazuli, agate, or jasper, and some of them were gilt.   The following were the most important :   L.† Isis. A. Horus.   J. Harpocrates.   L. A. Apis.   L. Scarabæus.   A. Frog.   L. A. Nilometers.   L. J. A.   Emblems of the Nile.   A. Sceptre.   A. Altar.   A. Pyramid.   A. Cross mounted on a heart.   This mummy also contained the Ethiopic stone in the form of two fingers. ‡

Necklaces are found upon males as well as females.   M. Passalacqua met with one at Thebes of large pearls in enamelled glass,§ from which a scarabæus in serpentine, with a human head and hands, was suspended.   At each angle of this beetle there was the head of a hawk, and on the reverse six lines of hieroglyphics engraved on it.   Another male had a necklace in fine stones and gold, and a scarabæus in jasper, also engraved with hieroglyphics.   Mr. Sams showed me a necklace entirely of gold, and of most excellent workmanship.   He could not tell whether it belonged to a male or a female mummy, but most probably the latter.

On the mummies of children necklaces of natural shells, or shells figured in gold, silver, precious stones, &c., are found.   They are, according to Passalacqua, chiefly met with on young girls. ‖

M. Passalacqua has given the description of a very fine female mummy

* Essai de Mumio-graphie, 12mo. Gothe, 1718, p. 55.

† The letters refer to the nature of the substances in which they are found.

‡ Plate IV. *fig. 5.*

§ In the manufacturing of glass the Egyptians excelled all other nations. This we have upon the authority of Strabo (Geograph. lib. xvi.), and it is supposed to have arisen from that country affording a superior kali, derived from the ashes of the *Mesembryanthemum Copticum*, which substance was necessary to render the material beautiful.   The breast of Dr. Perry's mummy was ornamented with a net-work of beads formed of earth, and covered with vitrified matter, several of which are in my possession, as well as a necklace composed of the same material. In the Museum of the London University there is a very fine specimen of mummy, the whole front of the body of which is covered with beads and bugles of this description.

‖ See Nos. 581, 585, 588, 596, of his Catalogue.

he met with covered with ornaments of considerable value. The hair of the
deceased was very tastefully plaited and ornamented with twenty spangles.
Three necklaces, composed of representations of the divinities, amulets, &c.,
in lapis lazuli, coral, and other precious stones, and in gold in the form of
rosettes, &c., displaying great taste and symmetry. Fine ear-rings of gold,
a ring (scarabæus set in gold) for the forefinger of the left hand. An elegant girdle around the body in gold, lapis lazuli, and coral similar to the
necklace, and a bracelet in fine pearls, precious stones, and gold on the left
wrist. With the exception of the two latter articles (which were stolen
from the possessor at Thebes) the ornaments detailed are in the collection
of M. Passalacqua at Berlin. Under the head of this mummy was a metallic mirror, and near to it a chest in enamel, which contained a necklace
curious in its construction, being composed of extremely small rings of
ivory, with pearls in gold, lapis lazuli, and coral ;* a square cistern in

---

* " The descriptions of golden ornaments and jewelled dresses might be considered over-rated,
if ancient testimonies did not exist to evidence that Mizraim (Egypt), under the Pharaohs,
abounded in precious metals and jewels. Of the immense quantity of gold which the Egyptians possessed, and their elegant manufacture of it, we possess abundant testimony. Diodorus,
describing a building he calls the tomb of Osymandyas, informs us that the exact sum of the
gold and silver dug from the mines of the Thebais, as inscribed on the walls, amounted to
3,000,000,000 of minæ, or £96,000,000 of our money. Another instance is the stupendous
circle of wrought gold, 365 cubits in circumference, which surrounded this tomb. From
Moses may be adduced the golden chain which Pharaoh placed around the neck of Joseph, and
" the exceeding riches in gold and silver" which Abraham carried out of Egypt : the multitude
of gold and silver vases, bracelets, and other golden articles offered to Moses by the Israelites
for the temple, were doubtless carried out of Egypt. Her treasures were so great that they
were made the subject of a prophet's promise to Nebuchadnezzar, as a reward to his whole
army for their incredible sufferings at the siege of Tyre. Much therefore of the Babylonian
treasures were derived from this source; yet in a very few years afterwards Cambyses found
Egypt again so opulent as to be almost incredible. From the mere cinders of the burning of
Thebes he had raked forth 300 talents of gold and 2300 talents of silver ; and at Memphis he
found such an immense treasure in bullion and ornamental vases, and statues of gold and silver,
as perhaps no palace ever before contained. We read of a golden vine in Persia, on whose
branches hung clusters of emeralds and rubies; but this was after the conquest of Egypt and
of Babylon. Under the Ptolemies the same profusion of wealth may be found ; and the veracity
of Athenæus can scarcely induce the mind to accredit the particulars he narrates of a religious
procession from his own ocular observation : it distances all the details of Peru, and surpasses

P

wood, supposed to be for washing the face; three small alabaster vases, one containing a liquid balm or perfume, a second some paint to tinge the eyebrows, with a bundle of cloth made like a brush to apply it: the third had also held perfume, but it was exhausted.

Mons. Becker of Leipsic has given an account* of two mummies, male and female, which were brought from Egypt by the traveller Pietro della Valle. They are Græco-Egyptian, and one was distinguished by a Greek inscription. Their antiquity cannot be dated further back than the time of the Ptolemies. They are in a high state of preservation; but the bodies have not been unrolled, on account of the beauty of the paintings on their coverings. These have, however, been pierced; and it is said that the bandages are more coarse exteriorly than interiorly, and from the perforations made down to the bones, the flesh appears to have been entirely destroyed by the process of embalming adopted. The male mummy measures five feet three inches (French) in length; the female three inches and a half less.

The outer covering of the male is of a fine byssus covered with a mastic varnish sufficient to receive and to fix the painting. It abounds with gilding and other ornaments. The Egyptian symbols are few in number. The colours of the paintings are yellow, green, red, brown, and black. All the figures are in relief. M. Becker does not recollect to have met with such a kind of relief on any coverings of mummies before. The gold has been laid on upon a red ground covering the mastic varnish.†

M. Passalacqua mentions the remains of apparently á soldier he found near to, but not within, the Necropolis of Thebes, and which he supposes, from its peculiar situation, to have been one to whom the rites of sepulchre had been denied. It was lying under five or six feet of ruins of stones. The

the wildest tales of the East. That military personages also wore and used such splendid appendages is evidenced by the accounts of Holofernes the Assyrian general, in the apocryphal book of Judith, whose reduction of Egypt, Lydia, Cilicia, Syria, and all Asia Minor, with the terror he impressed on these nations, prove him to have been no contemptible warrior; yet we find that the canopy of his bed was woven with purple and gold, and emeralds and precious stones, and silver lamps were carried before him."—*Note to Rameses*, vol. I. p. 323.

* Augusteum, ou Description des Monumens Antiques qui se trouvent à Dresde, fol. Leipzig. 1804.

† For a particular account of the paintings I must refer the reader to the " Augusteum."

means for providing honourable burial would appear not to have been wanting. The mummy was singularly rich in its ornaments; for there was a poignard described by M. Passalacqua as one of the richest ever found in the ruins of Egypt. This instrument was almost hidden in its scabbard, placed between his thighs, the point inclined towards his knees. There was also a hatchet and a pointed stone of a triangular form placed on the breast, and a large ivory bracelet on the left wrist. It is not a little singular that above the envelopes and within the coffin was a small vase containing a mineral matter with which, at the present day, the Coptic ladies paint their eyebrows. The case was covered with fine paintings.

The enamelled divinities and other amulets have holes pierced in them, and have been arranged as a necklace or collar round the necks of mummies. They are more frequently met with at Memphis and Hermopolis than at Thebes. The art of varnishing and baking the varnish was in great perfection among the Egyptians.

Scarabæi are found in basalt, in verde antico, in ivory, in bitumen, in serpentine, in steatite, in olive, brown, and in green jasper, in slate, in talc, in rock crystal, in amethyst, in silex, in glass, in baked clay, &c. Those with hieroglyphics are scarce.*

It is said that the Egyptians hung scarabæi round their necks when going to battle. They are sometimes found as a ring on the finger of mummies, or are placed within the left hand closed. Mr. Greaves had a specimen cut out of a magnet in the form and of the size of a scarabæus. It is remarkable that, notwithstanding its exceeding antiquity, it still possessed its attraction and magnetical virtue. The great scarabæi *with hieroglyphics* are almost always placed on the chest of mummies and on the flesh itself, as in Mr. Davidson's specimen. Sometimes they are found under the eyelids. The scarabæi *without hieroglyphics* are found within the bodies of mummies.

M. Henry has suggested† that the scarabæi with hieroglyphics being always placed without the body, and those without hieroglyphics within the

---

* Mr. Rogers is in possession of the largest and finest scarabæi with hieroglyphics I have seen. He also possesses a very fine coral necklace, and other beautiful and curious ornaments, taken from mummies.

† Lettre à Champollion, p. 189.

body, the former may be regarded as amulets recommending the deceased to the protection of some divinities, whilst the others were placed simply as amulets within the body, to sanctify the balm contained within for the preservation of the body. The scarabæus upon the body of Horseisi was however without any apparent characters.

According to Belzoni tablets in the form of an Egyptian temple are sometimes though rarely met with suspended on the breasts of mummies. These he supposed to be the breast-plates of the kings; but the inscription on the one obtained by this distinguished traveller from an Arab who was said to have discovered it in one of the tombs of the kings in Biban el Molouk, and which is now in the possession of Samuel Rogers, Esq., by whose permission I am enabled to give a representation of it, would not warrant the inference thus drawn. This tablet measures four inches in length and three inches in breadth, and is of black basalt. A scarabæus in *alto relievo* is in the centre of a boat, at the extremity of which are represented the goddesses Isis and Nephthys. See Plate VIII. *fig.* 1. On the reverse, *fig.* 2, is the hieroglyphical inscription, arranged so as to correspond with the shape of the scarabæus, and, at the extremities of the boat, figures of the goddess Isis. Mr. Rogers is also the fortunate possessor of another tablet of a similar nature to the one just mentioned. It was obtained at Rome, whither it had been brought from Egypt by Mr. Basseggio, and was said by him to have been found in a sepulchre at or near Thebes. He brought, together with this interesting tablet (which I have had figured in Plate VIII. *fig.* 3), a colossal head of Nephthys in red granite, of most beautiful execution, and a lion in calcareous stone, which were also found in the Thebaide, and which are both in the possession of Mr. Rogers. There is a tablet similar to that represented in Plate VIII., *fig.* 1 and 2, in the British Museum, which is likewise of black basalt. It is rather smaller than Mr. Rogers's specimen, but of the same shape. In the centre is the representation of the scarabæus (or rather the copris), the goddess Isis on one side and Nephthys on the other. On the reverse are hieroglyphics corresponding to the reverse of the beetle, and also running along the top and sides.* These are funeral

---

* Mr. Sams's collection contains three specimens of a similar nature to these, but differing entirely in the material of which they are composed. The largest, which measures four inches

tablets from the breasts of mummies, and are not the breast-plates of kings, as supposed by Belzoni. Mr. Wilkinson has kindly shown me a drawing of a tablet of this description (Plate VIII. *fig.* 4); it is not funereal. The emblem was suspended from the neck of king Osirei in Belzoni's tomb. The god Amunra (generator) wears a similar ornamental emblem at Kárnak.

In one of the tombs discovered by M. Belzoni, he saw a case over which was thrown a large covering, exactly like a pall upon the coffins of the present day. The cloth on the mummy contained in this case was exceedingly fine and very neatly applied. The mummy was ornamented with garlands of flowers and leaves, and over the heart was placed a plate of metal, soft like lead, covered with another metal, not unlike silver leaf. It had the eyes of a cow (the symbol of Isis) engraved on it, and in the centre of the breast was another plate with the winged globe. Both plates were nearly six inches long. Little besides the bones were to be found of the mummy.*

The four genii of the Amenti,† and other amulets and ornaments in *wax gilt*, are, according to M. Passalacqua, only found in Greek mummies. They are placed upon the chest and above the last envelope. The deities of the Amenti, together with the eye of Osiris,‡ have been found in the

by three and three quarters, represents Osiris seated, and receiving an offering and libation from a female figure standing before the deity. On the back-ground are the four deities of the Amenti, and the hieroglyphics by which they are distinguished. On the reverse of this funeral tablet is the Agathodemon, forming the upper part of the temple, and in the centre is seen a boat bearing (a scarabæus),§ and a deity on each side of it. The emblems of these deities (Isis and Nephthys, I presume) are not sufficiently distinct to be made out perfectly to one's satisfaction.

The second tablet in Mr. Sams's collection measures three inches and a half square, and is of vitrified earth. One side only is characterized by hieroglyphics, and represents the reverse of a scarabæus in a boat with a deity on either side. They are not sufficiently distinct to be made out. Of the third tablet two fragments only remain. These consist of a talcose rock, and the figures are coloured blue, green, red, and white. The remains of an Agathodemon, a figure of Isis, and a figure of Pthah Sokari Osiris, are to be seen. A line of hieroglyphics runs along the top of this tablet. The whole has been vitrified.

* Belzoni's Travels, p. 223.   † See Plate III. *fig.* 1, 2, 3, 4.   ‡ Plate VIII. *fig.* 5.

§ There can be no doubt that this was the subject represented, although it has fallen out. The whole tablet is composed of several portions, some of which are wanting. The substance of the tablet is serpentine rock.

bellies of mummies. The deities of Amenti with legs conjoined and separate, the latter rare.

The divinities are generally placed above or near to the mummies;* the representations of men and women within the cases, and sometimes over the heart of mummies outside the envelopes. The amulets of divinities in stone, as well as enamelled earth, are found in the cases; the larger specimens on the ground in the tombs or in niches. The bronze statues of divinities† are more frequently met with at Kárnak than any other place; they are very rare at Thebes, but are found at Memphis and Hermopolis. Amulets in gold and silver around the neck are always strung and in contact with the flesh. Gold is more commonly met with than silver. A small statue in wood was found by M. Passalacqua lying over the heart of a male mummy.‡ I have in the preceding chapter mentioned the finding of a bulbous root under the soles of the feet of a mummy. Dr. Giov. Bapt. Bonagente, a Venetian doctor, says he hath seen mummies often with an onion in their hands. This kind of onion, he says, is different from the ordinary sort and hath little taste.§

M. Passalacqua never found any money in mummies or in their tombs. The commerce of ancient Egypt was conducted by exchange: we are ignorant of money under the Pharaohs. The greatest commercial transactions were paid for in rings of pure gold of a certain weight and size, or in rings of silver, having a name and weight equally fixed.‖

The medals that have been found in small vases at Memphis and Lower Egypt have been struck under the Greeks, Romans, and Arabs. The first current coin of Egypt was struck by Aryandes, under the dominion of the

---

* Belzoni had some wooden cases from twelve to fifteen inches square, finely painted, and well preserved. They contained idols in wood (some of which he was so kind as to present to me), and were found by him in the mummy-pits at Gournou, near the mummies' cases. At a late sale of Egyptian antiquities by Messrs. Sotheby and son there were cases of a similar description, containing a great number of figures in baked and varnished clay, &c.

† See Plate VIII. *fig.* 6, a representation of Osiris in my possession.

‡ Catal. No. 123.

§ Observations made by Mr. Greaves in his Travels, extracted from his MSS. in the Savilian Library at Oxford.

‖ Champollion Lettres, p. 444.

Persians; and Sperling observes that they never had any great quantity of specie in circulation. M. De Pauw affirms * that what had been issued was entirely drawn back by the annual tributes; for the Arabs who search among the ruins of Egypt, and even sift much of the loose sand, have never discovered one single piece. None of the medals found · there are older than the reign of Alexander. They either belonged to the Ptolemies or to the Egyptian towns which were allowed the privilege of having their own coin under the dominion of the Greeks: these were Pelusium, Memphis, Abydus, Thebes, Hermopolis, and the great city of Hercules.† I am enabled, through the kindness of Mr. Abraham Kirkmann, of Lincoln's-inn, to figure a brass coin of Ptolemy which he purchased at the sale of M. Belzoni, and obtained by him from the wrappers of a mummy, the remains of which are visible, on *fig.* 1, 2, Plate XI. Some years since Mr. Kirkmann purchased another (also of one of the Ptolemies) of a dealer in Hamburgh, said to have been found under similar circumstances, and which he thinks he afterwards gave to Archdeacon Payne.‡ Mr. Burgon has also enabled me to represent in Plate XI., *fig.* 3, some leaden medals taken from a Greek mummy.

To perpetuate the memory of the deceased we find in the tombs the emblems of the profession or trade of the defunct. Thus we have pick-axes and various instruments for agricultural and mechanical purposes, the net of the fisherman, the razor and stone to sharpen it of a barber, cupping glasses, vases of perfumes, pottery,§ and wooden vessels of all kinds, baskets of fruits, seeds, &c. Loaves of bread near to the mummy of a baker, paints and brushes along-side of an artist, various instruments of surgery by the body of a physician, a bow and arrow by the side of a hunter, a lance by the soldier, a hatchet and a poignard by another, and the style and the receptacle for ink by the clerk. The distaff has been found in the cases of male mummies, which would appear to confirm the statement of Herodotus

* I 271.

† Vaillant, Hist. Ptolem. ad Fidem Numismatum accommodata, 104.

‡ Of the situation in which the coins were placed I know nothing; but common report assigns them either to the mouth, under the tongue, or beneath the chin.

§ On pieces of pottery and calcareous stone, fragments in the Enchorial, Greek, and Coptic characters are very often found. I have, by the kindness of Mr. Wilkinson, several specimens of these.

that the men were employed in the manufacture of the cloth, whilst the females were engaged in commerce. Combs, paints, mirrors, and other articles of the toilet, have been found with the mummies of females. In a box of wood placed in the neighbourhood of a mummy, almost entirely decayed, M. Passalacqua found nine instruments in silex, which he conceived to be knives for making the incision in the flanks of the dead. I have figured three of these in Plate IV. *fig.* 6, 7, 8.

The following list, although doubtless very imperfect, will yet enable the reader to form an idea of the extent of objects that have been found in the tombs:—

OBJECTS OF THE TOILET AND JEWELS.

Spangles, copper gilt.

Combs in ivory and in wood.

Necklace of glass of different colours.

Necklace of enamel of different colours.

Necklace of cornelian.

Necklace in form of shells.

Necklace of lapis lazuli.

Necklace of cornelian and gold.

Necklace of ivory.

Necklace of gold.

Necklace of lapis lazuli, cornelian, and ivory.

Necklace of gold, lapis lazuli, cornelian, and ivory, representing different divinities and sacred animals. (Thebes.)

Ear-rings in gold, in red and white enamel, in alabaster, in bronze, in crystal, and in coloured glass.

Bracelets in gold, in ivory, in iron, and in bronze.

Rings of gold, in cornelian, in bronze, in iron, in ivory, and in enamelled earth.

Various engraved stones, onyxes, amethysts, &c.

Pin for the head, ivory and wood.

Mirror of bronze.

Tweezers and scissars in bronze.

Vestments, tunics, sandals of wood and skin, and leaves of palm and painted cloth.   Shoes of similar materials.

Box containing black paint for the eyebrows, and brush for using the same.

VASES, SEALS, &c.

Vases in black basalt, in bronze, in alabaster,* in serpentine, in glazed earth, in terra cotta, in slate, in wood, and in calcareous stone.

Seals in terra cotta, in bronze, and in glazed earth.

Ball of skin.†   Mr. Sams has one composed of different colours like those now used as playthings by children.

Mallets in wood, nails in bronze, ladle in wood, little mortar in agate, moulds in calcareous stone for casting the figures of birds, &c.   Key in bronze, pillow for the head in wood, cistern in wood.   Knives in silex and in wood.   Spatulas, spoons, medicine-chests, baskets, stools, wooden bow, arrows of reed pointed with wood, hatchet in bronze, a musical reed or pipe, bells, sistrum, &c., &c., &c.

P. S. Since the preceding chapter was composed, I have seen two more funeral tablets taken from the breasts of mummies.   They belong to Mr. Burgon, to whom I am indebted for the leaden seals figured in Plate XI. *fig.* 3.‡   The largest tablet measures six inches by four inches and a half, and is composed of earthenware varnished and baked.   The shape is, like all the others, that of an Egyptian temple.   There is a space in the centre which I presume to have been supplied by a scarabæus that is now want-

---

* The alabaster vases are most frequently found at Eleithia, those of terra cotta at Memphis and Saccara.   These are the vases for the purposes of civil life.

† M. Passalacqua found a ball of this description in the case of a mummy of a little child. There were also different kinds of fruit.

‡ Mr. B. has kindly favoured me with the following note on the subject of these impressions.   "The outward covering of the mummy was sealed with wax in several places, but the impressions were effaced.   There were also appended at about equal distances down the back of the mummy, several leaden seals on twisted string, of which nine remained.   They were all impressed with the same representation of a naked bearded bust in profile, apparently a portrait, with the inscription ΚΟΠΡΗC.   The bust slightly resembles that of the emperor Hadrian as it sometimes occurs on his coins."   Mr. B. thinks he could assign more accurately a later period to the seals.

Q

ing; this would have occupied the centre of a boat, at the extremities of which are figures of Isis and Nephthys with their appropriate emblems, and their arms are extended towards the beetle. The boat is floating upon water represented green. At each of the upper corners are representations of the sacred eye of Osiris. On the reverse, painted in black, are the emblem of stability and a figure denoting the soul of the deceased. This tablet is of a white colour; the faces, arms, hands, and feet of the deities are painted red, the eyes of Osiris and other ornaments green.

The second tablet is similar to one of Mr. Sams's, but in better condition. It is of vitrified earth, of a bright green colour. There is a scarabæus in black in very high relief placed in the centre of a boat, on one side of which is Isis and on the other Nephthys. The reverse presents the reverse of the scarabæus covered with hieroglyphics, and on each side a figure representing, I presume, the soul of the deceased. These are of rude execution, and are merely marked, not engraven, on the tablet. The shape is like that of the other specimens of this kind I have described, and measures four inches and a half by three inches and a half. There cannot, I conceive, be any doubt as to these tablets being funeral emblems, and not the breast-plates of kings, as conjectured by Belzoni.

CHAPTER IX.

ON THE CASES AND SARCOPHAGI.

Mummy cases become rare—various kinds—1st, or linen cloth case—paintings and inscriptions upon them—splendour of the colours—subjects of the representations—description of the case of M. Cailliaud's Græco-Egyptian mummy—coffins of sycamore in human shape—description of the subject of a Papyrus MS. belonging to the Earl of Mountnorris—2nd, or sycamore case—sometimes painted—occasionally made of cedar, an emblem of eternity—history of Dr. Perry's mummy—sycamore-tree—description of it—stone sarcophagi—to hold the bodies of kings—tombs of black marble—sarcophagi of stone—marble—granite—pietro dura—Egyptian breccia—green basalt—Mr. Sams's marble sarcophagus with gilt hieroglyphics—the tomb of Alexander—the lover's fountain—alabaster sarcophagus found by Belzoni.

THE mummies being properly prepared and bandaged are ready to be placed in their cases or sarcophagi. The accounts given to us by travellers, however, teach us that all the bodies made into mummies were not enclosed in cases, but that some, after having been soaked in the natrum solution, were swathed in a bandage and then deposited in the tomb—so imperfect are the greater number of these that only the mere bones are to be met with, scarcely held together by the rotten condition of the cloths enveloping them.

Mummies in perfect cases are now rarely found, the remains of them alone are to be met with. It is only the rich who could have been so deposited, and according to the rank and importance of the deceased was the number of cases, sometimes two, three, or even four, in which the body was deposited. The Arabs have destroyed all of this description they could meet with, in search of the treasures supposed to be contained within them.

The cases are of different kinds and shapes. The first is generally composed of folds of linen cemented together; the others of sycamore, cedar, deal, or still more durable materials.

The first cases are made of many layers of cloth cemented together, and plastered with lime on the inside. They are as firm as a board, and require to be sawed through in order to get at the body. The cloths have been supposed to be dipped in sount, or gum of the acacia, and so pressed together that twenty folds would not yield a thickness beyond that of the third of an inch; their hardness and durability may be easily estimated by their density. The shape of the case corresponds to that of the human body without the arms or legs being rendered apparent.* On the head is represented a face, either male or female, and the whole figure terminates in a kind of pedestal, in shape somewhat resembling the feet when closed together. This case is always painted, and the subjects are deserving of particular notice. But before I proceed to these I would observe that the features of the face, either male or female, are depicted often in gold and colours. The countenance seems principally to have been formed upon a model and used for various individuals, rather than affording a resemblance of the deceased. They, however, do vary, but not in my opinion sufficiently so to mark them as being portraits of the deceased.† The case I am describing is called by the French the "Cartonage," from the resemblance of its composition to pasteboard. It must have been placed on the body whilst soft, and is found to be laced up the back‡ and along the bottom of the feet, by which a foot-board is secured. This part frequently contains the representation of some figure. In Mr. Saunders's mummy I found a very spirited delineation of Apis. Great care seems to have been taken that the body should not in any way be disturbed; for, in order to render it steady, small portions of wood and of cork have been found passing from the case to the side of the body to fix it, as well as the plaster with which the inside of the case was liberally smeared, and which generally, upon removal, is found to fall out in large dried portions.

Some of these cases are very handsome, I may fairly say splendid. The colours with which they are decorated have retained their liveliness and beauty in a most surprising manner. The green is the only colour that

---

* This inner case, together with the manner in which it is secured, is well represented in a front and back view in Plate IX. It contained Dr. Lee's mummy.

† For masks of mummies, see vol. V. Description de l'Egypte.　　　‡ Plate IX., *fig.* 2.

appears to have faded; it is sometimes confounded with the blue; the blue is metallic, the yellow vegetable; the nature of the white, which is most durable, has not been discovered; the red is very brilliant. Red, blue, yellow, green, white, and black, are the colours to be found both on the cases and on the walls of the tombs;* the drawings are in profile, the Egyptians being ignorant of perspective; their reliefs are, notwithstanding, full of vigour, life, and expression. An opinion has commonly prevailed that the subject of the representation upon the cases is a history of the life of the person embalmed within. Sufficient is known of the hieroglyphics not only to question this opinion, but to establish its inaccuracy. They are very similar in most cases, and usually commence with the same symbols. Mr. Davidson considers them as no more than a collection of homages offered by the deceased to Osiris, the deceased sometimes taking to himself the name of the god. There can be no doubt, I think, that an attentive examination of the characters and subjects will satisfactorily convince any one that the subject bears relation to the trial which the soul was to undergo, and the deities through whose intervention, or by whose intercession, it was to pass through the different stages of its progress towards another state of existence. This is well illustrated by a reference to the description of the inner case (a painting on cloth) of the Græco-Egyptian mummy brought from Egypt by Mons. Cailliaud.† It is as follows :—

At the upper part of the case is a sacred boat,‡ on which is the scarabæus or beetle, a symbol of Phtha, Tho, or Thore, father of the gods, upon the disk of the sun, to which the head of the deceased is consecrated; and the disk is encircled by a serpent, the emblem of Eternity, two deities without any characters attached to them being seated on each side of it. Near the feet is the same symbol of Phtha, their guardian; and beneath it are the emblems of Anubis, the keeper of the guardians, two jackals with the key

---

* At Kalabschi M. Champollion observed for the first time a violet colour employed in the -reliefs painted in the tombs. This colour, he says, formed a mordaunt, and was applied those parts which were intended to be gilt.—*Lettres d'Egypte*, &c., p. 158.

† Voyage à Meroé, Paris, 1827. Tom. IV., 8vo., p. 45, *et seq.*

‡ Bari (divine barge) guided by a steersman (πρωρεὺς) called by the Egyptians, in their own anguage, *Charon.* See also Plate III.

of Hades hanging from their necks. On each side of the lid the lower region is typified by a bunch of lotus flowers. Osiris Petempamentes,* *i. e.* the Western or Infernal, the true Egyptian Sarapis, is seated on his throne, beside his wife and sister Isis. An altar covered with flowers, loaves, fruits, and liquids is before them ; and Anubis, whose tiara marks his rank in the upper regions, presents the deceased as a suppliant before the judge of the Amenti (the West, *i. e.* the Infernal Regions). This is to represent the trial of his *corporeal* offences, as he appears here in his *bodily* form : the trial of his mental transgressions is represented on the other side, where Osiris, in the character of Phtha-Sacri or Socharis, indicated by a hawk's head, surmounted by the inner part of the tiara and two coloured plumes, is sitting as judge, and before the altar stands the soul of the deceased in the form of a hawk with human hands and head, on which the funereal cone and lotus are seen. The soul, thus symbolized, is pleading its cause, aided by Smé (Truth and Justice), represented by a female figure of a green colour, with a plume (the symbol of Smé) in the place of a head. The seven gates, guarded by seven genii, having a hawk's, baboon's, man's, jackal's, crocodile's, lion's, and vulture's head, are the Sbé Héth, or seven gates mentioned in the ritual (the funeral papyrus). These mystic dwellings were situated in the fields of Oën-ro, before the palace of Osiris. The guards are twenty-one in number ;† and one of them is the god Atmú, with the title of Hfé, *i. e.* the serpent, and the form of a winged dragon with human arms and legs. Inside of this case, near the head, is the hawk with expanded wings sailing through the starry sky, and bearing a red disk, *i. e.* Phré, the sun, symbolical of the spirit which gives life and action to the universe. Over the feet is the goddess Hathor (Venus), in the form of a yellow cow, couchant on an altar ; in an act of adoration before her is a bird with a human head crowned by a

---

* " Petempamentes (Πετεμπαμεντης, Letronne, *Recherches*, p. 345) is the Dionysius or Bacchus of the Greeks, and in Coptic P-ete-m-p-amente, signifies " he who belongs to the Amenti," " he who presides over Amenti." This is a very sufficient evidence that the Coptic was the vernacular language of Egypt, 150 years before the commencement of our era."— *Encyc. Met.*

† But this lid represented only eighteen.

disk, *i. e.* one of the purified spirits united with the sun, whose leader is Haroëris (Arueris), "the beneficent eye of the sun." This figure is probably meant to represent the soul of Ammonius (the name, as translated by Champollion, of the mummy enclosed in the case now being described) raised to that exalted rank in the course of its transmigrations. On the bottom of this case is Netphé, distinguished by the vase (*i. e.* the letter N) on her head, scated with her daughter Isis, and Hathor, in the Glebakh (*Persea*), pouring out streams of nourishment for the blessed. At her feet are the guardian jackals, emblems of Anubis. On the right side of the same coffin, the disk of the sun, in the centre of which is Ammon. Cnuphis (the intellectual sun), borne on a sacred bari, drawn by four jackals, and adored by four baboons *(cynocephali)*, the former referring to the solstices, the latter to the equinoxes. On the left side, the *bari*, accompanied as before, bears an image of the sun and moon united. The interior of this case has also astronomical symbols. In the centre is the goddess Tpé or Tiphé (the heaven personified) extending her arms and legs as if to occupy all space. Over her head rays of light issue from the sun placed in the sign of Capricorn, to indicate (January) the month in which Ammonius was born.* The serpent-headed beetles near the brow of Tiphé are still uninterpreted, but probably conceal some astrological mystery. Twenty-four female figures, twelve on the right and twelve on the left, each having a solar disk on her head, represent the twenty-four hours of the astronomic day; eight are painted yellow, eight green, and eight red, the meaning of which is not yet known.† On the wrapper round the body of Ammonius

* "Pet-amen-oph, or Petemenon (Ammonius), was born 12 Tybi (12 Jan.), A.D. 95, in the fifteenth year of Domitian, not in the fifth of Hadrian as M. Champollion (Cailliaud IV. 51) says. It may also be remarked that this zodiac is evidently astrological, as are all others hitherto discovered in Egypt, which all belong to the Roman period: astrology, as Letronne has justly observed (*Ecclaircissements*, p. 98), was a Chaldæan science, scarcely known among the Greeks before the beginning of our era, never much in vogue among them, but eagerly cultivated by the Romans so soon as they had any intercourse with the East."—*Encycl. Metrop.*

† "If the Egyptians subdivided their months into halves, these figures might represent the year, and then this triple division would indicate the three seasons; the green the first, red the second, and yellow the third, marked by a garden, a house, and water, in the hieroglyphic character. On other monuments the hours of night are represented as following a crocodile, the symbol of Darkness and the West (Horapollo, I. p. 70. 89)."—*Encycl. Metrop.*

the central figure is that of Osiris-Socharis, with his complexion, as usual, green; and near his head the *baris* or sacred boats of the sun and moon, symbolized by a right and a left eye. The god is adored by two images of the deceased, in the form of mummies only half-bandaged up. On the right and left are all the deities who take a part in the final judgment. On the right Osiris-Serapis and his wife Isis; on the left Anubis, crowned with the tiara, presents the deceased to the god. Further towards the right, Thoth is recording the sentence on his tablets, and, on the left, appears the Egyptian Cerberus, a compound of a crocodile, lion, and hippopotamus, the guardian of the palace of Osiris. Near him the four sons of Osiris, his assessors in Amenti, Amset, Hapi, Súmautf, and Keb'h Sniv, having blue, green, or yellow fillets in their hands, as if ready to bandage up the bodies of the deceased, whose intestines were considered as peculiarly their property.* In this mummy was also found a MS. on papyrus, of which I have given an account in the chapter on papyri, drawn from the observations of Mons. Champollion.

The most commonly-represented figures on the inner mummy cases are the four genii of the Amenti, the human, the dog-faced baboon, the jackal, and the hawk-headed; this is their constant order, but when they are placed *vis-à-vis* then the cynocephalus faces the human, and the hawk the jackal, as seen in Plate IX.

There are instances in which mummies have been placed in sycamore coffins or cases, without being previously enclosed in the description of case just described. These have generally been furnished with paintings on the face, chest, and body, accompanied sometimes by hieroglyphical characters and other writing. This was the case in the mummies belonging to Dr. Perry, Dr. Mead, and Captain Lethieullier.

Captain Lethieullier's mummy resembled that of Dr. Perry. It was enclosed in a case of sycamore, highly ornamented with hieroglyphical characters and emblems of the divinities. Upon this, which contained a male mummy, there was a representation of the embalming which is not an

* This account of the hieroglyphics upon the case of the mummy of Petemenoph has been drawn up by M. Champollion le jeune, and appended to the Voyage à Meroé, by M. Cailliaud. The mummy and cases are represented in the folio plates attached to that interesting and valuable work.

infrequent subject upon the inner cases. The body is stretched out upon a bier or table formed of the body of a lion, the limbs of which answer to the legs of the table. The embalmer holds a cup in one hand, and appears to be in the act of making the incision into the flank with the other. He is usually represented with the head of a jackal, and painted black. On this case there is also a representation of the judgment, similar to that so well depicted from a papyrus belonging to the Earl of Mountnorris, and published in the collection of hieroglyphics arranged by the late learned Dr. Young for the Egyptian Society (Plate V.) In this representation Osiris is seen seated, armed with his crook and flagellum. Before him is a kind of mace, around which is the skin of a leopard. On the left is a female Cerberus, and over her are resemblances of the four deities of the Amenti, having their proper denominations placed over them. Thoth, or Mercury, with the head of an ibis, holds in one hand a roll or tablet, and in the other a style, with which he has apparently commenced writing the judgment. Upon the balance behind him is seated a cynocephalus, probably in allusion to the nome* (Hermopolis) to which the deceased belonged, and under the beam, as representative of the good and evil genii of the deceased, are Cteristes and Hyperion, adjusting the balance by which the merits and demerits of the deceased are to be weighed. In one scale is placed a feather, the figure of Truth and Justice, and in the other a vase, supposed to contain and to represent the just actions of the deceased. The deceased is represented as standing with his left arm raised in token of respect between Rhea, the wife of the sun, who holds the sceptre of Isis, and another goddess, who holds up her right arm in token of respect, whose hieroglyphical name Dr. Young conceives to be a personification of honour and glory, and, perhaps, intended simply to signify " a divine goddess." Some of the tablets of this description are furnished with the judges, but they do not appear in this instance.

* But it must not be disguised that a different interpretation may be put upon this appearance of the cynocephalus. This animal is the symbol of the Egyptian Anubis, and may intimate watchfulness, or more probably be typical of time, which Anubis also represents, meting out the award upon its good or evil application in the life of the individual whose actions are thus weighing in the scales before the throne of the judge.

Some mummies have only a large envelope with a square piece covering the head, which is sometimes painted and gilt, and has been supposed to represent the person embalmed.

The second case is usually found of sycamore. In the instances in which the painting has been depicted upon cloth placed immediately upon and not enclosing a mummy, the sycamore case or coffin is generally hewn out of a solid trunk as in Dr. Perry's, Dr. Mead's, and Captain Lethieullier's mummies. When, however, the sycamore case encloses a painted one it is composed of several pieces glued together, and fastened as the single-trunk ones are with wooden pegs fitting into corresponding cavities, and thus closing the whole in the most perfect manner- Where the coffin has been scooped out of one trunk, the surface is found to be furnished with a kind of varnished plaster, upon which the representations of the divinities and the delineation of the hieroglyphical characters are affixed. In Dr. Perry's mummy the colour of this plaster is very dark brown, approaching to black, and the figures are all in yellow. In Captain Lethieullier's the ground is white and the characters are of various colours. Plate VI. *fig.* 4 is a reduced representation of the loculus feralis or coffin from Dr. Perry's work; it has been carefully compared with the original. The upper part of course presents the head, which, from the coiffure, one easily sees is intended for a female. Dr. Perry has made out (apparently to his own satisfaction) the history of the embalmed person who, from the richness of the ornaments, he infers must have been " an Ethiopian princess, or at least a person of very illustrious rank and condition."* He goes on to remark that in very early times a strict amity and commerce subsisted between the Egyptians and Ethiopians, and therefore presumes that she had come down to Egypt on a visit to some of her friends, and that, happening to die there, her remains were conserved in this pompous manner, either by order of her relations, or else by the care and affection of her friends whom she came to see. But to proceed with the case: Immediately below the neck is the ephod or breast-plate. This consists of ten semicircular compartments: the major part of these are merely ornamental; but the seventh, ninth, and tenth, are undoubtedly symbolical. In the first of

* Perry's View of the Levant, p. 472.

these is a string of the flowers of the lotus ;* in the second of the leaves of the persea,† and in the third of pendants or precious stones. Above the ephod, on each side, is represented the head of a hawk, supporting a fiery-coloured globe, which symbolizes Osiris, or the sun. Beneath the breast-plate is the goddess Isis in a kneeling posture, with her wings and arms expanded. Her head is bound with a vitta or riband. She supports a globe upon her head, and in each hand there is a knife for sacrifice. On each side there are four figures; on the right side there are human representations, but the fourth is a human body with a jackal's head upon its shoulders. On the left are the cynocephalus, the hawk, a human head, and a jackal, the four Amenti, all holding bandages in their hands. All the front part of the coffin, below the figure of Isis, and all the back part below the shoulders, are adorned with various hieroglyphical characters. The other kind of cases have usually the face carved out, and sometimes a row of hieroglyphics down the centre; occasionally they are found without any.‡ It is not unusual to find a figure painted in the inside of this case upon the bottom part.§

The third case I have observed to be more generally covered with hieroglyphics both inside and out, and Mr. Sams has an exceedingly fine specimen of this kind. This case is generally composed of sycamore.‖

* Nelumbium speciosum. Vide *Lancret Descript. de l'Egypte.* Antiq. I. p. 25.

† The persea was in a particular manner consecrated to the goddess Isis, because its fruit resembles a heart, and its leaves a tongue (*Plutarch de Iside et Osiride*). The *lébakh*, supposed to be the persea, is very common in Upper Nubia. Mons. Cailliaud (tom. III., p. 288) thinks that the tree consecrated to Isis was not the persea, but the baobab (*Adansonia digitata*).

‡ Plate X. *fig.* 1. This formed the outer case of Dr. Lee's mummy.

§ Plate X. *fig.* 2. The female figure thus represented is Netphé.

‖ An attentive examination of these cases has led me to suspect that those of sycamore consist chiefly of such as are scooped out into the human form, as in Dr. Perry's specimen, and that those in which carpentry has been employed to affix many pieces together are composed of a wood of a much harder nature. It is probably the *cordia myxa* of Linn., the *cordia Sebestena* of Forskal, and the *Sebestena domestica* of Prosper Alpinus. It is figured in the Description de l'Egypte (Plate XIX. *fig.* 1 and 2), and described by M. Delille (*Hist. Nat.* tom. II., p. 191). It is a tree growing to the height of thirty feet; its trunk is straight, cylindrical, and about a foot in thickness; the branches extend from ten to twelve feet. The wood is white and very solid. It is common in Egypt.

Some, however, of the second and third cases are found to be of cedar I have seen two instances of this sort. The outer case is generally painted yellow, the figures and hieroglyphics being blue, green, red, and black : the latter is seldom used. The whole is varnished. Cedar is, according to Pierius, an hieroglyphic of Eternity : it is esteemed the least corruptible of woods. The temple of Solomon, and the temple of Diana at Ephesus, were both constructed of it. The sycamore tree (*ficus fatua*) is described by Norden* as being of the height of a beech, and bearing its fruit in a manner quite different from other trees. The fruit, which is a kind of fig, shoots out from the trunk itself, suspended by little sprigs in the form of grape-stalks : they lie in clusters almost like bunches of grapes. The tree is always green, and bears fruit several times a year, without regard to certain seasons. The fruit has the smell of real figs ; but is inferior to them in taste, being of a disgustful sweetness. The colour of the fruit is a yellow, inclining to an ochre, shadowed by a flesh colour. Internally it resembles the common figs, except that it has a blackish colouring, with yellow spots. The tree is very common in Egypt,† and the people, for the greater part, live upon the fruit. They think themselves well regaled when they have a piece of bread, a couple of sycamore figs, and a pitcher filled with water from the Nile.

In the structure of the massy sycamore sarcophagi the ancient Egyptians appear to have been as anxious to afford protection and security to the preserved remains as by the processes adopted in embalming they had succeeded in making them durable. The bodies of their kings were in an especial manner protected ; for not only were they enclosed in linen and in wooden cases, but these were deposited in sarcophagi of a more durable material, as is evidenced by the specimens preserved in the collection of antiquities at the British Museum. The sarcophagi were also deposited in tombs constructed of various substances, and remain until this day, defying, as it were, the power of time. Diodorus Siculus speaks ‡ of their magnificence and of their wonderful sepulchres : their houses they called inns, and

* Vol. I. p. 50. Plate XXXVIII.

† Sycamore wood appears the most plentiful in the country, for not only most of the cases but various utensils are made of it.

‡ Lib. i.

bestowed little attention upon them, but the tombs they denominated Eternal Dwellings—Eternal Habitations. Strabo is not less laudatory in his description of the tumuli, near Syene, in the upper parts of Egypt.* The tombs were constructed of hard black marble, rendered very smooth and of a spherical figure: one was not less than twelve feet in diameter, and the whole of them not less than half that size. They were arranged on both sides of an even plain of considerable extent on the road from Syene to Philæ. Sarcophagi of stone, marble, and granite are mentioned by Abd' Allatif: Dr. Richardson and Mr. Wilkinson assure me that they have also seen sarcophagi of limestone and slate, the latter of a small size. It is not a little singular that the term sarcophagus should have been adopted for those receptacles chosen for the preservation of the dead, as it is derived from the Greek Σαρκοφαγος (*flesh-eater*), denoting a quality direct opposed to conservation.† The stone sarcophagi, which may fairly be called tombs, have usually other cases within them. They are sculptured out of one piece, and sometimes represent either a male or a female figure. Occasionally, like the sycamore cases, they are fashioned into the human shape; this was the case with one in pietro dura, discovered in the Nile at Boulac by Mons. Monge.‡ He says it was in the form of a mummy. Mr. Sams has one of a similar shape in white marble, upon which there are hieroglyphics gilt. All others that I have seen have been rounded at the head and square at the feet, and the image has been sculptured on the cover. I must refer the reader to two very fine specimens in red granite§ now lying in the court-yard

* Lib. xvii.

† The stones used by the ancients for tombs were supposed to have the power of consuming the flesh. The lapis assius was much used by the Greeks for this purpose, and it was said to be able to destroy a body (except the teeth) in forty days. All the ancient naturalists speak of it, and describe it as a reddish pumice-stone, having a saltish taste. The quarries whence it was obtained were at a place near the city of Troas, named Assum. Theophrastus speaks not only of its power of consuming the flesh placed within it, but also of a singular quality it possessed of turning into stone any thing that was put into it. This effect has been explained on the very reasonable supposition that a kind of incrustation might be produced from the water permeating the stone, and carrying along with it particles of its spar to be deposited upon the substances enclosed.

‡ See Description de l'Egypte, vol. V., Antiq.

§ The quarries of Philæ, Elephantine, and Syene, have been remarkable for the beautiful

of the British Museum. These have no hieroglyphics within. The bodies contained within these massy blocks are supposed with great justice to have been those of the kings of Egypt. They are of course very rare.

Mr. Hamilton states* that in the royal tombs where no sarcophagus is found there is always a large granite lid, placed over a hole or grave, cut in the rock, of from six to thirty feet deep. All the lids he found to have been removed or broken. The largest sarcophagus he saw measured eleven feet seven inches in length, six feet ten inches in breadth, two feet two inches thick, eight feet two inches in height, and the lid one foot six inches.

The British Museum contains two of the most magnificent specimens of sarcophagi in the world. Upon one of these a very learned and a very elaborate dissertation has been written by the traveller, the late Dr. Clarke, to prove that it was the tomb of Alexander,† removed from the mosque of St. Athanasius. The other was taken by the French from Cairo to Alexandria, whence it was brought to this country. It has been described by various travellers,‡ and was called the " Lover's Fountain." These precious monuments, which I presume to be familiar to all my readers, are rounded at the head and square at the feet, and are decorated within and without with numerous hieroglyphical characters. The material of which they are composed is a *breccia*,§ and formed out of a single block of this

oriental or rose-coloured granite. The chief part of it consists of felspar, varying in colour from a pale pink to that of a brick red; portions of mica and translucent quartz give it a shining appearance. Pliny calls it the Thebaic stone, from its frequent occurrence at that place, though there are no quarries of it in that neighbourhood. The hardness of this stone is very great; and in a climate like that of Egypt, where the air is of an almost uniform dryness, and no rain, its surface would suffer but little change from exposure during many ages.

* Egyptiaca, p. 155.

† That the body of Alexander may have been laid in this sarcophagus is exceedingly probable; but that it was made expressly for him the knowledge now possessed of the hieroglyphics most satisfactorily disproves. Mr. Wilkinson has pointed out to me the repeated occurrence of the name of Amyrteus upon the sarcophagus. He reigned from about 414 to 408 B. C.; whereas Alexander conquered Egypt 332, and died 323 years B. C., which so far, in my opinion, settles this part of the enquiry.   ‡ Pococke, Maillet, Niebuhr, and Browne.

§ See a particular account of this substance by Professor Hailstone in the 'Appendix to Dr. Clarke's Dissertation.

material. Lids of the same substance were doubtless applied to them as the grooves for their reception are apparent.

Alexander was worshipped as an Egyptian god; a superstitious veneration was paid to his tomb, and his image was worn as an amulet. Augustus did homage to his tomb, and had afterwards on his signet ring an engraved head of Alexander. This occurred three centuries after the death of Alexander, and thirty years before Christ. We have the authority of Dio Cassius that the Roman emperor saw and touched the body of the hero: " He saw the body of Alexander and touched it, so that a part of the nose, as they relate, was broken off."* And Suetonius adds that when the body was taken from the sarcophagus Augustus placed a golden crown upon it, and scattered flowers over it. A superstitious notion prevailed that whatsoever country possessed his body it should flourish most. Perdiccas would have sent it to the sepulchres of the Macedonian kings. Ptolemy arrested it in its passage to the Oasis, and conveyed it to Alexandria, the city of which he was the founder.† His tomb must be described in the words of Dr. Clarke: " This surprising sarcophagus is one entire block of green Egyptian *breccia*. There is not perhaps in the world another of such magnitude. We are not acquainted with the name which the ancients gave to this beautiful production of the Egyptian quarries: when their historians mention, that, from one entire emerald, columns and statues were constructed of a size that contradicts all our knowledge of the mineral kingdom, the stone thus named

---

* Lib. li. c. 16.

† Dr. Clarke's Dissertation, p. 45. Dr. Clarke quotes from Trebellius Pollio regarding the superstition of the Macrian family. " They had Alexander's portrait, as a talisman, in their ears, upon their hands, upon their clothes, and upon every article of external ornament, whether of their persons or their palaces. ' The men,' says he, speaking of that family, ' had Alexander the Great, the Macedonian, wrought in gold and in silver; the women in net-work, on their bracelets, their rings, and in all kinds of ornaments; so that the garments, embroidery, and matron vests of the family exhibit at this day the image of Alexander, with various elegancies. We have lately beheld Cornelius Macer, a member of the same family who gave a supper in the temple of Hercules, present to the high priest an electrinal patera, in the middle of which was Alexander's portrait, encircled by a representation of his whole history in minute figures, which he ordered to be carried round to all those who were his warmest votaries. I have mentioned this because they are said to be *benefited in all their actions who wear the portrait of Alexander expressed in gold or silver*." Dissert. p. 13.

has been sometimes supposed the green fluor. But none of the varieties of this substance are found in Egypt; and from the nature of their formation, as stalactites, they are not likely to appear any where in very large masses. From a frequent view of the materials used by ancient artists, and particularly those of Egypt, the country to which reference has been made for these pretended emeralds, I am disposed to believe it was the green *breccia.* The ancients used this substance only in their most sacred and sumptuous works; and the remains of it are extremely rare. In the whole city of Constantinople, adorned as it was by the munificence of its emperors, only two columns are found of this stone. They support a part of the seraglio, facing the sea, among several other columns of the beautiful green marble of Laconia, called by the Italians *verde antico.* I do not recollect it among the ruins of Greece, nor in any collection of the antiquities of Rome, either in that city or any other part of Europe. We have thus a proof that the stone used in this sarcophagus was of a rarity and price equal to that of the most precious materials of ancient art. The expense of working it could be undertaken only by sovereigns, who might procure, among the renowned artists of those times, talents and perseverance adequate to the achievement of such a surprising work. In these days, the substance itself, and the process by which it was wrought, being unknown, a notion of supernatural agency is excited in unenlightened minds ; while the refined part of mankind express their astonishment. If at any period in the history of the ancient world a work of this nature particularly corresponded with the genius of the age, and the wishes of the people, it must have been at that important crisis when the BODY OF THE DEIFIED ALEXANDER WAS RECEIVED BY PTOLEMY TO BE ENSHRINED AS THE SON OF AMMON BY THE PRIESTS OF EGYPT. That the construction of the tomb would demand every thing admirable in materials and in workmanship cannot be disputed; but upon this subject we have sufficient proof from the testimony of ancient historians. Diodorus, whose description of the funeral pomp seems to convey an adequate idea of the magnificence with which it was celebrated, represents it in magnitude and workmanship worthy the greatness and glory of Alexander."*

* Dissert. p. 41.

M. Champollion examined a third necropolis at Sais which had contained the remains of a person of quality, a keeper of the temples under Psammeticus II. In it there was a large sarcophagus of green basalt. Exteriorly and interiorly it was covered with fine sculpture in bas relief, and it is altogether described as an exquisite specimen. It is deposited in the Egyptian Museum of the Louvre.*

The most beautiful sarcophagus yet discovered is that in the possession of Sir John Soane. It was taken by M. Belzoni out of one of the chambers of the tombs (or rather gates) of the kings in the valley known by the name of " Biban el Molouk." The chambers in these tombs were very numerous, and extended to 309 feet, the whole extent of which had been cut out of the living rock. The walls or sides were as white as snow, and covered with paintings, all beautifully fresh,† *al fresco*, and abounding with hieroglyphics. The sarcophagus was within the innermost chamber, and measured nine feet five inches in length, by three feet nine inches in width. It is two feet one inch in height, and carved both inside and outside with hieroglyphics in intaglio, coloured dark blue, which are in great preservation. It is of alabaster or arragonite, very transparent, and sounds like a bell. It was placed over a staircase communicating with a subterraneous passage, leading downwards 300 feet. The tomb M. Belzoni conceived had been dedicated to Apis, as the remains of the carcase of a bull embalmed with asphaltum were found in the innermost chamber. I have some portions of the tomb, which correspond with this account: the hieroglyphics being in high relief. The walls of the tomb, I lament to say, have been literally knocked to pieces.

* Lettres écrites d'Egypte et de Nubie en 1828 et 1829, par M. Champollion le Jeune, 8vo. Paris, 1833. pp. 51 and 400.

† Mr. Salt says that the tints of the paintings were so resplendent that it was found scarcely possible to imitate them with the best water-colours made in England, and that they have been executed on a principle and scale of colour that would make them retain their lustre even by the side of a Venetian picture.—*Quart. Rev.*, No. 37.

CHAPTER X.

ON THE PAPYRI MANUSCRIPTS.

Papyri MSS.—erroneous opinion as to the nature of their contents—Cyperus papyrus—its history—mode of manufacturing it into paper—different kinds—situations in which the papyri are found—Egyptian literature—rosetta stone—labours of De Sacy—Akerblad—Young—his method of investigation—Champollion—his phonetic alphabet based upon the researches of Dr. Young—labours of Salt—Wilkinson—Burton—passage from St. Clement of Alexandria—Warburton—description of the characters—hieroglyphic—hieratic—enchorial—Reuvens' account of two bilingual MSS.—Champollion's account of the great funeral ritual—Græco-Egyptian MSS. at Leyden—papyrus of M. Sallier of Aix—Mr. Grey's Greek autograph—papyri at Turin.

THE Papyri constitute not the least interesting objects that have been found enclosed in mummies, or within cases placed near to them; and the researches of Dr. Young, M. Champollion, Signor Rosellini, Mr. Wilkinson, Mr. Burton, and a few others have rendered these documents of singular importance as it respects Egyptian history and antiquities. Mr. Madden has stated that all the papyri hitherto discovered have contained nothing of the religion or sciences of the Egyptians, that law processes, accounts, narratives of funerals, and title deeds have generally been the subjects of these MSS. This, however, is far from being the case, as a reference to the labours of those whose names I have just mentioned will satisfactorily demonstrate. But, further, M. Reuvens has shown* that of two bilingual papyri which he minutely examined the one treats of magical operations, and contains upwards of 100 chemical and alchemical formulæ, and the other relates to some of the mysteries of the ancient Egyptians. I allude here to the opinion expressed by Mr. Madden, be-

---

* Lettres à M. Letronne sur les Papyrus bilingues et Grecs, &c., 4to. Leide, 1830.

cause it does not rest upon his authority alone, for he expressly states *
that he had seen for the last two years every papyrus that had been found
in Egypt, and had the advantage of Mr. Salt's interpretation of them, and
that none of them contained any thing relating to the religion and sciences
of the Egyptians. Captain Caviglia, with whom Mr. Madden lived for
some months at Mr. Salt's, is stated also to be strongly of this opinion.
I have, therefore, thought it proper thus particularly to notice this assertion, which I believe to have been made upon imperfect information.

Previously to entering into any description or consideration of the papyri,
it will be proper to say a few words on the substance of which they are
composed, and the characters with which they are found to have been
impressed.

The papyrus plant, the cyperus papyrus, according to Champollion,† has
ceased to grow in Egypt. The ancient Arabs called it *berd;* it grew principally in marshy places, and its culture was a source of riches for the inhabitants of the borders of the ancient lakes of Bourlos, and of Menzaleh
or Termis. The baroness Minutoli says‡ that it is to be met with in the
environs of Damietta and on the banks of the lake Menzaleh. It is, however, exceedingly scarce. M. Savary states‖ that it is only to be met with
about Damietta and the lake Menzaleh, and observes that all the travellers
who have not visited this part of Egypt make no mention of the plant.
This author quotes from Strabo,§ who calls it biblos, and says that it is
indigenous to Lower Egypt; he describes it very clearly, and alludes to a
restriction of its growth to particular places. It grows abundantly in Syracuse,¶ and Captain Smyth has figured it, and described it with great

* Travels I. 361.   † Lettres, p. 444.   ‡ Recollections of Egypt, p. 194.   ‖ Lettres,I. 286.

§ Strabo, speaking of the environs of Alexandria, says, " Hoc in loco biblus non multa nascitur: non enim excolitur.   In inferioribus vero ipsius Delta partibus permulta est, alia dete-
rior, alia melior: Hieratica appellatur.   Nonnulli ut reditus augerent, Judaiacam versutiam
huc adhibuerunt, quam illi in palma caryotica, atque balsamo excogitaverant: non enim per-
mittunt multis in locis nasci: quo fit ut raritati pretium imponentes, reditum quidem augeant,
communi vero usui damnum adferant." Lib. xvii., p. 1134. Ed. Falconeri. fol. Oxon. 1807.

¶ Specimens of paper are made at this day at Syracuse from the papyrus plant, and sold to
travellers. The sheets do not extend beyond eight or nine inches in length, and five inches in

precision.* It floats as it grows; the principal root runs horizontally near the surface of the water, and throws out long filaments, which descend perpendicularly downwards, whilst numerous triangular green stems shoot upwards eight or ten feet, and bear on the crown a fibrous tuft of fine filaments, which, near their extremities, are again subdivided into others, bearing small seedy flowerets. This plant is supposed to have been sent from Egypt by Ptolemy Philadelphus as a present to Hiero. Paper is supposed to have been made of the yellow pellicle that surrounds the stem near the root; but Captain Smyth was more successful, by following the directions of Pliny, with the cellular substance of the whole stem cut thin, the slices laid over each other transversely at right angles, and well pressed. The ancients extracted sugar from this plant, and made cordage and canvas of its fibres. It served as a medicine for the sick,† as an article of food,‡ and also for fuel.§ The monopoly of this useful plant by the government of Egypt, alluded to by Strabo, probably occasioned its scarcity. M. de Sacy‖ quoting from an Arabic writer, whose MS. is in the Imperial Library, states that the Egyptians wrote on the paper of Egypt, and that it was made from a reed called *berdi*. Joseph is said to have been the first fabricator of this paper. The Greeks wrote upon silk, parchment, and other substances, and also on the paper of Egypt.

Pliny gives¶ a very full description of the mode of preparing the paper from the papyrus plant. He says, The stem of the plant is divided with a kind of needle into thin plates or slender pellicles, each of them as large as the plant will admit. These form the elements of which the sheets of paper are composed. The pellicles in the centre are the best, and they diminish in value as they depart from it. As they were separated from the reed, they were extended on a table and laid across each other at right angles. In this state they were moistened by the water of the Nile, and while wet were put under a press, and afterwards exposed to the rays of the sun.

---

breadth. The texture appears to be less uniform, and of a coarser description than that manufactured by the ancients.

* Travels in Sicily, p. 175.   † Dioscorides, lib. i. cap. 116.

‡ Guilandin (Melch) in C. Plin., 8vo. Lausanne, 1576.

§ Theophrastus, Hist. Plant. IV. 9.   ‖ Notes to Abd'Allatif, p. 109.

¶ Lib. xiii. cap. 11.

The water of the Nile was said to have a gummy quality sufficient to make the layers of the plant adhere to each other; but Mr. Bruce has shown that the plant itself is adequate to this from the quantity of saccharine matter it contains, and that the water of the Nile does not in any degree possess this property. Sometimes however, perhaps when the plant did not contain a sufficient portion of sugar, a kind of paste made of wheat flour was used for this purpose. The size of the paper seldom exceeded two feet, and it was frequently much less. Mr. Bruce made paper of the plant which he saw growing in Egypt and Abyssinia. The plant must formerly have been very abundant, for Cassiodorus* speaks of it as forming a forest on the banks of the Nile. "There (says he) rises to the view this forest without branches, this thicket without leaves, this harvest of the waters, this ornament of the marshes." Prosper Alpinus and Guilandin both saw it about two centuries since, and the latter remarks that the inferior and succulent part of it was eaten by the common people.

The papyrus, no less than the lotus and the fig, was consecrated to the god Osiris.† The purposes to which it was applied by the Egyptians, as well as the commerce sustained by it, were sufficient to gain for it this mark of respect. Bomare tells us ‡ that this paper was formerly called sacred or hieratic, and that it served only for the religious writings of the Egyptians. But it was taken to Rome, and there differently prepared, washed, beaten, and pressed, and this had the name of Charta Augusta. The Charta Augusta, so named from the Emperor Augustus, was so delicate and thin that it would scarcely admit the use of the reed upon it. It was also called Charta Livia, from Livia, the wife of Augustus, and Charta Fauniana, from Faunius, a Roman grammarian, who established a manufactory at Rome for the making of paper, and was celebrated for his mode of preparing it and glueing it together. Montfaucon § and Count de Caylus‖ have written at length upon this subject.

The Egyptian paper was manufactured principally at Alexandria, but also at Memphis and other Egyptian cities. At the close of the third century

---

* ‖Oper. Var. lib. xi., ep. 38.   † Martin, Religion des Egyptiens, p. 196.

‡ Dict. Hist. Nat. Art. Papier du Nil.   § Mem. de l'Acad. des Inscrip. VI. 592.

‖ Mem. de l'Acad. des Inscr. XXVI. 267.

the traffic in paper was very flourishing, and it continued until the fifth century, for St. Jerome says it was much in use during his time, although a very high impost was put upon it. This impost was abolished by Theodoric, king of Italy, who subdued the oppression in the sixth century, upon which Cassiodorus wrote a letter in which he congratulates the whole world on the removal of the impost from an article of traffic so essential to the convenience and improvement of mankind, and to the cultivation and prosperity of the arts, science, and commerce.

We have no means of ascertaining at what period the papyrus was first used. The ancients have left us in uncertainty upon this head. M. Henry* is disposed to think it was not much employed before the time of the Greeks in Egypt. Its use was superseded by the introduction of the Charta Bombycina (cotton paper), which was found to be better calculated for the purpose of writing. When papyri are met with in mummies, they are generally placed between the first and second layers of bandages, and usually between the thighs or legs, or on the insides of the arms. In other instances they have been found in cases of the human shape, made after the manner of the wooden sarcophagi : one of these is in the possession of my friend Dr. Lee, and measures twenty inches in length. M.Jomard† says that the tombs of Saccara have not yielded a single papyrus MS. Belzoni says that few papyri are met with among the lower class of mummies. If any, it consists simply of a small piece stuck upon the breast with a little gum or asphaltum. The same distinguished traveller also tells us‡ that " the mummies in the cases have no papyri; on the contrary, in those without cases they are often obtained; it appears (he says) that such persons as could afford it would have a case to be buried in, on which the history of their lives was painted ; and those who could not afford a case were contented to have their lives written on papyri, rolled up and placed above their knee." I quote this passage to prevent the error becoming current. Papyri have been frequently found in mummies that were contained in cases ; and, further, it is wrong to conceive that the life of the individual was pourtrayed

* Lettre à M. Champollion sur l'Incertitude de l'Age des Monumens Egyptiens, 8vo. Paris, 1828, p. 178.

† Descr. de l'Egypte. A. tom. II.   ‡ Travels, p. 164.

upon the case. I trust it has been shown * that the subjects painted on the cases do not bear any particular reference to the history of the individuals embalmed; but that they relate to the funeral rites practised, and the theological doctrine upon death and a future state professed by the Egyptians: that in short they specially apply to the trial the soul has to undergo, and refer to the deities through whose intervention it was to be enabled to pass to another stage of existence.

Having premised thus much as to the nature of the papyri and the mode adopted in their preparation, as well as the situations in which they are found, it will be proper to say a few words upon the characters of the MSS. impressed upon them, and then proceed to the subjects of which they have hitherto been found to consist.

The extraordinary magnitude and the permanency of the Egyptian monuments, the magnificent temples dedicated to their gods, and the splendid obelisks erected in honour of their kings, bespeak a people much advanced in the arts, and indicate a high degree of civilization. The learning of the Egyptians has been made known to us by the sacred historian. By this record we have been taught to believe in the political wisdom of this ancient people, and to feel astonishment at the nature of the institutions, the extent of the learning, and the perfection of the arts attained at so early a period. The records upon the monuments of ancient Egypt, but a few years since, appeared to be involved in impenetrable obscurity. The darkness which surrounded them had in vain been attempted to be dispersed, and it remained for British erudition and British industry to open the path of discovery, from which it now seems probable the ancient history and literature of Egypt may be brought to light. To decipher the characters impressed upon the monuments of the ancient dynasties of the Pharaohs and the Ptolemies, after the laborious but fruitless attempts of ages, is indeed a result far beyond the expectation of the most sanguine; and although those to whom we are indebted for the first-fruits of this glorious harvest are, alas! removed from us, it is satisfactory to reflect that there are a few others still behind who pursue the subject with an ardour commensurate to

* See chap. IX. on the Cases, Sarcophagi, &c.

their ability,* and nothing is now wanting but patronage on the part of the public to carry the work on to a complete and triumphal issue. It cannot be expected, in a work of the description of the present, that I should enter into any elaborate disquisition upon the Egyptian characters; it is sufficient for the present purpose, in accordance with the plan I have proposed to myself, and which I trust I have fulfilled, to bring together every thing connected with the subject of mummies as an interesting object of great antiquity, and I must refer the reader to the more learned and finished performances of other writers upon the branches of which they severally treat.

The attention of the public, and more particularly the learned world, has lately been drawn to Egyptian literature, and the labours of the late Dr. Young and the Rev. Mr. Tattam have satisfactorily shown that all that has come down to us of the language and literature of ancient Egypt is contained in the Coptic, Saaidic,† and Basmurico-Coptic dialects, and in the enchorial, hieratic, and hieroglyphic inscriptions and MSS. It is a point that cannot be too much insisted upon that a previous knowledge of the Coptic is absolutely necessary to a correct understanding of the hieroglyphics. Dr. Young regrets that the Coptic inscriptions, which are sometimes mixed with the Greek, have not been more generally copied by travellers, since it is only among these, he says, that we can hope to find any traces of the vernacular nomenclature derived from the Egyptian mythology; although, from the few specimens which have been hitherto examined, it seems probable that the introduction of the Coptic character was only coeval with that of Christianity.‡ M. Klaproth has pointed out the resemblance of a consider-

---

* I allude here particularly to the labours of my friend Mr. Wilkinson. See his Materia Hieroglyphica. This gentleman has detected a change in the mode of sculpturing the hieroglyphics in the time of Rameses III. He observed that the lower side was cut to a great depth, while the upper inclined gradually from the surface of the wall, till it reached the innermost part of the intaglio; so that the hieroglyphics could be distinguished by a person standing immediately beneath, and close to the wall, on which they were sculptured.—*Mat. Hierog.* p. 95.

† The word Saaid signifies the Upper Country (of Egypt).

‡ Suppl. to Encycl. Brit. Art. Egypt. p. 38. The Coptic language is compounded of the ancient Egyptian and Greek; the letters of its alphabet are copied from the latter, with the exception of seven, for whose peculiar sound new characters were formed, as the *sh, f, kh, h, g,*

T

able number of Coptic words to some of the dialects of the north of Asia and the north of Europe; but Mr. Tattam says* that if the remains which we possess of the Egyptian language be separated from the Greek, with which it has in some degree been mixed up, that it has no near resemblance to any one of the ancient or modern languages. Dr. Murray also states the Coptic to be an original tongue, deriving all its indeclinable words and particles from radicals pertaining to itself, and he adds that there is no mixture of foreign language in its composition, except Greek.†

The Key to the LOST LITERATURE OF ANCIENT EGYPT was found in the trilinguar stone of Rosetta; and it is highly flattering to our national vanity to know that after the almost vain and fruitless attempts of M. De Sacy and M. Akerblad, who had succeeded only in making some progress towards the identification of some parts of the sacred inscription, it was left to the erudite sagacity of Dr. Young " to convert to permanent profit a monument which had before been a useless though a glorious trophy of British valour." This stone, which is of black basalt, it may be right here to state, was discovered by the French when digging for the foundation of Fort St. Julian, near Rosetta, buried four feet beneath the surface of the ground. This monument, which affords to us the only known clue to the hieroglyphics and furnishes an example of the style of an Egyptian record or decree, may fairly be considered as one of the most interesting Egyptian antiquities in the world. It is deposited in the British Museum, and Mr. Hamilton tells us that when the claim was made for its delivery to the British authorities it was not given up without many remonstrances and deep regret on the part of the French.

The inscription on this stone is trilinguar or rather trigrammatic: hieroglyphic or sacred, enchorial or native character, and the Greek. This is, perhaps, almost the only hieroglyphical inscription in the world accompanied by a translation, and from the Greek we find that it is an inscription in honour of Ptolemy Epiphanes, and that the decree was ordered to be

---

another kind of *sh*, and a *d* or *t*. The names of individuals, though the language was coeval with Christianity, may still throw some light on those of the Egyptian deities, since we find many of the Christians bore the same as their heathen predecessors, as Ammonius, Isidorus, &c.

  * Compendious·Grammar of the Egyptian Language, p. 4.   † Bruce's Travels, II. 473.

engraved in three different characters, the sacred, the native, and the Greek. It was executed in the ninth year of this sovereign, or 196 B.C. The stone is unfortunately imperfect, being deficient of a part at the commencement of the first inscription, the beginning of the second, and the latter part of the third. It is deeply to be deplored that the labours of travellers directed to the recovery of the remaining fragments of this invaluable tablet have been unavailing; yet it is gratifying to know that enough is already possessed to permit of a comparison of the several parts with each other, and thus to establish their coincidence. In 1811, the Society of Antiquaries published an account of the Rosetta stone and translations of the Greek inscription into English by the Rev. Stephen Weston, and another into Latin by Professor Heyne, of Gottingen. To these were added some remarks by the late Mr. Taylor Combe.

M. De Sacy was, I believe, the first to compare the Greek inscription with the enchorial and hieroglyphic, and in two passages of the Greek, in which the proper names of Alexander and Alexandria occur, he recognized two well-marked groups of characters, very nearly resembling each other: these he justly considered as representing proper names. He made out also the place of the name of Ptolemy, but beyond this he could not proceed, and abandoned the research. M. Akerblad resumed the enquiry, established what M.-De Sacy had done, and endeavoured to construct an alphabet, but in this he completely failed. This failure has been attributed* to the notion which he and his predecessor had imbibed that the whole inscription was alphabetical, and partly from his expectation of finding all the vowels which the same words contain in the Coptic texts still extant. In 1814, Dr. Young directed his attention to this ancient monument, and the result of his unparalleled labours was given anonymously as an appendage to a communication made in 1815 by Sir W. Edward Rouse Boughton, Bart., to the Society of Antiquaries, entitled " Some Remarks on Egyptian Papyri and on the Inscription of Rosetta." The author, however, was soon discovered, and in 1815 he printed some " Extracts of Letters and Papers relating to the Egyptian Inscription of

Edinb. Rev., No. 89, p. 113.

Rosetta" in the Museum Criticum of Cambridge (Part VI.), a correspondence with M.M. Silvestre De Sacy and Akerblad, and in the following
year " Additional Letters relating to the Inscription of Rosetta ;" the first
addressed to the Archduke John, who had lately been in England, the
second to M. Akerblad (Museum Criticum, No. VII.) These letters were
printed and distributed in 1816 ; the journal was not published till 1821.
They announce the *discovery of the relation between the different kinds of
Egyptian letters or characters*—the basis on which the system of M. Champollion was afterwards erected.* A fac-simile of the inscription was published by the Society of Antiquaries, and has been copied into several
works. As it may be satisfactory to the reader to see a specimen of the
three characters, I have represented them in Plate XI., *fig.* 4, 5, 6.

In the article on Egypt, in the Supplement of the Encyclopædia Bri-
tannica, Dr. Young has told us of the manner in which he proceeded in his
investigation. First, attending to the enchorial text he verified the previous observations of M. de Sacy and M. Akerblad as to the names of
Alexander and Alexandria, and the application of the numerals. He next
observed a remarkable collection of characters, repeated twenty-nine or
thirty times in the enchorial inscription, and he found that nothing occurred so often in the Greek except the word *king* with its compounds,
which he found about thirty-seven times ; a fourth assemblage of characters he found fourteen times, and this agreed sufficiently with the name
of Ptolemy, which occurred eleven times in the Greek ; and by a similar
comparison he identified the name of Egypt, although it occurs much more
frequently in the enchorial than in the Greek, which often substitutes for it
country only, or omits it entirely. He then proceeded to write the Greek
text over the enchorial in such a manner that the passages ascertained
might also coincide as nearly as possible, and by this arrangement the in-
termediate parts of each inscription were found to stand very near to the
corresponding passages of the other.

Having succeeded thus far, Dr. Young proceeded to analyze and decipher the hieroglyphical text, and by a comparison of this with the encho-

---

* See Catalogue of the Works and Essays of the late Dr. Young.

rial and the Greek texts he ascertained the places of some most prominent names and words, as *Ptolemy* (which he found in one place occurred three times in the hieroglyphics, though only twice in the Greek), *God, king, priest, shrine,* by which he obtained a number of common points of subdivision; he then proceeded to write all the three inscriptions side by side, and was thus enabled to investigate the sense of the respective characters, and institute a minute comparison of the different parts with each other. At length he succeeded in arranging the results of his enquiry, and gave a vocabulary comprising upwards of 200 names or words, which he had succeeded in deciphering in the hieroglyphical and enchorial texts, and in the Egyptian MSS. This is given in the article on Egypt I have referred to, and has been justly pronounced to be " the greatest effort of scholarship and ingenuity of which modern literature can boast."*

The labours of M. Champollion succeeded to those of Dr. Young. The latter had shown the practicability of constructing an alphabet, and M. Champollion's attention appears particularly to have been directed to this important acquisition. He had the singular good fortune to meet with an interesting monument, the obelisk found in the Isle of Philæ, which contained also the name of one of the Ptolemies. This obelisk, it is said, was fixed to a basis bearing a Greek inscription, which is a petition of the priests of Isis at Philæ, addressed to King Ptolemy, Cleopatra his sister, and Cleopatra his wife. The developement of the hieroglyphic alphabet was principally effected by a comparison of the several signs entering into the names of Ptolemy and Cleopatra. The alphabet, which by the labours and ingenuity and perseverance of M. Champollion, based it must be acknowledged upon the previous researches of Dr. Young, was termed by Champollion the Phonetic alphabet, for a particular account of which the inquisitive reader is referred to the " Précis du Système Hiéroglyphique des Anciens Egyptiens." In this work the author endeavours to establish—

1. That the Phonetico-hieroglyphic alphabet is applicable to the royal hieroglyphic legends of every epoch in the history of Egypt.

2. That this alphabet is the true key to the whole hieroglyphic system.

3. That the ancient Egyptians constantly employed it to represent alphabetically the sounds of words in their spoken language.

* Edinb. Rev., No. 89, p. 114.

4. That all the hieroglyphic inscriptions are to a considerable extent composed of signs purely alphabetical.

5. That different kinds of characters, the nature of which he endeavours to appreciate, were simultaneously employed in the hieroglyphic texts.

6. That from all these propositions, each of which is supported by an immense number of applications and examples, he ventures to deduce a general theory of the graphic system of the ancient Egyptians.*

To the developement of these several propositions, and to the further elucidation of this interesting subject, I must direct the attention of the reader to the labours of Mr. Salt, and to the more recent and more valuable productions of Mr. Wilkinson and Mr. Burton. From an examination of these it will be seen how much has already been done by the most patient application, and we shall also learn how much there is still left behind for the exertions and skill of others to enable us to become versed in " all the learning of the Egyptians."

Herodotus tells us† that the Egyptians employed two kinds of characters, the hieratic or sacred, and the demotic or popular ; and Diodorus Siculus‡ confirms this statement, adding, that the knowledge of the former was confined exclusively to the priests, but the latter was common to all. I must not omit to refer to a celebrated passage of one of the fathers of the church bearing upon this subject, and which, though often variously misunderstood and mistranslated, is too singular a verification of the different modes of writing adopted by the Egyptians not to be inserted here.

" Ἀυτίκα οἱ παρ' Αἰγυπτίοις παιδευόμενοι πρῶτον μὲν πάντων τὴν Αἰγυπτίων γραμμάτων με-
θοδον, ἐκμανθάνουσι, τὴν ΕΠΙΣΤΟΛΟΓΡΑΦΙΚΗΝ καλουμένεν' δεύτερον δὲ, τὴν ΙΕΡΑΤΙΚΗΝ, ἤ
χρῶνται οἱ ἱερογραμματεῖς· ὑστάτην δὲ καὶ τελευταίαν ΙΕΡΟΓΛΥΦΙΚΗΝ, ἧς ἡ μὲν ἐστι διὰ τῶν
πρώτων στοιχείων κυριολογικὴ, ἡ δὲ συμβολική. Τῆς δε συμβολικῆς ἡ μὲν κυριολογεῖται κατὰ
μίμησιν, ἡ δ' ὥσπερ τροπικῶς γράφεται, ἡ δὲ ἀντικρὸς ἀλληγορεῖται κατά τινας ἀινιγμους. Ἥλιον
γοῦν γράψαι βουλόμενοι κύκλον ποιοῦσι, σελένην δὲ σχῆμα μηνοειδὲς, κατὰ τὸ κυριολογούμενον
εἴδος. Τροπικῶς δὲ κατ' ὀικειότητα μετάγοντες καὶ μετατιθέντες, τὰ δ' εξαλλαττοντες, τὰ δὲ πολ-
λαχῶς μετασχηματίζοντες χαράττουσιν. Τοὺς γοῦν τῶν βασιλέων ἐπαίνους θεολογουμένοις
μύθοις παραδίδοντες, ἀναγράφουσι διὰ τῶν ἀναγλοφῶν. Τοῦ δὲ κατὰ τοὺς ἀινιγμοὺς τρίτου εἴδους

---

* Précis, p. 11.   † II. § 36.   ‡ III. § 3.

δεῖγμα ἔστω τόδε· τα μὲν γὰρ τῶν ἄλλων ἄσπρων, διὰ τὴν πορείαν τὴν λοξὴν ὄφεων σώμασι ἀπει καζον, τὸν δὲ "Ηλιον τῷ τοῦ κανθάρου," κ. τ. λ.

Clementis Alexand. Strom. V. 647.   Potter.

"Those who are educated among the Egyptians learn first of all the method of Egyptian writing called *epistolographic;* secondly, the *hieratic,* which the hierogrammatists employ ; and, lastly, the most complete kind, the *hieroglyphic,* of which one sort is kuriologic, by means of the first elements, and another sort is symbolic.   Of the symbolic, one represents objects properly by imitation ; another expresses them tropically ; the third, on the contrary, suggests them by means of certain allegorical enigmas. Thus, according to the method of representing the proper form of objects, the Egyptians make a circle when they wish to indicate the sun, and a luniform figure to denote the moon.   According to the tropical method they represent objects by means of certain agreements which they transfer into the expression of those objects, sometimes by modifications, most frequently by complete transformations—thus, when they transmit the praises of their kings in their theological fables, they describe them by means of anaglyphs.   Of the third kind of symbolical writing, which is enigmatical, let this serve as an example : they assimilate the oblique course of the other stars to the bodies of serpents, but that of the sun to the body of a scarabæus," &c.

Porphyry has also a passage much to the same effect.*   In " The Divine Legation of Moses demonstrated," the profound Bishop Warburton discussed with his great learning and consummate ability the different texts relative to the Egyptian modes of writing, distinguishing the several kinds of characters employed; and he ventured to draw a conclusion which has now received a complete verification, that the hieroglyphics or sacred characters were not so denominated as being employed solely for sacred purposes, but that they absolutely formed a real written language, applicable to the purposes of history and common life, as well as to those of religion and mythology.

The graphic system of the ancient Egyptians may be classed as follows:

* De Vit. Pythag, cap. 11, 12.

I. Hieroglyphic. II. Hieratic. III. Enchorial.

I. The Hieroglyphic is the sacred character, and is expressed either alphabetically, figuratively, or symbolically.

1. The alphabetical is what M. Champollion and some others have called the phonetic. These, like the letters of any other alphabet, may be combined so as to form words and express certain sounds corresponding to those in the vernacular language of Egypt, and they form the largest portion of the hieroglyphics.

2. The figurative represent the object meant literally to be expressed.

3. The symbolic expresses an idea by the representation of a physical object bearing a relation either near or remote, direct or indirect, to the idea intended to be expressed.

II. The Hieratic is the sacerdotal, descended from the hieroglyphic, and all the manuscripts in this character simply exhibit a tachygraphy of the hieroglyphical writing, and appear to have been employed only in the transcription of texts or inscriptions connected chiefly with sacred subjects.

III. The Enchorial or vulgar, the native character, is called also the demotic or popular, and the epistolographic. As the hieratic has descended, probably for the sake of despatch, from the hieroglyphic, so the enchorial has been derived from the hieratic, and a comparison of the different kinds will speedily convince any one of the correctness of this assertion. The enchorial admits alphabetic, figurative, and symbolic characters. The alphabetic are the most frequent in occurrence, the figurative the least employed; the symbolic are admitted to express ideas connected with the Egyptian theology.

With respect to the subjects of the papyri hitherto found, I have already mentioned* that M. Reuvens has discovered two of the bilingual MSS to relate one to chemistry, or rather alchemy, the other to the mysteries of the ancient Egyptians. Dr. Young, M. Champollion, and others, have also reported the contents of various papyri. Dr. Young has expressed an opinion† that there is little chance of our discovering any astronomical records of importance among the profusion of hieroglyphical literature which is still in existence, and he quotes from Herodotus, who tells us that

---

* p. 131. † Suppl. to Encyc. Brit. p. 51.

the Greeks derived their acquaintance with astronomy from the Babylonians, though they were supposed to have learned the elements of geometry from the Egyptians, and that it is well known that Ptolemy, the astronomer, who lived at Alexandria, and who must have had easy access, as well as Eratosthenes before him, to all the knowledge of the Egyptian priests, refers to no Egyptian observations, but employs the Babylonian records of eclipses which had happened a few centuries before his time—records which, as Pliny informs us, were preserved on a particular kind of bricks, the same perhaps that have been brought to Europe in our own times, as undeciphered specimens of the nail or arrow-headed character. Dr. Young adds that a degree of geometrical knowledge can scarcely be denied to a people who had made very considerable progress in sculpture and architecture at a time when all Europe was immersed in the profoundest barbarism, and who must necessarily have had frequent occasion for the employment of agragrian measurements. The Egyptians must also have been good practical chemists, so far at least as was required for the preparation of brilliant and diversified and durable pigments : and even their devotion to alchemy must have led them to make some little progress in experimental philosophy, although neither their manufacturers nor their magicians would have any right to boast of solid acquirements in genuine science. The same learned author has also told us* that there is scarcely any one of the inscriptions which we are not able to refer to the class either of sepulchral or votive— astronomical and chronological, he says, there seem to be none, since the numerical characters, which have been perfectly ascertained, have not yet been found to occur in such a form as they necessarily must have assumed in the records of this description. Of a historical nature he could only find the triumphal, which are often sufficiently distinguishable ; but they may also always be referred to the votive, since whoever related his own exploits thought it wisest to attribute the glory of them to some deity, and whoever recorded those of another was generally disposed to intermix divine honours with his panegyric.† The sepulchral inscriptions, in the

* P. 72.

† This cannot apply to the sculpture of the temples and public buildings in Egypt, since

U

opinion of Dr. Young, appear, on the whole, to constitute the most considerable part of the Egyptian literature which remains, and they afford us, upon a comparative examination, some very remarkable peculiarities. Their general tenour is, as might be expected from the testimony of Herodotus, the identification of the deceased with the god Osiris, and probably of a female, with Isis;* and the subject of the most usual representations seems to be the reception of this new personage by the principal deities, to whom he now stands in a relation expressed in the respective inscriptions Of this description I have already given examples, and shall, therefore, proceed to notice that which appears to me to be of by far the most frequent occurrence in the papyri found in mummies—namely, the great funeral ritual of which M. Champollion has given so particular an account.

This author says that anterior to the conquest of Egypt by the Persians it was the constant practice to place near an embalmed body a copy, more or less carefully prepared, of a work entitled DJOM-aN-ROOU-NA-HORT-heM-HROU-RE, i. e. *The Book of Gates concerning the manifestation to Light.* This consisted of a collection of formulæ relative to the embalming, the conveyence of the dead into the tombs, and a series of prayers addressed to all the divinities who were able to decide upon the lot of the soul whether in the Amenti where it was judged, or in the mystic regions it was doomed to inhabit before it should recommence the course of its

---

many of the subjects there relate to the conquests of the Pharaohs, and distinctly state the nations they conquered. We must certainly use the word historical in reference to those series of compartments that point out the order of march, the successive battles with the enemy, and the respective position of each nation; the triumphal are those where the offerings of thanks, and of the captives to the deity of the temple are introduced. That astronomical subjects are met with in some of the temples and tombs cannot be denied; nor would any one, after an inspection of the monuments in Egypt, allow that the most considerable part of Egyptian literature consists of sepulchral inscriptions.

* Men and women were both represented after death under the form and name of Osiris, but not of Isis. Osiris Mr. Wilkinson supposes to signify, in his character of judge, the lenity of the deity, and to this unity or original essence man returned after death, but man collectively, and no distinction of sex was maintained after the soul had quitted its material envelope.

transmigrations. A copy of this M. Champollion says is found either in the bandages or in the coffin of the most ancient mummies either in whole or in part—sometimes there will be found the first and second parts, in others the second and third, and in some the whole.

The more modern the mummy, the more rare the MSS., and the more careless the execution of them. A tomb in the necropolis of Thebes contained the bodies of an ancient Græco-Egyptian family of rank. One of the members, Soter, son of Cornelius Pollius Soter, filled the office of archonte, i. e. *the chief magistrate of the city of Thebes.* The Royal Museum of the Louvre possesses the MSS. drawn from this tomb ; the leaves are of small dimensions : M. Champollion has given an account of them.*

I shall now refer to the MS. which was found in the mummy, the rich case of which I have already spoken of.† It appears that the MS. belonging to this mummy contained invocations addressed to the principal forms of the sun, the chief of the visible gods ; then to Osiris, the king of the souls and of the dead, and then to the ministers and gods of his family. " Grand est le Dieu RE par ses diadèmes (ou dominations)! Grand est Atmou par ses productions ! Grand est OSIRIS-Pethempamentes (l'habitant de l'Occident) par son sceptre (gherov) de Pas-sou-Re ! soyez lui propices, ô vous qui gardez les portes de la contrée occidentale, vous, les deux gardiens des mères divines de la demeure de Siou, vous, gardiens des portes de la demeure divine où sont les lotus, l'eau et la bari divine ; sois-lui propice, toi, Anubis, fils d'Osiris, gardien des gardiens des portes des deux divins générateurs de la demeure de Siou ; soyez-lui favorables, vous, dieux des régions de Matos, assistans d'OSIRIS, assistans de la demeure de Oskh (la demeure de la moisson), des dieux divines Vérités dans les champs de Oen-RO ; sois-lui favorable, déesse HATHOR, qui es la déesse NEITH dans la contrée orientale, et la déesse SME dans les lotus et les eaux . . . . de la contrée occidentale ; soyez-lui propices vous, dieux de la demeure de Siou, votre domaine ; soyez-lui propices, dieux qui veillez auprès d'OSIRIS ! Il est grand votre père le SOLEIL ! L'épervier du monde (l'esprit actif du monde) qui vous a manifestés avec lui dans les demeures

* Voyage à Meroé, par M. Cailliaud, tom. IV. p. 25, et seq.   † p. 117.

de Sop ! Grand est HORUS, le fils d'ISIS, le fils d'OSIRIS, qui est sur .... sa demeure à toujours ! Grand est HAR-OERI, seigneur des esprits solaires, l'œil bienfaisant du soleil," &c. &c. There are, however, MSS. more complete than this, and they present eight forms of invocation addressed to the god Thoth, under the name of the god A, to recommend the soul of Petaménoph to the divinities of the eight regions over which this god presides.

M. Champollion gives a very curious account of a MS., from the contents of which it appears that the different parts or members of the body were supposed to be under the influence of particular deities. This is extracted from a Great Funeral Ritual, or Book of the Manifestations, and by a careful collation of MSS. M. Champollion has been able to form a kind of table of theological anatomy. It is too curious to be omitted here :—

The hair belongs to Pemoou (the celestial Nile, the god of the primordial waters, and the father of the gods).

The head to Phrè (the Sun).

The eyes to Hathor (Venus).

The ears to Macedo (god with the head of the jackal, guardian of the Tropics).

The left temple to the living spirit in the Sun.

The right temple to the spirit of Atmou in the dwelling of Siou.

The nose and lips to Anubis, in the dwelling of Sakhem.

The teeth to the goddess Selk.

The beard to Macedo.

The neck to Isis.

The arms to Osiris.

The knees to Neith.

The elbows to the god of the region of Ghel or Gher.

The back to Sischo.

The genitals to Osiris and the goddess Koht (Leontocéphale of Memphis).

The thighs to Bal-hor (the eye of Horus).

The legs to the goddess Netphe (the Egyptian Rhæa).

The feet to Phtha.

The fingers to Uræus.

The Museum of Egyptian Antiquities, attached to the University of Leyden, is said to be one of the most valuable and interesting in Europe. It is formed of the celebrated Anastasy* collection, which was purchased by the Netherlands' government in 1828; of the private collections of M. de l'Escluze, a merchant of Bruges, and of Signora Cimba of Leghorn. To these have been added a great number of specimens either by donation or purchase, forming altogether a very extensive and important museum. In Græco-Egyptian MSS. it is said to be the richest of any known. There are 147 papyri, fifteen of which are purely Egyptian, and in the highest state of preservation. Twenty-three are in Greek, and three bilingual. Professor Reuvens, whose attainments in Egyptian archæology are very considerable, has devoted his particular attention to the illustration of two of the bilingual MSS.,† and has added much to the knowledge already possessed upon the subject. Of the labours of Professor Reuvens it has been justly observed that " by a happy concentration of numerous scattered rays, scarcely discernible by an ordinary eye, he has succeeded in throwing a powerful and steady light on several points which were previously involved in mystery and darkness, and particularly in detecting the real source of those theosophistical extravagances which, engrafted on Christianity, constituted the Gnosticism of the first ages of the church.‡ The writer of the article from which the preceding quotation is taken justly laments that Professor Reuvens has neglected or rather omitted to improve and extend the enchorial alphabet and vocabulary, and to add to our knowledge of the demotic characters and groups. It appears that the MS., numbered sixty-five in the collection, is, for the most part, in the hieratic character, but contains interlinear transcriptions in Greek letters of Egyptian words, according to the demotic form of writing. Towards the end of the MS. there are several demotic transcriptions of words in hieratic, and in the body of the text numerous demotic letters mixed with the hieratic, and isolated

---

* The Chevalier Anastasy was Swedish Vice-Consul at Alexandria.

† Lettres à M. Letronne sur les Papyrus Bilingues et Grecs, et sur quelques autres Monumens Græco-Egyptiens du Musée d'Antiquités de l'Université de Leïde, 4to. Avec un Atlas en folio. à Leïde, 1830.   ‡ Edinb. Rev. June, 1831, p. 372.

words in demotic in some few instances containing hieratic letters. Perhaps in no MS. has this mixture of characters been so extensively employed, and it is, therefore, to be hoped that the Professor will turn his attention more especially to this matter, the improvement of which is so much to be desired, and upon which Egyptian scholars are so anxious for further information.

Mons. Sallier, of Aix, is reported by M. Champollion* to be in possession of a papyrus the subject of which is not funereal. It is said to be in a bad state, but written in a fine hieratic character, and relates to astrology. M. Sallier has also two rolls containing a kind of ode or litany in praise of one of the Pharaohs, and another roll (which is imperfect) but which contains a laudatory account of the exploits of Rameses the Great, in the form of a dialogue between the gods and the king. There is a date attached to the MS.:—" L'an IX au mois de Paôni," of the reign of this monarch.

George Francis Grey, Esq., of University College, Oxford, put into the possession of Dr. Young a box containing several specimens of writing and drawing on papyrus. They were chiefly in hieroglyphics and of a mythological nature, but two of them to which the Doctor's attention was particularly directed contained some Greek characters written apparently in a pretty legible hand. These had been purchased of an Arab at Thebes in January 1820. They are lithographed in the collection of hieroglyphics published by the Egyptian Society. The contents of one of these MS. are very remarkable, and as they relate to the sale of a portion of the collections and offerings made from time to time on account, or for the benefit, of a certain number of mummies of persons described at length, in very bad Greek, with their children and all their households, it will, I conceive, not be out of place here to transcribe the translation. I must premise, however, that the price is not very clearly expressed; but as the portion sold is only a moiety of a third part of the whole, and as the testimony of sixteen witnesses was thought necessary on the occasion, it is probable that the revenue thus obtained by the priests was by no means inconsiderable.†

* Lettres écrites d'Egypte et de Nubie en 1828 et 1829.
† Young's Discoveries in Hieroglyphical Literature, p. 60.

Dr. Young's Translation of Mr. Grey's Greek Autograph.

Copy of an Egyptian Writing respecting the Dead Bodies in Thyn. having been ratif . . . .

" In the xxxvith year ; Athyr 20, after the usual preamble, this writing witnesses : that the dresser among the servants of the great goddess (Isis ?) Onnophris, the son of Horus, and of Senpoeris (aged about) forty, lively, tall, of a sallow complexion, hollow-eyed, and bald, has ceded voluntarily for the price of . . . . to Horus, the son of Horus and Senpoeris, one moiety of the third part of the collection for the dead lying in Thynabunun, on the Libyan side of the Theban suburb, in the Memnonia: likewise one moiety of the third part of the services or liturgies and so forth : their names being Muthes the son of Spotus, with his children and all his household ; Chapocrates, the son of Nechthmonthes, with his children and all ; Arsiesis, the son of Nechthmonthes ; likewise Petemestus, the son of Nechthmonthes ; likewise Arsiesis, the son of Zminis ; likewise Osoroeris, the son of (Horus) ; likewise Spotus, the son of Chapochonsis ; likewise Zoglyphus : from which there belongs to Asos, the son of Horus and of Senpoeris 'thy' younger brother, one of (or, the younger brother of) the same dressers ? a moiety of the aforesaid third part of the services and fruits, and so forth. He has sold it to him in the year xxxvi ; twenty Athyr, in the reign of the everlasting king, for the completion of the third part. Also a moiety of the fruits and so forth of the other dead bodies in Thy. that is to say, Pateutemis with his children and all ; and a moiety of the fruits belonging to me from the property of Petechonsis the milk bearer, and from a place on the Asiatic side, called Phrecages, with the dead bodies in it ; of which a moiety belongs to the same Asos : all these things I have sold to him. They are thine, and I have received their price from thee, and I make no demand upon thee for them from this day : and if any person disturb thee in the possession of them, I will withstand the attempt, and if I do not (otherwise) repel it, I will use compulsory means. Written by Horus the son of Phabis, the writer of the (priests) of Amonrasonther, and the other gods of the temple. Witnesses : Erieus the son of Phanres. Peteartres, the son of Pateutemis. Petearpo-

crates, the son of (Horus). Snachomneus, the son of Peteuris. Snacho-
mes, the son of Psenchonsis. Totoes, the son of Phibis. Portis, the son of
Apollonius. Zminis, the son of Petemestus. Peteutemis, the son of Arsiesis. Amonorytius, the son of Pacemis. Horus, the son of Chimnaraus.
Armenis, the son of Zthenaetis. Maësis, the son of Mirsis. Antimachus,
the son of Antigines. Petophois, the son of Phibis. Panas, the son of
Petosiris. Witnesses sixteen.

Copy of the Registry. In the year xxxvi; the ninth of Choeak (iv).
Transacted at the table in Diospolis, at which Lysimachus is the President
of the twentieth department; in the account of Asclepiades and Zminis,
farmers of the tax, in which the subscribing clerk is Ptolemaeus; the purchaser Horus, the son of Horus the dresser? a part of the sum collected by
them on account of the dead bodies lying in Thynabunun, in the Memno-
nian tombs of the Libyan suburb of Thebes, for the services which are
performed. Bought of Onnophris the son of Horus, pieces of brass 400.
Z... The end.

Lysimach. subscribes.

The Royal Museum of Turin is rich in papyri obtained from M. Dro-
vetti's collection. M. Champollion examined them, and described them as
remarkable for their beauty, their size, their whiteness, and their perfect
state of preservation. Nearly the whole of these are written in hieroglyphics, adorned with designs, and are only extracts, more or less extensive,
of the grand funerary ritual: they have all been taken from mummies,
which perhaps accounts for their uniformity. The length of one of these
exceeds perhaps that of any other known MS. on papyrus. The one in
the king's cabinet, described in the great French work on Egypt, and
which was taken from between the thighs of a mummy in a cave in the
interior of the mountain behind the Memnonium temple on the plain of
Thebes, is exceedingly voluminous, and measured I believe twenty-two feet
in length.* This was regarded as the complete funeral ritual of which
other funerary manuscripts, hieroglyphic or hieratic, contained portions
either longer or shorter, according to the rank of the person for whom they

---

* It is figured in vol. II. Antiquités, pl. 61. to 65. Description de l'Egypte.

were made. M. Champollion had, however, remarked that the designs on the beautiful mummy cases, which presented scenes and texts so analogous to those of the funerary ritual, likewise afforded some which were not to be found in the great MS. of the king. He therefore supposed that there existed a still more extensive copy of this ritual, a conjecture which has been confirmed by one of the papyri at Turin, which is also the funerary ritual, and measures nearly sixty feet in length. In this MS. M. Champollion has discovered some very curious scenes, as well as the method of classing strictly in their order the various extracts from this ritual, which the other funerary papyri contain.

At Turin M. Champollion applied himself to the most beautiful MSS., and those in best preservation. He put aside about twenty parcels of papyri, blackened and corroded by time, doubled square, of different sizes, without designs, each enveloped in a piece of cloth. Fatigued by the perpetual recurrence of the funerary ritual, which the best preserved and most beautiful papyri presented to him, he cast his eye upon one of the rejected packets, and found that it was written in hieratic, and the first line disclosed to him the name and the prenomen of the great Sesostris! He saw this repeated eight or ten times in the MS. Connecting together no fewer than fifty fragments, which composed this MS., he was convinced that it contained either a portion of history or a public act of the reign of Sesostris. Another MS., which upon bringing the fragments together he found to form a sheet of more than two feet, M. Champollion ascertained to be the plan of a royal catacomb. The design, he says, is very fairly done, and some improvements have evidently been made of a very pale colour, as if done with a black-lead pencil. The catacomb is that of king Ramses-Meïamoun, who built the magnificent palace of Medinet-Abou, of which fact these are the proofs. The commission of Egypt has drawn plans of many tombs, and one of those published corresponds exactly with that on this papyrus: it is the fifth of Biban-el-Molouk, westward of Thebes, and the basso-relievos on this tomb discover very frequently the name of Ramses-Meïamoun. The great hall in the plan, upon the papyrus, represents a bird's-eye view of a sarcophagus in rose granite; the lid is ornamented with three personages with different attributes, and it is moreover precisely of the form, in every particular, of the lid, also in rose granite,

x

taken from this same tomb to the west, brought away by Belzoni, and presented to the University of Cambridge, which bears the name and prenomen of Ramses-Meïamoun. The correspondence of the plan on the papyrus, M. Champollion justly observes, suggests some observations not destitute of interest. It is remarkable that the contours of the mountain shown upon the two plans agree perfectly, and that every corridor, every chamber, of the plan upon the papyrus bears an hieratic inscription, succeeded by cyphers, giving very varied numbers. These are doubtless the dimensions of each part of the royal excavation; and, the commission having given these very details in *metres*, we have thus a new element of the great question respecting Egyptian measures.

One other papyrus of this collection, regarded by M. Champollion as *unique*, must be noticed. He considers it to be a genuine *chronological picture, a royal canon*, the form of which reminded him of that of Manetho, and the fragments of which, when joined together, furnished him with a list of more than 100 kings. Here, then, is an invaluable supplement to the celebrated genealogical table of Abydus, as well as a motive to redouble our zeal in the search for Egyptian papyri: a subject of great hope, if this search be encouraged by Government and the approbation of the friends of letters.

CHAPTER XI.

___

ON THE PHYSICAL HISTORY OF THE EGYPTIANS.

Varieties of complexion and figure among mankind—difficulty of the subject—present natives of Egypt descended either from the Arabs or the Copts—Egyptian physiognomy—opinion of Jomard—no trace of Negro descent—opinion of Volney—Browne—resemblance of the modern Copts to the ancient mummies, paintings, and statues—the Barâbras—opinions of Legh—Prichard—Madden—measurement of the heads of mummies, Copts, and Nubians— opinion of Larrey—Blumenbach's arrangement of the varieties in the national physiognomy of the Egyptians—configuration of the skull—methods adopted by Camper, Blumenbach, and Cuvier, to determine the diversities—description of the skulls of mummies—peculiarity in the formation of the teeth—hair of mummies—stature of the ancient Egyptians—circum- cision practised by the Egyptians.

WITHIN the whole range of objects embraced by natural history, there is no one capable of exciting an interest superior or even equal to that which results from a consideration of the variety, both of form and complexion, among mankind. Deeply interesting as this enquiry must be, and im- portant in the highest degree as it certainly is in the physical history of man, it is remarkable that little of any value has, until very recently, been elicited on the subject. The errors and falsehoods which abound in the earlier writers have been dissipated by the laborious researches and accurate information of later naturalists, who have much enriched our store of knowledge in this department. It is not my intention, and it would be foreign to the purpose of the present work, to enter into a consideration of the causes which have been assigned for the varieties of complexion and figure observable in the human species. The difficulties attendant upon such an enquiry have been attempted to be solved by numerous hypotheses, forming subjects of curious speculation. The natural history of our species is now daily receiving additional elucidation ; but sufficient information has hardly yet been obtained to form a regular and systematical view of the subject. Much has already been accomplished, but more remains to be done, and it will only be achieved by a diligent and laborious examination of all the circumstances connected with this interesting and important enquiry.

The present natives of Egypt are considered to be either the descendants of the Arabs, who overran the valley of the Nile in the early part of the seventh century, or of the Copts, who are regarded by some as the only remains of the genuine Egyptian race. Various opinions have prevailed, and still continue to prevail, as to the primeval race of the Egyptians. By some they have been regarded as of the Negro race, by others as having relation to the Chinese, and some have considered them as allied to the Copts of Cairo. The character of the physiognomy of the Egyptian race is distinctly preserved in the mummies. These, according to Jomard,* resemble neither the Copts, Chinese, nor Negro. The Arabs and the inhabitants of Upper Egypt present more resemblance to the mummies and the ancient sculptures than any beside. This has been particularly observed by the author I have just referred to, and it has been confirmed by the opinions of several of his fellow-travellers:—" Plus nous avons cherché à la vérifier," says he, " plus l'experience l'a confirmée." The Negro frequently appears as a captive in the sculptured figures of the Egyptian tombs : his sable complexion, flat lips, and woolly hair, are well delineated. The character most commonly represented is of a race very different in appearance, and distinguished by a sharp countenance, a swarthy complexion, the hair curled, but not woolly. It has been remarked† that in the more ancient, as well as the modern sculptures, the leading figures, the heroes of the design, are almost invariably the furthest removed from the Negro expression of countenance, and that they sometimes approach to that character to which we are accustomed to assign the praise of manly beauty. The paintings are said to confirm this view; the pure and uncompounded colours used by the Egyptian artists enabling them to distinguish, if not nicely, yet with sufficient clearness, between the different races which they represent. The still more unexceptionable testimony of the mummies is equally strong.

* Descr. des Hypogées, p. 28.   † Quarterly Rev. No. 85, p. 130.

Those of the upper orders reveal the almost living lineaments of a people, tawny, not black, with long and sometimes lank hair, and with features which bear no trace of Negro descent.

The celebrated Volney has endeavoured to prove that the original inhabitants of Egypt were Negroes, and that, accordingly, the world is indebted to that sable race for all the arts and sciences which are generally considered as having been transmitted to us by the ancient Egyptians, and for the erection of those stupendous and magnificent monuments the remains of which have so strongly excited the admiration of all ages. The testimony of Herodotus* is rather in favour of this opinion, μελάγχροές καὶ ουλότριχες, " black in complexion, and woolly headed." Mr. Browne† thinks this may apply to the greater or less degree of blackness and crispature of the Egyptians as compared with the Greeks to whom the author was addressing himself, and he corroborates this interpretation of the passage of Herodotus by a reference to a similar one from Ammianus Marcellinus‡ in which that author says that the Egyptians are *Atrati*, a term of equally strong import wrth the μελάγχροες of Herodotus, but, like it, evidently applied in a comparative sense; for, in the very next sentence, he says, *erubescunt*, they blush, or grow red. It is true, indeed, as Mr. Browne says, that Negroes suffer a certain change of countenance when affected with the sentiment of shame, but it would be rather a bold assertion that the word *erubescere* can ever be applied to characterize the effect of that feeling on a Negro. It may also be urged as a strong evidence against this that ancient writers preserve a complete silence as to the Negro character of the Egyptians. In this absence of historical testimony, therefore, we are compelled to recur to the sculptured figures found on the ruins of the temples and tombs, and these, as I have already noticed, are in opposition to such an opinion. The small statues of Isis and other deities in which the hair is frequently represented of length, goes also very far towards contradicting it. It might be supposed that the appearance of the mummies would place this matter beyond doubt, but the mode of embalming, and the substances employed in the operation, tend much to obscure the matter, and it is not possible, in my opinion, to draw any satisfactory conclusion as to the precise colour of

* Lib. ii.   † Travels, p. 163.   ‡ Lib. xxii.

the skin of the ancient Egyptians from those preserved specimens of the race.

The present Copts are by M. Niebuhr, Mr. Browne, and others, supposed to be the genuine descendants of the ancient Egyptians, and to preserve the family likeness in their dusky brown complexion, their dark eyes and hair, often curled, their lips sometimes thick, but the nose as often aquiline, and other marks of a total dissimilitude between them and the Negro race. Mr. Browne particularly remarked* the resemblance between the modern Copts and the ancient mummies, paintings, and statues. Mr. Legh† bears his testimony to the similarity of the visage and appearance of the modern Copts to the paintings found in the tombs of Thebes. He remarks, however, that the inhabitants of the island of Elephantine are nearly black, whereas the Barâbras, who live so much further to the south, are considerably fairer in their complexions. But, notwithstanding their colour, the females of Elephantine are conspicuous for their elegant shapes, and are, upon the whole, the finest women he saw in Upper Egypt. The appearance of blacks at Elephantine is certainly curious, and Mr. Legh thinks may, perhaps, be explained by the removal of a tribe of Negroes from the west, and the settlement of a colony in this neighbourhood. Dr. Prichard has arrived at nearly a similar conclusion. In a letter with which he has favoured me, he says that, after examining all the evidence that he could collect, he drew the inference that the Egyptians were a people " rather resembling the Berberins or Barâbras of the Upper Nile, who are a red or copper-coloured race, with hair not woolly, than like the Negroes."

Mr. Madden‡ believes the ancient Egyptians to have had swarthy complexions and wiry hair, not like the negroes, but like the modern Nubians. He bestowed some pains in the examination of a great number of the heads of mummies to ascertain this point, and he has given a comparative table of the measurements of the heads of twelve mummies divested of their integuments, of twelve living Copts divested of their hair, and of twelve living Nubians divested also of their hair: from these observations he concludes that there is no affinity between the head of the Egyptian mummy

---

* Travels, p. 72.　　† Ibid. p. 104.　　‡ Ibid. II. 89.　　§ Ibid. II. 95.

and that of the Copt, and he tells us that the great distinction between the mummy and Copt, in a line drawn right across the orbits, from one external angle of the eye to that of the other, is in the greater space of the Copt across the eyes, in every skull that he measured, the line across the orbits of the Copt being half an inch longer than in the same line of the mummy In this respect, likewise, the Nubian skull differed nothing from the latter. He describes the old Egyptian skull as extremely narrow across the forehead, and of an oblong shape anteriorly. He supposes he must have seen several thousands of mummy heads; but he says he never found one with a broad expanded forehead. It is among the Nubians, Mr. Madden thinks, we are to search for the true descendants of the Egyptians; a swarthy race, with wiry hair, surpassing, in the beauty of their slender forms, all the people of the East; living on the confines of Egypt, where probably their ancestors had been driven by the Persians; and possessing a dialect some-what mixed with Arabic, but which he observed no Arab understood.*

In examining the paintings which still retain so much freshness in the temples at Philæ, Mr. Madden was more struck here than elsewhere by the different complexions given to the two sexes in their pictures; the males were always painted red, and the females yellow. "The few colours," says Mr. Madden, "known to the Egyptians, enabled them to approach no nearer to the real complexions of their race. If a painter had now only the use of the primitive colours, he would find that red would be the nearest approach to the swarthy complexion of the male Nubian, and yellow to the female, whose tint is so much lighter from the less exposure to the sun.† But what struck me as the greatest proof I met with in Nubia of the identity of the Nubian race and that of the Egyptian is the strong resemblance of the former to the features of all the Egyptian statues. The length of the eye, and the peculiar softness of the mouth, are the two distinguishing characteristics of Egyptian physiognomy, such as their sculpture has transmitted; and these are the very points which are most remarkable in the Nubian countenance. One must have seen the people of Nubia to

* Travels II. 95.

† In confirmation of this I may state that the painted *cartonage* of male mummies have the face invariably of a red colour, whilst that of the female is yellow.

understand how beautiful is that elongation of the eye which is peculiar to them and to the Egyptian figures."*

Baron Larrey considers the Copts to be the true descendants of the ancient Egyptians. He collected a number of the skulls of this people, and compared them with those of the Abyssinians and Ethiopians, and found them to differ very little from each other. He describes the Abyssinian in the following terms : " L'Abyssin a les yeux grands, d'un regard agréable, et l'angle interne en est incliné chez lui ; les pommettes sont plus saillantes ; les joues forment, avec les angles prononcés de la mâchoire et de la bouche, un triangle plus régulier ; les lèvres sont épaisses sans être renversées, comme chez les nègres, et, ainsi que je l'ai déjà dit, les dents sont belles et moins avancées ; les arcades alvéolaires sont moins étendues ; enfin, le teinte des Abyssins est cuivré."†

Professor Blumenbach conceives that we must adopt at least three principal varieties in the national physiognomy of the ancient Egyptians: 1. The Ethiopian cast; 2. The one approaching to the Hindoo; 3. The mixed, partaking, in a manner, of both the former. The *first*, he says, is chiefly distinguished by the prominent maxillæ, turgid lips, broad flat nose, and protruding eyeballs, such as Volney finds the modern Copts ; such, according to his description and the best figures given by Norden, is the countenance of the Sphinx ; such were, according to the well-known passage of Herodotus on the origin of the Colchians, even the Egyptians of his time ; and thus hath Lucian likewise represented a young Egyptian at Rome.

The *second*, or Hindoo cast, is characterized by a long slender nose, long and thin eyelids, which run upwards from the top of the nose towards the temples, ears placed high on the head, a short and very thin bodily structure, and very long shanks. As an *ideal* of this form Professor Blumenbach adduces the painted female figure upon the back of the sarcophagus of Captain Lethieullier's mummy in the British Museum, and which, he thinks, most strikingly agrees with the unequivocal national form of the Hindoos, which is so often to be seen upon Indian paintings.

The *third* sort of Egyptian configuration, he says, is not similar to either

* Travels II. 117.   † Notice sur la Conformation Physique des Egyptiens, p. 3.

of the preceding ones, but seems to partake something of both, which must have been owing to the modifications produced by local circumstances in a foreign climate. This is characterized by a peculiar turgid habit, flabby cheeks, a short chin, large prominent eyes, and rather a plump make in the person. This is the structure most frequently to be met with.*

The configuration of the skull offers the most important diversities in the human form, and the attention of Professor Camper, Professor Blumenbach, and the Baron Cuvier, has been principally directed to this point. Each of these eminent naturalists and physiologists has proposed various methods to arrive at a precise knowledge of the different appearances, and adopted peculiar modes of classifying them, and reducing them to general principles. Anatomists cannot fail to observe the great variety which exists in crania belonging to different nations; and although these are sufficiently constant to mark the national peculiarities of the class to which they belong, yet so gradual are the changes or shades leading to this variety to be traced, that it is with much difficulty they are rendered perceptible.

As the most remarkable difference in the heads of man and other animals is principally observable in the relative proportions of skull and face, it has been proposed to ascertain the nature and extent of these by the application of what is called the *facial line*. Professor Camper was, I believe, the first to adopt this method, and his plan consisted in drawing a line from the most prominent part of the forehead to the most projecting part of the upper jaw : this he called the facial line. Another being drawn from this latter point in a horizontal direction, and extended to the opening of the external ear, enabled him readily to take the angle formed by the two lines, and thus he endeavoured to determine the degree of intellectual character of the individual, by marking the relative proportion between that part of the skull in which the brain is contained and that of the face, which is known to be the principal seat of the organs of sense. He thus considered the form of the skull principally with reference to the varieties of expression imparted to the countenance by the diversity of its configura-

* Philos. Trans. 1794, p. 191.

Y

tion, and to the supposed connexion of this formation with the character of the mind.

That the mode proposed by Camper will, to a certain degree, point out the general character of animals, and manifest the extent of docility or instinct possessed by them, is unquestionably true, and founded upon anatomical and physiological knowledge; for Professor Seommering has long since very satisfactorily shown* that in proportion to the size of the brain exceeding that of the rest of the nervous system, do animals approach in a greater or less degree to what we term reason. The face is the chief seat of the organs of sense, as the cavity of the skull is of intellect, and the devolopement of each is correspondent to the character of the animal. Man has by far the largest skull, properly so called, and the smallest face; and, in proportion as other animals deviate from this condition, do they also manifest their stupidity and ferocity. But the facial angle is insufficient to exhibit the characteristics of the skulls of different nations; it is chiefly applicable where varieties in the form or prominence of the jaws are most remarkable, and it has been justly remarked that crania of the most different nations, which differ *toto cœlo* from each other on the whole, have the same facial line, and, on the contrary, that skulls of the same nation, which agree in general character, differ very much in the direction of this line.† Reference to the Decades Craniorum of Professor Blumenbach will abundantly prove this position.

The facial angle of man varies from 65° to 85°.‡ In the representation of their deities and heroes, the masters of Grecian art carried this angle to 100°, and every one must have been struck with the high and elevated character of their ancient statues. This practice is, therefore, in strict accordance with the principle of Camper. The facial angle, however, will only give us the dimensions of the skull in one direction; and should its capacity vary essentially, either posteriorly or laterally, we acquire no in-

* Diss. Inaug. de Basi Encephali et Originibus Nervorum Cranio egredentium, 4to. Gott. 1778. Vide lib. v.

† Lawrence's Lectures on Physiology, Zoology, &c. p. 333.

‡ Dr. Granville gives the facial angle of his mummy at 80°. M. Jomard states it to be from 75° to 78° in those he examined in Egypt.

formation of this condition by the method of Camper. Baron Cuvier felt this deficiency, and endeavoured to supply it by proposing two sections of the skull and face, one vertical and the other longitudinal. By these means we are enabled to ascertain with precision the relative proportions of the skull compared with those of the face: thus the extent of the intellectual and sensitive structures become apparent.* Professor Blumenbach felt also strongly the difficulty of adopting any one mode by which the variety of appearances in the conformation of the skull could be shown, and he was induced to employ a method different from either that of Camper or Cuvier, and by which he conceived that, at one glance, he could distinguish the greater number of distinctive marks of the skulls of different individuals and nations. This method is also founded upon the comparative magnitude of the jaws, thus based upon the relative proportions of skull and face. His method was to place various skulls upon a table in a row, and contemplate them from behind. By this means he obtained a good knowledge of the breadth or narrowness of the skull, and according as the face projected or receded he obtained a view of its relative magnitude or diminutiveness. This is, I think, the best method that has been adopted.

Blumenbach classes the heads of the Egyptian mummies in his first grand division—the Caucasian variety, a class which, as Mr. Lawrence has said, "includes all the human races in which the intellectual endowments of man have shone forth in the greatest native vigour, have received the highest cultivation, and have produced the richest and most abundant fruits in philosophy, science, and art, in religion and morals, in poetry, eloquence, and the fine arts, in civilization and government, in all that can dignify and ennoble the species."†

The assertion of Volney, that the ancient Egyptians were Negroes, is not supported by the examination of the mummies. The heads of mummies are, however, far from displaying a uniformity of appearance, and the situation of Egypt has been observed to favour the notion of a mixed population,

---

* The proportions thus obtained are curious and worthy the attention of the reader; they may be found in the Leçons d'Anatomie Comparée of M. Cuvier.

† Lectures, p. 338.

emanating at various times from different quarters of Africa, Asia, and Europe. The communication with Arabia and India by the Red Sea, and with Africa from the south and west, may account for some of the varieties afforded among mummies, and in the representations of the painter and sculptor. No distinctly or unequivocally Negro skull has, I believe, been found among the mummies; the one most approaching to that character by the projection of the jaws and the reclining forehead was in the mummy of Mr. Saunders, now in my possession; but this differs in many respects from the skull of the Negro.

Blumenbach has figured three skulls from mummies in his Decades Craniorum, Nos. 1, 31, and 52. No. 1 represents the head of an Egyptian mummy purchased of a Dantzic merchant in 1779. The skull is compressed at the sides, chiefly towards the top. The forehead is small, but rather elegantly arched. The eyebrows are very prominent and the orbits large. The cheek bones appear large from the malar fossæ being much sunk. The lower jaw is large and strong; the crowns of the incisor teeth are described as thick, cylindrical, or obtusely conical, rather than lancet-shaped. "Coronæ crassæ, cylindricæ magis aut obtuse conicæ quam scalpriformes."* The hinder part of the head projected greatly. The Professor sums up his description by declaring the skull to possess the same character as that which the great works of ancient Egyptian art aspire to. " In universum hujus cranii habitus eundem characterem præ se ferre videtur quem et ingentia Egyptiacæ artis veteris opera spirant, non quidem elegantem et pulchellum est magnum."

No. 31 is the skull of a male, and is less compressed at the sides than the preceding, and the cheek bones are a little narrower, and the eyebrows not so prominent. The same appearances of the teeth presented themselves in this as in the former skull. The incisors in each jaw, but particularly the upper one, were not wedged like lancets, bent on the inside, and terminating in a transverse point, as is the case with teeth destined by nature for cutting or dividing the food; but thick, obtuse, and towards the outermost rim obliquely truncated on its broad face.† Professor Autenrieth, of Tubingen,

* Decas I. p. 13.

† " Quam vero alias jam ex professo tetigi mirandam et vere anomalam dentium incisivorum

presented to Professor Blumenbach an impression from a copper-plate en_
graving representing the jaws of a mummy, the teeth of which so perfectly
corresponded with those above described that, Professor Blumenbach says,
you would imagine they had been drawn from those belonging to his skull.
I have observed the same description of teeth in three heads of mummies.
The same has been remarked by Dr. Middleton in the Cambridge mummy; †
by Bruckmann at Cassel,‡ and something similar by Storr, in a mummy
preserved at Stuttgard.§ This appearance of the teeth, however, is not
found in other specimens. Professor Blumenbach could not observe it in
the Gottingen mummy, nor in two that he examined at the British Museum;
but he found this peculiar structure in the mummy of a child about six
years old, belonging to John Symmons, esq.

Of No. 52 no description is given, and I lament this the more as the
skull simply noticed as " Mumiæ Ægyptiacæ Tertiæ" differs from the two
already noticed, and corresponds to that of my Græco-Egyptian mummy.
A front view only is given : there is no lower jaw, and the incisor teeth are
wanting.

Professor Soemmering has also described three heads of mummies. In
one of these he notices a larger space marked out for the temporal muscle ;
but in no other respect does it appear to partake of the Negro character.
The other two are distinctly mentioned as not differing from the European
formation. ‖ I can state the same of the greater number of skulls in my
own collection, or that I have been able to examine elsewhere. Baron
Cuvier examined more than fifty heads of mummies, and he says that not
one of them presented the characters of the Negro or Hottentot.¶ I have

conformationem, in tot jam mumiis (ex eorum nempe numero quæ bitumine vere obduratæ,
non vero mollibus tantum fasciis byssinis laxius obvolutæ sunt) observatam, etiam in hoc
egregio specimine luculentissime cernere licet. Sunt enim utriusque maxillæ, præsertim vero
superioris incisores, si modo incisores eos appellare licet, non scalprorum in modum cuneati,
intrinsecus sinuati et in transversam desinentes actem, ut dentibus ad secandum a natura pa-
ratis, convenit, sed mirum in modum crassi, obtusi et versus extimum marginem latiori facie
oblique truncati."—*Decas* V. p. 5.

† Miscell. Works, IV. 170.   ‡ Account of this Mummy, Brunswick, 1782, 4to.
§ Prodromus Methodi Mammalium, Tubing. 1780, 4to.
‖ De Corp. Human. Fab. I. 70.   ¶ Mémoires du Museum d'Hist. Nat. III. 173.

seven heads of Egyptian mummies in my collection, and with the exception of one specimen, that of the mummy of T. Saunders, esq., there is not the slightest approximation to the Negro character.

Herodotus has stated the skull of the Egyptian to be remarkably thick. This observation has not been confirmed by any other writer, and it is denied by many. I have seen the skull exceedingly thin, although the individual to whom it belonged had not attained an advanced age.

The hair of the mummies, as has already been noticed in the chapter on embalming, varies much in its character. In some instances it is long and smooth ; this was the case with the mummy described by Denon, in another by Belzoni, and is also noticed in the large French work on Egypt. Mr. Wilkinson brought me three heads from Thebes, and one of these exhibited a profusion of dark brown hair upwards of a foot in length, and at the back part was plaited in three distinct portions, exactly as it is done in this country and in Egypt by the females at the present day. In my Græco-Egyptian mummy and in Dr. Lee's mummy the hair was very short and smooth ; in Mr. Saunders's mummy it was short and curled. The head of Horseisi, as is the case with all the priests, was shaven close. It is difficult to say any thing precise with respect to the general colour, which appears frequently to be affected by the process of embalming : in the greater number of instances it has obtained a reddish hue, but I have frequently seen it quite black and occasionally grey.

The stature of the ancient Egyptians would, from the measurements I have taken and collected of different mummies, appear to have been somewhat diminutive. In no instance have I been able to meet with a mummy that even enveloped in its bandages would measure more than five feet six inches. The following collection will demonstrate this subject :—

1. *Male Mummies in their Bandages.*

	Feet.	Inches.
1. Græco-Egyptian Mummy . . .	5	6
2. Mummy at Dresden	5	3
3. Captain Lethieullier's mummy at the British Museum	5	2
4. Mummy at the British Museum (varnished specimen)	5	2

		Feet.	Inches.
5. Mummy at the Museum of the London University		5	2
6. Mummy of a Youth at the British Museum	.	5	0

II. *Female Mummies in their Bandages.*

1. Dr. Mead's Mummy*	5	5
2. Mummy in the Museum of the London University	5	1
3. Mummy at the British Museum . . .	5	0
4. Mummy at Dresden	4	11½
5. Dr. Perry's Mummy	4	10

III. *Unrolled Male Mummies.*

1. Mummy belonging to the Royal Asiatic Society at the Museum of the King's College . .	5	5
2. Græco-Egyptian Mummy	5	4
3. M. Cailliaud's Græco-Egyptian Mummy . .	5	3½
4. Mummy of Horseisi at the Museum of the Royal College of Surgeons	5	3½

IV. *Unrolled Female Mummies.*

1. Mr. Davidson's Mummy	5	2
2. Dr. Granville's Mummy	5	0 $\frac{7}{10}$
3. Dr. Lee's Mummy	4	11

The following table of the relative measurements of various parts of the body may not be unacceptable.

	King's Col.		Gr. Egypt.		Horseisi.		Mr. Davidson.		Dr. Lee's.	
	ft.	in.	ft.	in.	ft.	in.	ft.	in.	ft.	in.
Top of the head to the angle of the jaw .		7¾		7½		7		7¼		6½
Neck		3½		3		3½		3		2½
Shoulder to trochanter	1	10	1	7	1	10	1	10	1	6
Trochanter to the knee	1	3½	1	5	1	3	1	3½	1	2
Knee to foot	1	6	1	5½	1	5	1	4½	1	2
Arm	1	0	1	0	1	0		11½		10½
Fore-arm		11		11		11		10½		10
Hand		7½		7		7½		7¼		7
Foot		9		9		9½		9		8

* This so much exceeds all the instances I have measured that I am disposed to think there has been some mistake in the statement.

Herodotus* and other authors acquaint us that circumcision was generally practised among the Egyptians. The Ethiopians also performed this rite, and the Phœnicians and Syri of Palestine took the custom from the Egyptians.† The Colchians were supposed by Herodotus to be of Egyptian origin, and he says that he believed them to have belonged to the army of Sesostris. Not only from their conformation, their black colour, and curly hair does he draw this inference, but more especially from their having from time immemorial practised circumcision. From the Colchians, he says, the Syrii‡ (Cappadocians) learnt the practice. The Phœnicians having intercourse with Greece, he tells us, refrained from circumcising their new-born children. Whether circumcision be of Ethiopian or Egyptian origin is not quite clear. It probably belongs to the former, as it appears not unlikely that Upper Egypt was peopled by the Ethiopians. Perhaps the practice originated in a regard for health and cleanliness. All Egyptians were not obliged to submit to the operation, the priests only were compelled to undergo it, or those wishing to be initiated into the mysteries, or to obtain a knowledge of the sacred sciences.§ Females underwent a similar operation, as we learn from Strabo and others ; and a modern traveller, M. Labate, says that he has observed traces of this operation in women. My Græco-Egyptian mummy had not been circumcised. Mr. Madden states that for one Egyptian mummy bearing the marks of circumcision there are fifty that do not.

---

* Euterpe, lib. ii. § 36.   † Ibid. § 104.   ‡ See Schweighaeuser.   § Wesseling.

CHAPTER XII.

ON THE SACRED ANIMALS EMBALMED BY THE EGYPTIANS.

Numerous animals held sacred and embalmed by the Egyptians—worship throughout Egypt of the bull, dog, hawk, and ibis—origin of the worship of animals—difficulty of the enquiry—no one principle adequate to the explanation of it—Dr. Prichard's opinion— Egyptian mythology—elucidation by Porphyry—sacred animals maintained at great expense—ridicule of the worship of animals by Anaxandrides—decline of mythological learning and superstitions—worship of Osiris and Isis—table of the sacred animals—mummies of animals not to be found in human tombs—catacomb of birds—Cailliaud's opinion on the mode of embalming the sacred animals.

Quis nescit Volusi Bithynice, qualia demens
Ægyptus portenta colat? Crocodilon adorat
Pars hæc, illa pavet faturum serpentibus Ibin,
Effigies sacri nitet aurea Cercopitheci,
Dimidio Magicæ resonant, ubi Memnone chordæ.
Atque vetas Thebe centum jacet obruta portis.
Illic cæruleos, hic piscem fluminis, illic
Oppida tota canem venerantur, nemo Dianam :
Porrum et cepe nefas violare ac frangere Morsu,
O sanctas gentes, quibus hæc nascuntur in hortis
Numina ! lanatis animalibus abstinet omnis
Mensa, nefas illic fœtum jugulare expellæ,
Carnibus humanis vesci licet.

Juvenalis Satyr. 15.

WE have already seen upon how extended a scale the ancient Egyptians practised the art of embalming the human species, and our asto-

nishment will not be less excited by an examination into the tombs that
have been devoted to the reception of the prepared and preserved bodies
of various kinds of animals respected and even worshipped by this people:
quadrupeds, birds, amphibia, fishes, insects, nay even plants, have been
in particular parts of Egypt and at different times the objects of religious
superstition.*

Egypt has ever been regarded as the principal seat of idolatry and superstition, and this has arisen from the attention paid to various animals and
the respect shown to their remains. Historians, mythologists, orators,
poets, and painters have vied with each other in displaying the worship of
animals by the Egyptians. Certain animals were supported at the public
expense. The people offered up presents to the animal representing the
divinity to whom they were addressing their prayers, to render their suppli-
cations fruitful. Animals of the lowest character, even vile insects, have
been fostered in their temples, nourished by their priests, embalmed after
death, entombed with pomp, and received all kinds of honours. Those
who either by accident or design have occasioned the death of any of these
animals have even paid the forfeit of their lives as the penalty of the offence. " He who has voluntarily killed a consecrated animal," says Diodorus Siculus,† " is punished with death; but, if any one has even invo-
luntarily killed a cat, or an ibis, it is impossible for him to escape capital
punishment; the mob drags him to it, treating him with every cruelty,
and sometimes without waiting for judgment to be passed. This treatment inspires such terror that if any person happens to find one of these
animals dead he goes to a distance from it, and by his cries and groans
indicates that he has found the animal dead. This superstition is so deeply
impressed on the minds of the Egyptians, and the respect they bear these
animals is so profound, that at the time when their king Ptolemy was not

---

* M. de Pauw supposes that Europe possesses very few animal mummies taken from catacombs situated beyond the twenty-sixth degree of north latitude. The true cause of the
scarcity of embalmed animals in Thebais he attributes to the difficulty of procuring a sufficient
quantity of drugs of the best quality, such as the cedria and bitumen of Judæa.

† Lib. i. § 83.

as yet declared the friend of the Roman people, when they were paying all possible court to travellers from Italy, and their fears made them avoid every ground of accusation, and every pretext for making war on them, yet a Roman having killed a cat, the people rushed to his house, and neither the entreaties of the grandees whom the king sent for the purpose, nor the terror of the Roman name, could protect this man from punishment, although the act had been involuntary. I do not relate this anecdote on the authority of another; for I was an eye-witness of it during my stay in Egypt."

Did the Egyptians really regard these animals as divinities? Strabo says that the worship of animals obtained throughout Egypt for the bull, the dog, the hawk, and the ibis; but that in various parts other animals were the objects of the superstitious veneration of particular cities. The people of Sais and the Thebans adored the sheep; those of Lycopolis the wolf (or jackal); those of Hermopolis the ape (or monkey). Herodotus tells us that the animals esteemed as sacred in one city were held in abhorrence and detestation in another, and that these varieties of opinion were frequent sources of quarrel and dispute. Thus the Ombites fought against the Tentyrites on account of the sparrow-hawks, and the Cynopolitans against the Oxyrhynchites from disputes about dogs and pikes. The people of Mendes honoured the goat, but immolated the sheep. The inhabitants of Thebes worshipped Jupiter Ammon under the figure of a ram, and offered to him goats in sacrifice. Herodotus ascribes the veneration of the ibis to its utility, and Cicero appears to have been of the same opinion, for he says, " Ipsi qui irridentur Ægyptii nullam belluam nisi ob aliquam utilitatem consecraverunt, velut ibes maximam vim serpentium conficiunt. Possum de ichneumonum utilitate, de crocodilorum, de felium dicere: sed nolo esse longior."* It is quite natural to trace the origin of the worship of animals to the benefits supposed to be derived from their services, or as being typical of their powers and properties—the ox tills the land, the cow yields milk, the sheep affords wool, the dog exhibits vigilance and gives protection, the hawk destroys serpents, &c. &c. Mr. Wilkinson conceives

* D e N atura Deorum, lib. i.

the multiplicity of objects of Egyptian worship to have been owing, in some measure, to the " indiscriminate admission of whatever was considered beneficial to mankind, or in which the least resemblance could be traced of the .properties of those deities already worshipped."*

The Abbé Banier† thinks the reason assigned by Herodotus and Cicero may have tended to keep up the worship of these animals ; but he does not conceive it to have derived its origin from such causes. " Je scais bien," says this author, " à la vérité, que le reconnoissance et la crainte ont intro-duit plusieurs Dieux dans le monde ; je ne discouviens pas aussi des grandes utilitez qu'on retire de plusieurs animaux, et je n'ignore pas jusqu'à quel détail est descendu sur ce sujet Gérard Vossius dans son traité de l'idolatrie; mais cette seule raison auroit-elle suffi pour ériger des monstres et de vils insectes en autant de Divinitez?   N'attribuons pas à un peuple sçavant et cultivé des exces dont il ne fut jamais capable.   Toute culte n'est pas un culte religieux, et encore moins une vraie adoration ; et tout ce qui est placé dans les temples pour être l'objet de la vénération publique, n'est pas au rang des Dieux.   Cela étant, je crois que le culte que les prêtres Egyp-tiens rendoient aux animaux, étoit purement relatif, et qu'il se terminoit aux Dieux dont ils étoient les symboles."

In support of the proposition thus advanced, the Abbé goes on to show that the bull was the symbol of Osiris and of Isis, and that these divinities themselves were merely symbols of the sun and moon : the worship of the bulls Mnévis and Apis, the former being the emblem of the sun, the latter of the moon, as we learn from Porphyry, Ælian, Ammianus Marcellinus, and others. The inhabitants of Mendes rendered worship to Pan, and represented him under the figure of a goat ; and this, according to Diodorus Siculus, was typical of the fecundity of nature.   The dog is the most vigilant of animals, and Mercury has been painted with the head of a dog.   It would appear, then, that the worship rendered to animals was only a relative one, and that they received divine honours only as typical of the divinities themselves.   It is easy to conceive how the mass of the people in succeeding times would lose

* Materia Hieroglyphica, Part I., p. 13.

† Memoires de l'Academie des Inscriptions, tom. III. p. 89.

sight of the original of this worship, and transfer to the animals themselves the adoration intended to be far otherwise bestowed.

It would be a task of no little difficulty to assign the reasons or motives which gave rise to the worship of animals among the Egyptians. To account for the worship of such strange gods ; for the respect and veneration paid to some of the meanest objects of creation are still desiderata in mythology. No one principle is adequate to explain the subject. The worship was not confined to the useful animals, nor did it include many that could be ranged in that class: on the contrary, it embraced many of the most noxious and destructive. Lucian has looked upon the sacred animals as types or emblems of various constellations or figures of groups of stars in the heavens; but this is insufficient to explain the mystery. The attributes of the deity expressed by the qualities of various animals have, in the opinion of others, given rise to the worship of animals. There is probably somewhat of truth in all these conjectures, though, taken altogether, it must be confessed they are inadequate to the solution of the question. Dr. Prichard conceives the true explanation of this worship to be deeply rooted in the principles of the Egyptian mythology, and perhaps better elucidated by Porphyry than any other author. In support of his opinion he quotes the following passage:—" The Egyptian priests (says Porphyry)* having profited by their diligent study of philosophy, and their intimate acquaintance with the nature of the gods, have learnt that the divinity permeates not human beings only; that man is not the only creature on the earth possessed of soul, but that nearly the same spiritual essence pervades all the tribes of living creatures. On this account, in fashioning images of the gods, they have adopted the forms of all animals, and have sometimes joined the human figure with those of beasts, at others have combined the shapes of men and of birds ; for some of these images have the form of a man up to the neck, with the face of a bird or a lion, or some other creature. Others, again, have the head of a man, with the remainder of the body, either the upper or lower parts, shaped like some other animal. On this account the lion is adored by them as a god, and there is a part of

* De Abstinentia, lib. iv. cap. 9.

Egypt which is called the Leontopolite nome, another is called the Busirite, and a third the Cynopolitan; for they adore, under these semblances, the universal power which the gods have severally displayed in the various forms of living nature." In this passage Dr. Prichard perceives the doctrine of *emanation*, which he has endeavoured to trace among the fundamental principles of the Egyptian philosophy,* and he sums up the whole in the following manner:—" We have seen that all the operations of nature were ascribed by the Egyptians to certain demons or spiritual beings, who were supposed to animate different portions of the universe. All these were emanations from the universal deity or soul of the world. This doctrine was extended still further; and it was imagined that the soul or vital principle in every living being is an emanation from the same source, that it is a divided portion of the divine nature, and derived either primarily or secondarily from the fountain of divinity. Accordingly, in men and animals, and even in plants, they adored the indwelling portions of the same essence."†

" Certain effluxes or eradiations from the essence of the gods were believed to be embodied in all living creatures, and it was to these indwelling portions of the divinity that the people addressed their adorations. Being possessed with this idea, they were led to look out for symptoms of the mystical indwelling power in the outward qualities of animals; and hence the absurd stories so current among the ancient priests. Every instinct was regarded as a mysterious allusion to some fable in the mythology. It was natural that noxious creatures should be regarded as manifestations of the destructive power, and those which are most friendly and serviceable to man of the productive or beneficent. Still the gratitude of men, for the services rendered them by the latter, was not the first principle which led to the deification of animals."‡

" The Egyptians believed that the souls which had emanated from the

---

* I cannot do better than refer the reader who is anxious to obtain information on this abstruse and difficult subject to Dr. Prichard's " Analysis of the Egyptian Mythology." See particularly Book II. chap. 1, " On the Philosophical Doctrine, Cosmogony, &c., of the Egyptians."

† Analysis, p. 336.   ‡ p. 338.

primitive source transmigrated through various bodies; nor was this change of forms confined to emanations of a lower or secondary order. As the souls of men transmigrated through different shapes, so the higher orders of spiritual agents could, as occasion required, assume any form they chose; and sometimes the gods appeared in the world under the disguise of bulls, lions, eagles, or other creatures of the like description." *

The sacred animals were maintained at great expense in sacred parks, and persons were appointed to nourish them with the greatest care. Bread, milk, honey, meat, birds, fish, &c., all according to the nature of the animals, were supplied. The most beautiful of their kind were associated to perpetuate the race, and great sorrow was manifested at the death of any of them. They were embalmed and interred with great pomp and splendour. The persons having the care of the animals bore upon their persons the resemblance of the species to which their care was devoted, and the people paid marks of respect to them as they passed along.

In the famine that afflicted Egypt, although the people were driven to eat human flesh, the sacred animals were respected.

Dr. Prichard has quoted a fragment from a comedy, entitled ' The Cities,' by the comic poet of Rhodes, Anaxandrides, in which the devotion to animals by the Egyptians is treated with keen and humorous derision, although the Greeks originally borrowed the fables of their own mythology from this ancient people. I subjoin the translation of this fragment:

> " Tis plain that you and I can ne'er agree,
>   So opposite are all our ways and rites.
> Before a bull, four-legged beast, ye bend,
> With pious terror smitten: at the altar
> I offer him a victim to the gods.
> You fancy in the little eel some power
> Of dæmon huge and terrible: within
> We stew it for our daintiest appetite. The flesh
> Of fatted swine you touch not: 'tis the best
> Of all our delicate meats. The yelping cur
> Is in your creed a god: I whip the rogue
> Whene'er I catch him stealing eggs or meat.

* Analysis, p. 338.

Our priests are whole in skin from foot to head :
Not so your circumcised and shaven seers.
You cry and wail whene'er ye spy a cat
Starving or sick : I count it not a sin
To hang it up, and flay it for its skin.
Ye say the paltry shrew-mouse is a god."*

The ancient Egyptians painted the images of their sacred animals, and affixed the representations to the heads of their spears, and thus carried them as standards before their troops.†

When the Egyptians went to return thanks to the gods whose assistance they had invoked for the relief of the diseases of their children or relatives, they cut off the hair of the convalescents, and gave to those who had the care of the sacred animals its weight in gold.

The decline of the power of the Egyptian hierarchy may be dated from the reign of Psammeticus, who first encouraged the intercourse of his subjects with foreigners, and thus endangered the influence of those superstitions which, during some thousands of years, had maintained the character impressed by ancient priestcraft on the people of Egypt.‡ Under the persecution of Cambyses the system must have received great checks and innovations. Under the Ptolemies, who were so desirous of gaining the affections of the native Egyptians, the ancient system may have recovered some of its lost splendour; for it must not be forgotten that the Greeks acknowledged Egypt to have been the cradle of their own mythology. From this period the mythological learning and superstitions underwent a gradual decline. As late as the time of Strabo, however, the old Egyptian gods were still fed in their temples—serpents and crocodiles were still worshipped notwithstanding the ridicule of the Greeks. Whilst the whole Egyptian people participated in the rites offered to Osiris and Isis, each particular province or nome, as it was called by the Greeks, had its own peculiar superstition, and directed their devotions to particular deities. The worship of Osiris and Isis was the worship of the sun and the earth, or nature in general,§ and may

* Anaxand. in Civitat. apud Athenæi Deipnos, lib. vii. p. 299.   † Diod. Sicul. lib. i. c. 6.
‡ See Dr. Prichard's " Analysis of the Egyptian Mythology,"
§ Macrobii Saturnalia, lib. i. cap. 21.

be regarded as forming an important part of the national religion of the Egyptians. The most intelligent of the ancient writers who have alluded to this subject have assured us that the principal objects of Egyptian worship were those physical agents whose operative energy is the most conspicuous in the phenomena of nature. They considered every part of the visible universe as endowed with an inherent life, energy, and intelligence; they worshipped the intelligent and active cause of the phenomena of nature, as it is displayed in its most striking and powerful agencies, but without accurately discriminating the cause from the effect; or they believed, as men seem naturally prone to imagine, that the elements themselves were animated.*

Dr. Prichard has given the legend of Isis and Osiris, and its interpretation according to the most ancient writers on this enigmatical story, and from a close examination of these authorities the following conclusion has been derived :—

" Osiris was not simply the sun or the Nile, but every part of nature in which productive qualities are displayed. Osiris clearly seems to have represented the active energy of nature, the beneficent or generative influence of the elements, wherever exhibited; Isis, the passive cause, or the prolific powers of nature, in the sublunary world. Hence Osiris was sometimes worshipped in the sun, whose rays vivify and gladden the earth, and at whose return, in the vernal season, all its organized productions receive a new generation; and sometimes in the Nile, whose waters bestow riches on the land of Egypt. Isis was the earth, or sublunary nature in general; or, in a more confined sense, the soil of Egypt, which is overflowed by the Nile; or the prolific or genial principle, the goddess of generation, and all production. Considered jointly, Osiris and Isis are the universal being, the soul of nature, corresponding with the Pantheus or masculo-feminine Jupiter of the Orphic verses."†

Mr. Wilkinson has remarked that the principal office of Osiris, as an Egyptian deity, was to judge the dead, and rule over that kingdom where the souls of good men were admitted to eternal felicity.‡

According to Plutarch, Serapis was the name by which Osiris was called after he had changed his nature, or had descended into the infernal regions.

* Analysis, pp. 27—34.   † p. 78.   ‡ Materia Hierog. p. 19.

2 A

This could only have been after the introduction of the god of Sinope into Egypt by the Ptolemies, Serapis not being in reality an Egyptian deity.

Jablonski* considers Isis as simply denoting the moon. Diodorus Siculus says, Osiris and Isis represent the sun and moon; so also Diogenes Laertius, and others. Io was the common term for moon in the Coptic language. The general acceptation is, however, more prevalent, and the moon is regarded as the chief seat of the genial goddess of nature.

As Osiris represented the *productive* power, so Typhon was symbolical of the *destructive*. Plutarch tells us† that " whatever is turbulent, or noxious, or disorderly, in irregular seasons, or a distempered condition of the air, or in eclipses of the sun and moon, are incursions and representations of Typhon." And again, " every thing that is of an evil or malignant nature, either in the animal, the vegetable, or the intellectual world, is looked upon in general as the operation of Typhon, as part of him, or as the effect of his influence." ‡

Nor are Isis and Nephthys, the consorts or passive representations of Osiris and Typhon, less opposed to each other than Osiris and Typhon. Isis represents *fertility*, Nephthys *sterility*. §

The preceding observations on the Egyptian mythology will, I trust, be found useful preparatory to an investigation into the nature of the properties of the sacred animals, and the rites that have been established in their worship. I shall now present the reader with a table of the animals and vegetables which, as far as I have been able to collect, were regarded as sacred by the ancient Egyptians, and which have received the honour of being embalmed :—

I. *Mammalia.*

		Worshipped ‖ at
1. Monkey tribe	. . . .	Hermopolis.
2. Dog	. . . . .	Cynopolis.

---

* Pantheon Egypt.   † De Iside et Osiride, § 45.   ‡ Ibid. § 50.

§ I must here, once for all, refer the reader who may be desirous of gaining information on the subject of the Egyptian Pantheon to the labours of Mr. Wilkinson. See Materia Hieroglyphica, Parts I. and II., and Appendix. Malta, 1828. Also, Extracts from several Hieroglyphical Subjects, 8vo. 1830.

‖ I fear that the word " worshipped" is not applicable to all the animals enumerated in this table ; many were embalmed for sanatory reasons. The owl, the eagle, the swallow, the toad, &c., are probably of those animals to whom no religious feeling was attached.

Worshipped at.

3. Cat	. . . . . .	Bubastis.
4. Lion	. . . . . .	Leontopolis.
5. Wolf	. . . . .	⎫
6. Jackal	. . . . .	⎬ Lycopolis.
7. Fox	. . . . .	⎭
8. Hyæna	. . . . .	⎫ Papremis.
9. Bear	. . . . .	⎭
10. Ichneumon	. . . .	Heracleopolis.
11. Shrew-Mouse	. . .	Atribis, Boutos, Cynopolis.
12. Deer	. . . . .	Coptos.
13. Goat	. . . . .	Mendes.
14. Ram, sheep, lamb	. . . .	Sais, Thebes.
15. Bull, cow, calf	. . . .	⎡ All Egypt.
Apis	. . . . .	⎢ Memphis.
Mnevis	. . . .	⎢ Heliopolis.
Basis	. . . . .	⎣ Hermonthis.
16. Hippopotamus	. . . .	Papremis.

II. *Aves.*

1. Vulture	. . . . .	Thebes, Eleithyia.
2. Eagle	. . . . .	Theban nome.
3. Falcon	. . . .	⎰ Apollonopolis, Tentyris, Her- ⎱ mopolis, Philæ.
4. Hawk	. . . . .	⎰ All Egypt, particularly Ten- ⎱ tyris.
5. Owl, hobby	. . . .	Thebes.
6. Ibis	. . . . .	⎰ All Egypt, particularly Her- ⎱ mopolis.
7. Goose	. . . . .	Thebes?
8. Swallow	. . . . .	Do.

III. *Amphibia.*

1. Crocodile	. . . . .	Coptos, Arsinoë, Ombos.
2. Toad	. . . . .	Thebes.

Worshipped at.

3. Lizard (monitor)	Thebes?
4. Coluber	⎰All Egypt, particularly Ele-
5. Adder, Asp, Serpents . . .	⎱ phantine.
6. Cerastes	Thebes.

IV. *Pisces.*

1. Carp, lepidotus ?	Lepidotum.
2. Pike ?	Oxyrhynchus.
3. Sir (joël?)	Thebes ?
4. Mœotis	Elephantine.
5. Variole (perch ?)	Latopolis.
6. Sparus	Syene.

V. *Insecta.*

1. Scarabæus ⎱	All Egypt.
2. Copris ⎰	
3. Cantharis ⎱	Thebes ?
4. Buprestis ⎰	

Vegetables.

Lotus ⎫	
Persea ⎬	Egypt.
Sycamore ⎭	
Onion	Sethroite nome.

The sacred animals of which the foregoing table is composed have all been, under various circumstances, found embalmed. Most of them had their own proper sepulchres consecrated and appropriated to their species only; but they were frequently found mixed with others.* Scarcely ever

---

* The variety of embalmed animals is much greater in the Thebais, and particularly at Thebes, than in any other part of Egypt. There are tombs there containing mummies of oxen, sheep, cats, dogs, ibis, hawks, eggs, snakes, &c., in great numbers. In a note in p. 170, I have quoted an opinion from M. de Pauw, that few animal mummies are found beyond the

have any animals been found in a human tomb. It has been asserted that this never occurred; but Belzoni, upon whose veracity every reliance may be placed, states that he examined some tombs in which the mummies of human beings and those of animals were intermixed, and he expressly names as having seen in the same tomb mummies of bulls, cows, sheep, monkeys, foxes, bats, crocodiles, fishes, and birds. Idols of them often occur. Belzoni has opened all these sorts of animals. Of the bull,* the calf, and the sheep, the head only is covered with linen, and the horns project out of the cloth. The body of the animal is represented by two pieces of wood, eighteen inches wide and three feet long, in a horizontal direction, at the end of which is another, placed perpendicularly, two feet high, to form the breast of the animal. The calves and sheep are of the same structure, and large in proportion to the bulls. The monkey is in its full form, in a sitting posture.† The fox‡ is squeezed up by the bandages, but in some measure the head is kept perfect. The crocodile§ is left in its own shape, and, after being well bound round with linen, the eyes and mouth are painted on the covering. The birds are squeezed together and lose their shape, except the ibis, which, according to Belzoni, is formed like a fowl‖ ready to be cooked, and bound round with linen like the rest.¶ The same author observes, however, that no mummies of animals are to be met with in the tombs of the higher sort of people.**

The catacomb of birds is distinct from the catacomb of human mummies. One bird only is enclosed in each earthen pot,†† and Perry says‡‡ that he found an infinite number of pots in good order; that is, whole and sealed, and of these he adds, " a man might bring away hundreds if he would." The hot nature of the materials with which they had been embalmed had, however, dried up the greater number to powder. Upon the possession of Egypt by the French upwards of five hundred mummies of the ibis were

26th degree of north latitude; but it must be observed that the latitude of Thebes, according to Mr. Wilkinson's observations, is 25° 43′, and the difficulty of procuring drugs from the north would of course be easily remedied by the ready communication offered by the Nile.

* See Plate XII. *fig*. 6. † See Plate XII. *fig*. 7. ‡ See Plate XII. *fig*. 4.
§ See Plate XII. *fig*.8, 9. ‖ See PlateXIII. *fig*. 4. ¶ Belzoni's Travels, p. 168.
** Ibid. p. 169. †† See Plate XIII. *fig*. 5. ‡‡ View of the Levant, p. 321.

discovered in the catacomb of birds.   According to Jomard, animals have been found equally well embalmed as human beings.   Passalacqua found at Thebes a packet of embalmed animals all mixed together; little birds, rats, mice, toads, adders, beetles, and flies.   How singular that, in the city where the cat was so greatly respected and cherished, rats and mice should also be found embalmed!*   No amulets have ever been found upon the mummies of animals.

Mons. Cailliaud thinks† that before embalming much of the flesh of the animals was removed, as he found among the sacred animals scarcely any thing remaining beyond the bones.   This may perhaps be accounted for by the mode of embalming, for M. Rouyer tells us‡ that animals are chiefly prepared by natron.   The ibis and the hawk appear to have had most care bestowed on them, for resin and asphalt are frequently found within their envelopes. Birds in general having been wrapped round in their bandages have then been placed in an earthen urn‖ and deposited in the tomb ; but in some instances they were left in their bandages alone § (these are the best preserved), and the hawk and the ibis have been found preserved in a human form.¶   The mummies of birds are done up conically, the quadrupeds cylindrically or quadrangularly.

* This custom seems to have originated in a sanatory regulation tending to prevent the noxious effluvia arising from the putrefaction of decayed animal matter, and was consequently extended to all animals.

† Voyage à Meroé, I. 13.

‡ Descript. de l'Egypte.   ‖ See Plate XIII. *fig.* 5.   § See Plate XIII. *fig.* 7, 8.

¶ See Plate XIII. *fig.* 2, 6.

CHAPTER XIII.

ON THE SACRED ANIMALS—THE MAMMALIA.

The monkey tribe worshipped by the Egyptians—Hermopolis the chief seat of this worship—mummy of a human monster—the dog—Cynopolis the principal place of the worship of Anubis—different accounts of this worship—number of embalmed dogs seen by Abd'Allatif—the cat principally worshipped at Bubastis—food of the consecrated cats—account of the embalming of cats by Diodorus Siculus—the wolf—the jackal—the fox—Lycopolis celebrated for the worship of these animals—the ram sacred at Thebes and Sais—the goat worshipped at Mendes—the bear and hyæna held sacred at Papremis—also the hippopotamus, a symbol of Typhon—the ichneumon worshipped at Heracleopolis—shrew-mouse held sacred at Boutos—the bull consecrated to the sun and moon—characters of the sacred bull—Apis, the Epaphus of the Greeks—the worship of Apis principally at Memphis—Mnevis chiefly adored at Heliopolis and had the same rites as Apis—cows never killed in sacrifice.

Simia—Monkey Tribe.

In the collection exhibited a few years since in London by the lamented Belzoni was the specimen of an embalmed dog-faced baboon from the sepulchre of Thebes, in which the character of the animal was exceedingly well preserved, and the hair remained attached to the skin in great perfection. This animal is represented in Plate XII. *fig.* 7, and was improperly called an ape. It is the *Simia Cercopithecus Cynocephalus* of Linnæus, and described by Hasselquist* as *Simia Egyptiaca cauda elongata, clunibus tuberosis nudis.*

Hermopolis was the chief seat of the monkey worship. M. de Pauw states† that two kinds of monkey were worshipped at Babylon, near Memphis, at Hermopolis, and in an anonymous town of Thebais, and that they were brought from the interior of Ethiopia. The same authority observes, ‡

---

* Itin. 189. † Phil. Diss. 148, ‡ Ibid. 149.

that it is not known whether the cebus or the cynocephalus gave rise to the error of Porphyry, who pretends that the Egyptians had a particular temple, where they adored a living man. As this was undoubtedly false, it follows that one or other of these monkeys had been taken for a human being, by voyagers who were either deceived or wished to impose on the Greeks; for their curiosity is insatiable, says Heliodorus, with regard to whatever concerns the Egyptians.

M. Geoffroy St. Hilaire made a communication to the Royal Academy of Sciences, in 1826, relative to the mummy of a human monster which had been submitted to his notice by M. Passalacqua, who had previously regarded it as a mummy of the cynocephalus. M. St. Hilaire says that its characters were so distinct that it occasioned him no difficulty in detecting its real nature.* He thought the subject worthy of being laid before the Academy, and he has described it as belonging to the class of ANENCEPHALE, characterized by the want of the brain and spinal marrow. The position of the monster is curious. It was seated, the feet joined together, and the hands placed under the knees. It was deposited along with the embalmed monkeys in the catacombs of Hermopolis, not among the human mummies. It is worthy of remark, also, that near to this mummified monster was observed an amulet in baked earth and enamelled, an exact copy of a cynocephalus, and the posture of this animal corresponds with that in which the mummy was found. " La forme de ce symbole (says M. St. Hilaire) exprime-t-elle l'intention d'une comparaison entre l'inferiorité organique accidentale de la monstruosité embaumée, et l'inferiorité normale de l'être le plus dégradé parmi les animaux à face humaine?" The figure of the cynocephalus placed near to the mummy shows clearly that the embalmers were quite aware of its nature, as in no instance, I believe, has any amulet or divinity been found situated near or attached to the mummy of any animal.

THE DOG.—ANUBIS.

THE city of Cynopolis was the principal seat of the worship of Anubis, or Anoubis, a worship highly venerated by the Egyptians in general. It was

* To any one familiar with the Philosophie Anatomique this will not be a matter of the least surprise.

also common to the Greeks and Romans, and the rites of Anubis are to be found conjoined with those of Isis. We learn from Strabo,* and other authorities,† that dogs were held sacred at Cynopolis in the Lower Thebais, supported at the public expense, and reared in temples. There is considerable obscurity as to the attribute of Anubis. Plutarch, and after him Jablonski, conceived that the Egyptians understood by Anubis the horizontal circle which divides the invisible from the visible part of the world; and the latter authority has endeavoured to support the opinion by referring to the etymology of the name, which he derives from the Coptic word *nub*, " gold," or *annub*, " gilt," signifying " golden." Dr. Prichard has justly observed that this epithet would be more aptly applied to twilight, the harbinger of day, than to the horizontal circle.‡ An able writer, in a foreign work of considerable merit,§ has endeavoured to explain this in the following manner :—" The inferior is to the superior hemisphere what the shade is to the light, death to life, the earth to the heavens. Anubis is here identified with the crepuscule, twilight, when day is no more, and night is not yet come—the confines of light and darkness. This state, which results from the diurnal movement of the earth, would appear to the primitive people parallel to a bad and a fine season, to long and short days, to great heat and piercing cold—the result of the annual movement. The god who represented the horizon, the mutual limit of the two hemispheres, would also represent the limited period between the day and the night." The writer I have referred to considers Anubis to be the god who presided over the embalmed, who committed to the incorruptible tomb the sacred remains of Osiris, who assisted Isis in recomposing the body of the deity; hence he concludes that Anubis is a god of the lower regions. He calls him *Le Dieu Transition*, and considers him as presiding over that period in which is to be found the passage from life to death, from time to eternity, from the physical world to that of ideal and incorporeal existences—over that period which separates light from darkness (as in genealogy he bears equal relation to Osiris and Typhon,

---

* Lib. xvii.   † Herodotus, Diodorus Siculus, Clemens Alexandrinus, Lucian, &c.

‡ Analysis, p. 124.

§ Biographie Universelle Ancienne et Moderne, Partie Mythologique, Paris, 1832. Tom. LIII.

being begotten by Osiris and Nephthys), and that at the moment of the departure of the soul from the body he conducts the spirit to the regions of the Amenti.

The deity Anubis is always represented with the head of a jackal, and in one of his characters Anubis answers to the Hermes or Mercury of the Greeks. In the Egyptian mythology he certainly appears to have been concerned in the office of conducting the souls of the dead to their place of destination.

The etymology given by Jablonski has been treated with contempt, and it has been contended that Champollion le jeune has given the true one in the following forms, as seen upon hieroglyphical legends at the present day: " Anbô," " Anébô," " Anébou," and that these names bear no relation whatever to " Nub," " Noub," or " Annub."

Greek authors, erroneously supposing that Anubis bore the head of a dog, have conjectured this animal to be an emblem of that deity, and that the worship of it was owing to the discovery and preservation of the mutilated portions of the body of Osiris after he had been massacred by Typhon. The dog conducted Isis to the spot where the murder had been perpetrated, and where the fragments remained hidden. To celebrate the fidelity of this animal in the ceremonies dedicated to the honour of Isis, a dog was made to march at the head of the procession. Plutarch says* that it is not literally the dog that they honour under the name of Mercury, but his qualities: his vigilance, his good faith, his sagacity in distinguishing a friend from an enemy, which, to use the words of Plato, have rendered this animal a fit symbol of that god who is the immediate patron of reason. And Larcher† quotes from Servius‡ in confirmation of this opinion, " Quia canino capite pingitur Anubis, hunc volunt esse Mercurium, ideo quia nihil est cane sagacius." When a dog died in a house, all the inmates shaved their heads and bodies. This was, agreeably to Larcher,§ because the dog was consecrated to Anubis, who was represented with the head of a dog. Virgil‖ and Ovid¶ call this god " Latrator Anubis," and Propertius** and

---

* De Iside et Osiride, p. 355.   † Note to Euterpe, § 138.   ‡ Æneid, lib. iii. ver. 698.
§ Note to Euterpe, No. 66.   ‖ Æneid, lib. viii. ver. 698.
¶ Metamorph. lib. ix. ver. 692.   ** Lib. iii. Eleg. XI. ver 41.

Prudentius,* "latrans Anubis." Plutarch† tells us that greater honours were paid to the dog than to any other animal, although Cambyses having caused the bull Apis to be killed, and no other animal being found to touch the body but the dog, the latter sunk much in the estimation of the Egyptians. From Herodotus, however, we learn that the dog was still held in great veneration, and a war was even waged against the Oxyrhinchytes by the Cynopolitans,‡ for having killed a dog and eaten it. When Cambyses returned from his unsuccessful and disastrous expedition against the Ethiopians, he found the inhabitants of Memphis rejoicing ; and, imagining this to have been produced by his ill success, he became enraged, and sent for the magistrates, who assured him that it was occasioned by a manifestation of the god Apis. Suspecting that they were deceiving him, Cambyses applied to the priests, and from them received a similar account. He then ordered the god to be brought before him, when, as Herodotus reports,§ " Cambyses, like a maniac, grasping his dagger, and intending to strike the belly of Apis, wounded him in the thigh : then, bursting into laughter, he said to the priests, ' You scoundrels, are there gods such as this, of blood and flesh, and sensible of steel ? A deity this worthy, indeed, of the Egyptians ; but you shall not, of a truth, laugh at me, at any rate with impunity.' When he had so spoken, he charged those whose office it was to scourge the priests, and to put to death whomsoever of the rest of the Egyptians they might catch celebrating the festival ; so that the festival of the Egyptians was put an end to, and the priests were punished. Apis, after being wounded in the

*Apotheos. V. 196.　　　　　　　　† De Iside et Osiride, p. 368.

‡ " Pliny records the dissensions between the inhabitants of Hieracopolis and Arsinoë, also those of Cynopolis against Oxyrhinchus. Similar dissensions were multiplied throughout Egypt, and the respective deities were brought into combat; but it should be ever remembered that this was when the priesthood, the real lever which acted upon and guided the Mizraim race, were scattered and destroyed, Egypt in bondage, and their wisdom extinguished. But, under the beneficial sway of the Pharaohs, these feuds are not so apparent; as there are manifest traces of the priests recognizing a superior power, or energy, that governed even the seeming evil, so as to become part of its own essence, and a ray of its own power.—*Note to Rameses*, vol. III. p. 305.

§ Thalia, § 29.

thigh, pined away, lying in the temple, and, having died in consequence of the wound, the priests buried him, unknown to Cambyses." The authority of Herodotus is unquestionably superior to that of Plutarch on this point. Herodotus (as Larcher observes) was born but forty-one years after this event, and during his stay in Egypt might have conversed with persons who were actual witnesses of it. Plutarch did not live till nearly six hundred years afterwards. It is, therefore, most probable that Apis was not devoured by dogs, but that he received the rites of burial and the customary process of embalming.

Dogs would appear to have been held in greater veneration by the Egyptians than cats, if we are entitled to draw a conclusion from the manner in which their loss was mourned. If a cat died, the owner of the house shaved off his eyebrows ; but if a dog, died, he shaved his whole head and even his body.

The dead dog was delivered to the embalmer of animals* to be prepared and deposited in the proper tombs, previously to which it was wrapped in linen, and the by-standers manifested their grief by beating themselves on the breast and uttering doleful cries.

Abd'Allatif says he saw heaps of bodies of dogs consisting of 100,000 and more.

In M. Passalacqua's collection there is a specimen of a dog embalmed. He is at his full length.†

The Cat.

We have already seen‡ that it was unlawful to kill a cat, and that capital punishment followed the act. The utility of this animal, separate from other reasons, might appear to be sufficient cause to put it under the protection of the law, and this was indeed most rigidly maintained.

The cat was principally an object of worship in the city of Bubastis or Bubastos, and a celebrated temple was dedicated to the goddess Bubastis, who is said to have assumed the form of a cat to avoid Typhon. Most of the cats that died in Egypt were embalmed and buried at Bubastis,§ a city of

---

* Ælian. Hist. Animal. lib. x. c. 19.   † No. 363.   ‡ p. 171.
§ Herod. Euterpe, § 67.

Lower Egypt, now called Tel-Basta, but many are found in other parts of Egypt. The representation of the cat in connexion with the sistrum of Isis* has been referred to the common opinion relative to a certain mysterious sympathy between this animal and the moon. This goddess was invoked by parturient women, over whom she was supposed to preside, like Diana or Lucina of the Greeks and Romans.

The consecrated cats were fed upon fish† kept in reservoirs for the purpose. M. De Pauw says it was a species of *silurus*. Three species of this fish are found in the Nile, not one of which has scales.

Mons. Champollion‡ saw in the desert valley near to Beni-Hassan a small temple excavated in a rock. According to its decorations it was commenced by Thouthmosis IV. and continued by Mandouei of the eighteenth dynasty. The decorations were in very fine coloured bas-relief, and dedicated to the goddess Pascht or Pépascht, who is the Bubastis of the Greeks as well as the Diana of the Romans. This accords well with the position that geographers have marked out as the scite of the grotto of Diana, and this temple, which presents only images of Bubastis, is surrounded by different tombs for sacred cats, some cut in the rock, one of which was constructed under the reign of Alexander the Great. Before the temple, under the sand, there was a large mound of mummies of cats folded in mats, and mixed with those of dogs ; and further on in the desert plain were two large collections of mummies of cats in packets and covered with ten feet of sand. The cat is much altered in its character when enveloped in the bandages, but the head is well preserved.§ They are frequently enveloped in bandages of different colours,‖ and Belzoni saw a a tomb which was filled with cats, carefully folded in red and white linen, the head covered by a mask representing the cat and made of the same linen. Passalacqua's collection contains two specimens of the cat mummied and placed in cases of wood.¶ Diodorus Siculus affords testimony to the

* Denon saw in one of the temples at Dendera, dedicated to Isis, on the capitals of the columns supporting the hall, four figures of that goddess, represented with the ears of the cat. Tom. II. 34.　　　　　　　　　　† Ælian. Hist. Animal. lib. xii.

‡ Lettres écrites d'Egypte, &c., p. 85.　　§ See Plate XII. *fig.* 5.

‖ Passalacqua Catalog. Nos. 369 à 376. Mr. Wilkinson kindly presented me with a specimen of this description.

¶ Ibid. Nos. 377. 378.

embalming of cats: "When one of these animals," says he, "happens to die it is wrapped in linen, and after the by-standers have beaten themselves on the breast, uttering doleful cries, it is carried to the Tarichæa, where it is embalmed with cedria and other substances which have the virtue of preserving bodies, after which it is interred in the sacred monument.*

The Wolf—The Jackal—The Fox.

HERODOTUS describes the wolves of Egypt as being very small, a little larger than foxes, and congregating together in great numbers, which circumstance is quite true of the jackals to this day, which find a retreat in the catacombs where their cry is so lugubrious at night, and so much resembling the melancholy howl of the Arabs, that Mr. Madden says† he has frequently mistaken it for the common lamentation of the women at the moment of a death. It has been asserted that there are no wolves in Egypt, but Prosper Alpinus‡ gives his testimony in support of their being in that country in his time. Aristotle§ and Pliny‖ confirm this statement, and mention their diminutive size. Sonnini says¶ that it is of the jackal that we are to understand all that authors have said of the wolf, and even of the fox of Africa; for, admitting that these animals have, to a certain degree, a relation to each other, it is, however, well known that there are neither wolves nor foxes in that part of the world. Upon this authority Mr. Larcher has made some observations which deserve attention. Granting that there are neither wolves nor foxes in Africa, he suggests** that it is not improbable that some of these animals might have entered Egypt by the isthmus of Suez, but that, stopped by the mountain which lies towards the west, they could not penetrate into the rest of Africa. Herodotus also, he thinks, being an Asiatic, ought to have been acquainted with the jackal, an animal common throughout Asia Minor, and which is probably the same that he designates by the name of "thos."†† The wolf could not have been less familiar to him. Added to these are the confirmations of the statement by Aristotle

---

* Lib. i. § 83.   † Travels, II. 24.   ‡ Hist. Nat. Ægypt. lib. iv. cap. 9.
§ Hist. Animal. lib. viii. c. 27.   ‖ Hist. Nat. lib. viii. c. 22.   ¶ Travels, vol. I. p. 140.
** Notes to Euterpe, § 67.   †† Book iv. § 192.

and Pliny, and Prosper Alpinus. The pains which the former took to perfect his History of Animals is well known, and in his time Egypt was as well known to the Greeks as Greece itself. The learned commentator on Herodotus from whom I have just quoted strengthens his argument still further by referring to a passage from Eusebius,* in which he expressly says that wolves were honoured, in Egypt because they bear a considerable resemblance to the dog, and because formerly, as the Egyptians say, Isis with her son Horus being on the point of encountering Typhon, Osiris came from the infernal regions to their succour under the form of a wolf. Others say that the Ethiopians having undertaken an expedition against Egypt were put to flight by a vast multitude of wolves, and that this circumstance gave to the nome in which it occurred the name of Lycopolis. Mr. Wilkinson found the mummy of a wolf at Lycopolis. He has kindly presented me with the head. He has also given to the British Museum a specimen of this animal, and informs me that he has seen hundreds, and shot great numbers, in Egypt.

Siout, the ancient Lycopolis, was celebrated for the worship of the jackal. These animals are found embalmed entire at this place, and are very numerous. In the Description de l'Egypte (vol. II. Antiq.) there are representations of portions of embalmed jackals that have even been gilt. Osiris assumed the form of the jackal and also that of the wolf, to assist Horus in his war against Typhon.

M. De Pauw ridicules the statement of Ælian that the inhabitants of the great Lycopolitan prefectory took care to pluck up entirely that species of aconite vulgarly called *wolf's-bane*, lest it should injure any of the objects of their veneration. Wolves were surely never permitted to run at liberty in the provinces. Belzoni saw mummies of the fox, the form of which is generally much compressed by the bandages. It is represented in Plate XII. *fig.* 4.

THE RAM—THE GOAT—THE SHEEP.

THE ram was sacred at Thebes in Upper Egypt. Also at Sais in the Delta. Kneph was represented in the form of a ram, or a human figure with the head of that animal, and worshipped in the Theban nome. He represents the sun in the sign Aries.

* Præparat. Evang. lib. ii. § 1. p. 50.

Denon * observed at Esneh, the ancient Latopolis, a temple in the interior of the city; the portico alone remains, the other parts of the buildings are buried in ruins. The capitals of the columns of the portico are, according to this traveller, beautifully executed, and most elegant. The temple was dedicated to Ammon, and the hieroglyphics and the paintings represent sacrifices offered to this god. The goats were mostly the antelope oryx; the Egyptians included these and the gazelle under the general denomination of " mountain goats."

The temple of Eleithias seems to offer the most ample field for the study of the Egyptian mythology. Here are to be found representations of nearly all the superstitions of the ancient Egyptians. " The most conspicuous figure over the entrance into the adytum of the temple is Osiris with a ram's head and the horns of Ammon. On each side of him are four priests in the posture of adoration, with clasped and lifted hands. A priest is piercing a man with his spear at the foot of Osiris Ammon, and Isis lunata, i. e., crowned with the globe and lunar horns, exactly corresponding to the appearance of the new moon, when under a clear sky the obscure disk is just perceptible. Another priest is dancing with great agility before the same deity, accompanied by Isis leonata, or with the head of a lioness. Three figures, one with the head of Osiris in the human character, the second disguised as Osiris Ammon, and the third with a lion's head, are drawing together a large net in which are caught a quantity of fish and waterfowl, and which is fastened at the other end to the sceptre of Isis. A crocodile is seated on an altar, viewing a table placed before him covered with fruits and other delicacies, while a priest is on his knees and presenting him a crux ansata, a sistrum, and the sceptre of Osiris. A priest is presenting offerings to a procession of four rams, each with the horns of Ammon. In a group of monsters is a lion with the head of a crocodile, and the forepart of a serpent for his tail. In one place Osiris is seen with the head of an ibis, and above is the crescent and dark disk of the moon. There is also a serpent with two female heads, and a tree growing out of its back."† Mendes or Pan was worshipped in the form of a goat : he represents capricorn, and was typical of animal reproduction.

* Voyage, tom. II. p. 20.   † Hamilton's Egyptiaca, p. 107.

Passalacqua's collection contains two embalmed heads of the ram (Numbers 322 and 323). They are enveloped in bandages, and the horns are apparent. One of these (322) is figured in Plate XII. *fig.* 3. The same rich collection has also the head of a lamb enveloped in its bandages.*

Mr. Wilkinson tells me that though the sheep is sometimes represented in the tombs of Thebes, it never occurs among the animals slaughtered either for sacrifices or for private use.

The Bear—The Hyæna—The Hippopotamus.

Bears and hyænas were held sacred at Papremis. So also was the hippopotamus ; and it is probable they were buried here, as the town was dedicated to Typhon or the evil principle, who was supposed to be appeased by the worship rendered to the hippopotamus, the symbol of the Typhonian character. M. De Pauw† has asserted that this animal, at the present day, never descends below the cataracts of the Nile. In ancient times the race must have been much more numerous than at present.

The hippopotamus was an emblem of the western pole, the Ζοφος, or dark region, which swallows up the sun and the other celestial bodies. He was seen figured in this view in the temple of Apollonopolis, standing with open jaws, and gaping upwards to engulf the descending lights of heaven.‡ The crocodile was also, according to Horapollo, a symbol of the West; and the tail of this animal was the hieroglyphic character which expressed darkness in the sacred sculpture of the Egyptians.§ The crocodile and the hippopotamus are the true Typhonian animals, and are emblems of blackness and destruction.‖ At Edfou there was a temple dedicated to Typhon, and the ornaments exteriorly and interiorly are characteristic of the evil genius. The hippopotamus was an object of horror to the Egyptians. The paintings in this temple represent the triumph of the hippopotamus.¶

* No. 324.　　† II. 108·　　‡ Prichard, p. 80. Euseb. Præp. Evang. lib. iii. c. 12.
§ Horapoll. Hierog. lib. i. c. 69, 70.

‖ Or " the black colour, *Chame.*" The tail of the hippopotamus was thence chosen as the hieroglyphic for Egypt, Khemi.

¶ Denon, II. 18.

The Ichneumon.—Viverra Ichneumon, *Linn*.

THE ichneumon, or mangouste of Buffon, a species of weasel inhabiting Egypt, and abounding particularly on the banks of the Nile, has been classed among the sacred animals of Egypt. It was frequently called Pharaoh's rat, and was nourished with the greatest care, and treated with the utmost tenderness. Lands were appropriated to its support, and it was fed on bread and milk, and fish of the Nile. It was embalmed after death. These honours have been paid to it, it is supposed, from its power in checking the numbers of the crocodile, by destroying the eggs of that animal. M. Blanchard says* that he breaks the eggs without profiting by it, for that he does not eat them. " Hors d'intérêt, il agit par un instinct, pour délivrer, autant qu'il est en sa nature, l'homme des dangers auxquels l'exposeroit la multiplication de ces animaux, si tous ces œufs venoient à bien." It is not now domesticated in Egypt, as it destroys poultry. It is common in parts of Egypt where the crocodile is not now found, and rare in Upper Egypt, below the cataracts, where this animal abounds. A species of tortoise, called Thirse, Tarsèh, or Tirsèh, is employed in effecting the destruction of the crocodile. As soon as the young one is hatched, and reaches the river, he is attacked by the tortoise and devoured. Sonnini has treated of the ichneumon somewhat at length.† He states that the animal, with great dispositions to familiarity, is yet not altogether domestic in Egypt. When he visited that country none were reared by this people, nor had they even the recollection of their ancestors' having reared any. But Belon, and Prosper Alpinus, assert that they had seen them domesticated, which can only be accounted for by supposing that they had seen some preserved by some individuals, rather from motives of curiosity than utility. Its destruction of poultry would more than counterbalance its good in the destruction of rats and mice, so easily effected also by the cat.

* Mem. de l'Acad. des Inscrip. vol.   , p. 28.   † Vol. I. p. 295.

I have never seen an embalmed ichneumon, nor is there a single specimen in the collection of M. Passalacqua, or any other that I am acquainted with. The animal was worshipped at Heracleopolis, and the feuds and animosities excited between the inhabitants of this place and those of Arsinoë are well known, arising naturally out of the exercise of the destructive power of the ichneumon upon the eggs of the crocodile, this latter animal being there an object of worship.

SHREW-MOUSE.

THIS animal was worshipped at Boutos, near the Sebenytic mouth of the Nile. The temple of Latona, whence the oracles of this goddess were delivered, is described by Herodotus as having been very magnificent, and furnished with porticos forty cubits in height, and a shrine of one solid stone, having equal sides, each forty cubits in length; and Latona is described as denoting night or darkness. The goddess assumed the form of the mygale or shrew-mouse to avoid the pursuit of Typhon, and the Egyptians held this animal sacred from its supposed blindness, and regarded it as an emblem of primæval night or darkness. M. De Pauw says* that the shrew-mouse was revered at Atribis and embalmed after death in a sepulchre for the purpose at *Butos*, although the distance between the two places was more than fifty miles. Herodotus mentions† the city of Buto as the place of sacred sepulture for this animal.

Two specimens of Sorex (musaraigne) are in Passalacqua's collection embalmed. They were found at Thebes.‡ It is curious, and the testimony of M. Geoffroy St. Hilaire places the matter beyond dispute, that although this class consists of the smallest known species of mammiferous animals, yet these specimens are the largest of the kind known, and much beyond the size of that named by St. Hilaire as the *Sorex Indicus.* M. Passalacqua's collection has also twenty-five specimens of another species of musaraigne (vulgaris?). Strabo speaks of a part of the Cynopolitan nome consecrated to these animals.

* II. 103.   † Euterpe, § 67.   ‡ Nos. 396, 397.

The Bull—Apis.

———

" Quos dignetur agros, aut quo se gurgite Nili
Mergat adoratus trepidis pastoribus Apis."*
Statii Sylvarum, lib. iii. carm. 2. ver. 115.

———

Apis, the bull, was consecrated both to the sun and moon. This animal, when having certain peculiar marks,† was affirmed by the priests to have been begotten by celestial influence, and was supposed to contain the soul of Osiris. He consequently received great honour from the Egyptians. The characters‡ of the sacred bull were that he should be of a black colour, having a square white mark upon his forehead, the figure of an eagle upon his back, a lump under his tongue resembling a beetle, and a white spot in the form of a crescent on his right side. To these were added that the hairs of his tail should be double or cleft. His black colour was symbolical of the sun, the action of which would render bodies black; the square white spot on the forehead belonged to the moon, so also the crescent on the right side. The following note of M. Larcher§ is deserving of attention here :—" Ælian‖ says that the god Apis was recognized by twenty-nine marks,¶ and that the Egyptians did not admit those mentioned by Herodotus

* " Say in what meads the god-like Apis deigns
    To browze before the crowd of suppliant swains,
    Till, headlong mid the sacred waters hurl'd,
    Sated with life, he quits the grieving world ?"

† Strabo, XVII. 1.

‡ In the tomb of Osirei, the father of Rameses the Great, exhibited by M. Belzoni, there was a representation of Apis answering precisely to the description I have given, and also the ceremonial of the sacrifice of a bull in honour of Psammis.

§ Herodot. Thalia, § 38.   ‖ De Nat. Animal. lib. xi. cap. 10. p. 617.

¶ The twenty-nine marks alluded to by Ælian, he says, had all the same mystical import, not easy to be understood by the profane. One was a symbol of the increase of the Nile; a second was a microcosm of the world; a third was an allusion to the darkness of chaos, &c. &c.

and Aristagoras. At the time when Ælian wrote, the religion of the Egyptians had fallen into disuse, and the sacred language was entirely forgotten. The testimony of Herodotus, therefore, is of greater weight than that of a compiler, who was not characterized by the most solid judgment. Ammianus Marcellinus affirms* that this bull should have the figure of a crescent marked on his side. Our historian may have forgotten this mark; or in his time it might not have been thought necessary."

Apis was called by the Greeks EPAPHUS; but the Egyptians affirm that Apis was prior to Epaphus by some hundreds of centuries.† Larcher has endeavoured to account for this disagreement. "We know very well," he says,‡ that the Greeks, from a casual resemblance of a name, or even of one syllable of it, forged vain genealogies, and attributed to their own heroes the origin of almost all other nations and their gods. They had learned in Egypt that the mother of Apis was rendered fruitful§ by a ray from heaven, by a flash of lightning, by a ray of the moon, says Plutarch, or, as the Egyptians sometimes express it, ἐπαφῇ τῆς Σελήνης, by the contact of the moon. This expression Ἐπαφὴ, which bears some analogy to the Epaphus, has perhaps occasioned them to identify the two. The worship of Apis was most prevalent at Memphis. The soul of Osiris was supposed to reside within the body of the bull, bearing the marks that have been described; and, as Osiris was zealously devoted to the improvement of agriculture, the bull became the symbol of it. Alexander, Germanicus, Augustus, Titus, Adrian, Septimus Severus, and others, consulted and worshipped Apis. There can be little doubt but the marks were contrived by the priests, who secretly reared the bull intended for Apis. His birth was announced as the consequence of celestial influence, and the feasts in honour of it were called Theophania, and continued during seven days in each year. Ælian says,‖ they built a temple to the new god, facing the east, in pursuance of the order of Mercury, and nourished the young calf with milk for four months. After this time, and at the new moon, he was visited by the priests, and saluted by the appellation of Apis. He was then conducted with great pomp and splendour to Nilopolis, where he was kept for forty

---

* Lib. xxii. cap. 14. p. 257. † Ælian, Hist. Nat. lib. xi. c. 10.

‡ Herodot. Thalia, § 27. § Herod. lib. iii. § 28. ‖ Hist. Animal. lib. ix.

days, during which time women only were suffered to visit him.   Thus inaugurated, he was conveyed to Memphis, and became sacred to all the world.   He was placed near to the temple of Vulcan,* which was of great splendour, and surrounded with columns and statues of colossal dimensions. Pliny says† that he was furnished with two beds, or apartments, and that good or ill was augured according to the selection of these which he made upon being consulted.‡   He gave responses to individuals by taking food from their hands; and refusing that which was offered by Germanicus, it is said, that prince died shortly after.   " Responsa privatis dat, è manu consulentium cibum capiendo.   Germanici Cæsaris manum aversatis est, haud multo post extincti."§

The priests occasionally exhibited him to the people, and the animal was allowed to indulge in a meadow specially allotted to him.   He might be seen at all times through a window; but once a year a solemn sacrifice of a heifer was made to him, having similar marks to those with which he was adored.   The priests, as we learn from Plutarch, gave the Apis his water from a well particularly set apart for this purpose, restraining him entirely from drinking of the Nile; not that the river was regarded by them as impure (for nothing could be held in greater veneration by the Egyptians than the Nile), but because the waters of that river were remarkable for their tendency to fatten and nourish, and this was a condition they studiously endeavoured to prevent; for we are told that they were studious that their bodies might sit as light and easy about their souls as possible, and that their mortal part might not oppress and weigh down the more divine and immortal one.

Pausanias describes ‖ the mode of worship to Apis.   Those who came to consult the god burnt incense on an altar in the evening amidst numerous lighted lamps.   A piece of money of copper of the country was placed on the altar to the right of the statue: the applicant then applied his mouth

---

* According to Aratus (Phœnom. in Capricor.) it was in this temple the kings were crowned, and initiated into the most profound mysteries of their religion.

† Hist. Nat. lib. 8.

‡ " Les prêtres, en le ramenant du pâturage, le laissaient entrer du côté qui lui plaisait davantage."—*Biog. Univ.* tom. LIII. p. 249.　　§ Lib. viii. cap. 46.　　‖ Lib. viii.

to the ear of the deity to make his interrogation. The worship offered to Apis was very solemn; oxen were sacrificed to him. Yellowish or red bulls were permitted to be immolated, those being the colours of Typhon who massacred Osiris, and whose members were placed in the body of a cow, some say a heifer of wood, by Isis. The city of Busiris took its name from this circumstance, and there was to be found the tomb of Osiris.

But the days of Apis were numbered, and the priests, multiplying the number five by itself, gave the number of letters in the Egyptian alphabet, and at the termination of twenty-five years the bull Apis was drowned in the fountain of the priests, according to Pliny,* or in the Nile. It has been inferred that Apis was the tutelary divinity of the solar year, which consisted of 365 days, and of the cycle of twenty-five years, and it has been well conceived by M. Savary that the priests, by fixing the course of his life to twenty-five years, and by making the installation of a new Apis concur with the renewal of this period, had probably perceived, as the result of long meteorological observations, that this revolution always brought about abundant seasons. Nothing was better calculated to procure a favourable reception of this emblematical divinity from the people, since his birth was a presage to them of a happy inundation, and of all the treasures of teeming nature.† After death the body was embalmed and deposited in the temple of Serapis at Memphis. Should he not have survived the period of twenty-five years, his death was announced to the people by the priests who mourned his dissolution, and shaved their heads, until another animal, having the proper marks, should be produced. The people also mourned for the defunct bull. In short, his death occasioned general consternation throughout Egypt. The priests hastened to find another bull, and to perform the funeral ceremonies to the defunct animal. We are told they began by opening the two brazen gates of Memphis, the noise occasioned by which was exceedingly great. These gates were named Cocyte and Lethe, the gates of groans and forgetfulness, in reference to the mourning for the dead Apis, and to the joy at the acquisition of the new one. The expenses of

---

* Non.est fas eum certos vitæ excedere annos, mersumque in sacerdotum fonte enecant.—Lib. viii. c. 46.

† See Savary, Lettres sur l'Egypte, tom. II. p. 192.

the entombment of Apis were very great.   Diodorus Siculus relates* that
the priest to whom the duty was consigned expended not only a considerable
sum amassed expressly for this purpose, but also fifty talents of silver
which were borrowed from the royal treasury on this occasion.   This was
in the time of Ptolemy the son of Lagus.

All the mystic phenomena that attended the birth, growth, character,
death, and worship of Apis, bore an obvious reference to the agriculture of
Egypt, and the fertility occasioned by the inundation of the Nile.†

The sacred bull was called Apis at Memphis, Mnevis at Heliopolis, and Basis
at Hermonthis.‡   Father Martin§ makes a distinction between Apis and
Mnevis: the former, he says, was the sanctuary of the soul of Osiris, and his
living image, as well as that of Isis; whilst the latter merely represented Osiris.
The worship of Mnevis was principally at Heliopolis, and he had the same
rites as Apis.   M. De Pauw tells us‖ that Pharaoh Bocchoris conceived the
idea of removing Mnevis from Heliopolis, and by that means he lost entirely
the esteem of the people, among whom such animals had been worshipped for
a greater length of time than the Roman empire had existed.   From the same
author we learn that Apis did not disappear altogether from Memphis until
the reign of Theodosius; and, according to M. Jablonski,¶ the first had been
consecrated 1171 years before our present era.   Thus a regular succession
had taken place during a period of at least 1550 years; probably longer,
as Jablonski has been guided in this sentiment by Eusebius rather than
Manethon, whose authority would have been preferable.   The late Dr.
Young has stated** that the sacred characters denoting Apis are pretty
clearly determined by the triple inscriptions; the enchorial name, he says,
is perfectly so.   If, however, any doubt remained on the subject, the learned
Doctor thinks it would be removed by an examination of the inscriptions on
four vases found by Paul Lucas at Abousir,†† the Busiris of the ancients;

* Lib. i. c. 6.   † See Rees's Cyclopædia.   Art. *Apis*.   ‡ Strabo, lib. xvii.
§ Explication de Divers Monumens Singuliers qui ont rapport à la Religion de plusieurs
Peuples, 4to.   Paris, 1739, p. 190.
‖ Philos. Dissert. II. 141.   ¶ Pantheon Ægyptiac. lib. iv. cap. 2.
** Art. *Egypt*, Suppl. to Encycl. Brit. p. 58.
†† Voyage dans la Turquie, 2 vols. 12mo.   Amst. 1720. Tom. I. p. 346.

that is, the BE OSHIRI or sepulchre of Osiris, as Diodorus translates it. Lucas established the truth of the tradition of the worship of Apis at this place by finding the mummy of a bullock in the catacombs. Now, Dr. Young tells us that all the inscriptions on the vases end with a bullock, preceded by this character, though the angles are turned in a different direction from those of the inscription of Rosetta, so that the two forms of the character seem to have been used indifferently. With this latitude Dr. Young has no difficulty in identifying the name, as it occurs in almost every line of the inscriptions on the great sarcophagus of granite formerly at Cairo, called the Lover's Fountain, and now in the British Museum, which there is some reason to suppose, from the frequency of this name, may have been intended for receiving a mummy of the bull Apis. The candour of Dr. Young, however, leads him to confess that in several other monuments the names of the deities are introduced in a manner somewhat similar, with an evident relation to the designation of some human being whom they are intended to commemorate.

Paul Lucas, I have mentioned, says that he saw in the catacombs of Abousir several heads of a bull, and also a case containing an embalmed bull.* Father Sicard, according to the authority of Hassalquist, sent a specimen of this kind to Paris. The French Commission discovered near Saccara a case full of embalmed portions of the bull, which proved by a comparison of the bones to be of the same species as our domestic ox.

In the hypogæa near Abousir, Mons. Cailliaud also saw the bull bandaged with great precision, but the limbs formed only a mass with the body. The head preserved its natural form, and the eyes were painted on the cloth. On the top of the head was the spot characteristic of Apis. The horns were surrounded with bandages. Mons. Cailliaud observed that sometimes branches of the date tree were placed in these mummies to preserve their form. The dust contained within them was of a yellowish colour, and offensive; it was very penetrating, and probably consisted of the residue of the flesh mixed with the natron and other embalming materials. After being enveloped in the bandages, they were bound with cords made of the

---

* Voyage fait en 1714, tom. II. p. 136.

2 D

bark of the palm-tree and of hemp.   Mons. Cailliaud saw eight chambers of these mummies; they were placed over each other.   I have figured an embalmed bull in Plate XII. *fig.* 6, from Belzoni.

Cows were never killed in sacrifice, nor was their flesh permitted to be eaten by the Egyptians.   This custom of abstaining from the meat of cows was owing no doubt to the paucity of those animals in Egypt, and the fear of exhausting their small number.   Porphyry says* that both the Egyptians and Phœnicians would rather partake of human flesh than of that of a cow. When dead they were committed to the sand, river, or taken to a burying-place at Atharbechis, whither their bones were brought in boats; but the bulls were buried in the suburbs of the city where they died, with their horns projecting from the ground, where they remained until putrefied, when their bones were collected together and conveyed to Prosopitis, an island of the Delta, where they were all buried.

* De Abstinent. ab esu Animal. lib. ii. § 11.

CHAPTER XIV.

ON THE SACRED ANIMALS—AVES.

Nahamou the goddess characterising the vulture—worshipped at Thebes—falcon—several species found embalmed—the hawk—an emblem of Osiris—worshipped throughout Egypt, but particularly at Philæ—the eagle held sacred in Thebais—the screech-owl at Sais—the swallow found embalmed at Thebes—the ibis—consecrated to Thoth—worshipped throughout Egypt, but especially at Hermopolis—innumerable mummies of the ibis to be found in Egypt.

Vulture—Eagle—Hawk—Hobby—Owl—Swallow.

Nohemouo, or Nahamou, is the goddess characterising the vulture. This is the companion to Thoth, and from the legends accompanying the emblem appears to preside over the preservation of offspring. A worship was rendered to this goddess in the same temple as that in which Thoth was adored. The vulture was a most useful bird in Egypt in removing much of the carrion infecting tne atmosphere, and it was a capital offence to destroy it. Mr. Madden states that at this day some religious people at Cairo make a merit of feeding them daily.

A specimen of the large vulture embalmed is in M. Passalacqua's collection (No. 365—Thebes).

Falcon: Several species of falcon are mentioned by Passalacqua: Falco subbuteo (*Hobreau*), Falco nisus (*L'Epervier*), Falco gallinarius (*Le Grand Epervier*), Falco hypogeolis (*Aigle pecheur*). All these embalmed are in M. Passalacqua's collection.

The representation of Osiris with the head of the hawk is of most frequent occurrence, and has been already noticed as common in the tombs and on the cases of mummies. In the tomb exhibited by Belzoni he was to be seen in almost every part, and Dr. Young described him as representing

Arueris, the son of the sun, appearing as the tutelary genius of Egypt, in intimate union with Osiris, to whom the hawk was dedicated, and of whom this figure was probably viewed as an essence and emanation.

M. De Pauw says* two towns, known by the name of Hieracopolis, fed sparrow-hawks; but a different species brought from Ethiopia, and not hitherto ascertained by naturalists, was consecrated in the temple of Philæ. The eagle was revered in Thebais, and the screech-owl at Sais; the vulture, the ibis, the tadorne, the stork, and the puet, were universally sacred, although they had no temples. The sacred hawks were kept in the island of Philæ in granite shrines or cages, some of which remain to this day. Herodotus tells us that whoever killed a hawk or an ibis could not by any means escape capital punishment. Although the worship of the hawk was common to all Egypt, yet it was most respected at Philæ. It was a larger species than ours, and delivered the country from the scorpions. It is said that a hawk carried to Thebes a book attached to it by a red thread, which contained an account of the ceremonies of the worship of the gods, and that in memory of this event the registrars of the temples carry on their heads a red turban and a portion of the wing of the hawk.

In Plate XIII. *fig.* 2, I have represented a hawk bandaged up and with envelopes, giving to it a human face and appearance. The drawing has been taken from M. Passalacqua's collection. Plate XIII. *fig.* 1 is the representation of an embalmed hawk from my own collection.

Owl.

M. Passalacqua obtained three specimens of embalmed owls, one of which was the great owl, with short tufts of feathers on his head, and which was named *Ascalaphus* by M. Savigny, who was the first to describe this species. It was found at Thebes. It is represented in Plate XIII. *fig.* 3.

Hirundo—Swallow.

Sixteen specimens of this small bird were found embalmed by M. Passalacqua. They were obtained at Thebes.

* II. 111.

THE IBIS.

THIS bird was consecrated to Thoth* or Theuth, who is regarded as Mercury as well as Anubis. The Greek and Latin writers have uniformly associated Thoth with Hermes, or Mercury. To this god all the science and all the learning of the Egyptians were attributed; and the books containing this knowledge were called the Hermetic books. In the description of the paintings upon the cases containing mummies, I have already noticed the representation of Thoth the Egyptian Mercury, and the part of Scribe which he appears to sustain in the scene of judgment. Next to Osiris this deity, perhaps, is the most commonly figured of the whole Egyptian mythology, and he is repeatedly seen with the head of the ibis. This bird on a perch constitutes his hieroglyphical name; in the manuscripts a feather has been found to represent this deity. It is said that, when the gods were pursued by Typhon, Mercury eluded his research by assuming the form of the ibis. Hermopolis was the nome principally devoted to the worship of this bird. It was, however, prevalent throughout Egypt, and of no other animal are there so many mummies to be found. It has been remarked that the ibis, when viewed in a particular position, sitting with its neck bent forwards, and its head concealed under its wing, resembles the form of a heart.† The heart was looked upon by the Egyptians as the seat of the intellect, and in this way it has been attempted to explain the attribute of this bird, which was no less than to preside over and inspire all sacred or mystical learning of the Egyptian hierarchy. Horapollo describes the Egyptian Hermes as " the president of the heart, or a personification of that wisdom which was supposed to dwell in the inward parts."

This bird was esteemed so sacred by the Egyptians that if any one

* Plato in Phædro, vol. III.   Horapollo Hierog. lib. i. c. 10 and 36.   Ælian. Hist. Animal. lib. x. c. 29.   † Horapollo—Ælian.

voluntarily killed it he was put to death. Should the death of the animal have been occasioned by accident, the penalty was reduced by the priests, provided the individual displayed his grief, to a pecuniary fine. Porphyry remarks* upon the practice of the Egyptians to wash themselves three times a day in cold water; on getting out of bed, before eating, and immediately before retiring to rest; and Plutarch says† that those of the priests who observe the law most strictly use, for the purpose of purifying themselves, pure water, of which the ibis has drank; for this bird, so far from drinking any water that could occasion disease, or might contain poison, will not even approach it.

Two species of ibis were known in Egypt, the black and the white; the latter, according to Herodotus, was a domesticated bird, the former the enemy of the serpents, and dwelling in the deserts. Linnæus and Buffon were ignorant of the true Egyptian ibis; Bruce saw it and described it as the Abou-hannès or father John. M. Savigny has treated of the natural and mythological history of this bird at considerable length.‡ He says that he has studied the bird along with the white ibis found embalmed in a very perfect state, and that it was impossible to ascertain the slightest difference between them. The late lamented Cuvier gave also his attention to this subject, and has figured in the Annales du Museum d'Histoire Naturelle (tom. iv.) the Numenius Ibis, which he conceives to be the true Egyptian ibis. He examined two mummies taken from the pits at Saccara, and found the bones smaller than those of the Tantalus Ibis of Linnæus; they were only of the size of the curlew, the beak of which resembles that of the ibis. The plumage is white with the wing-feathers tipped with black according to the ancients. Dr. Shaw's account corresponds with that of M. Cuvier. The left humerus of an ibis examined by Cuvier had been fractured and re-united, which would not, in all probability, have been the case, had the bird been in its wild state. This M. Cuvier regards as a proof of its domesticity in the Egyptian temples. He has compared the skeleton of the ibis with that of the curlew, and given a table of the same.§ The following are the conclusions drawn by this most talented naturalist and his de-

* De Abstinent. ab esu Animal. lib. iv. § 7.   † De Iside et Osiride, p. 381.

‡ Savigny (J. C.) Hist. Nat. et Mytholog. de l'Ibis, 8vo. Paris, 1805.   § Annal. p. 122.

scription of the bird: "L'ibis des anciens n'est point l'ibis de Perrault et de Buffon, qui est un *tantalus*, ni l'ibis d'Hasselquist, qui est un *ardea*, ni l'ibis de Maillet, qui est un *vautour;* mais c'est un *numenius* ou *courlis* qui n'a été decrit et figuré au plus que par Bruce sous le nom d'*abou-hannès*. Je le nomme Numenius Ibis, *albus, capite et collo nudis, remigum apicibus, rostro et pedibus nigris, remigibus secundariis elongatis nigro violaceis.*" *

Cuvier states that he found in an embalmed ibis the remains of serpents of which the skin and scales had not been digested. This circumstance is put forth in support of the opinion entertained by the ancients as to the power of the bird in destroying and feeding upon these reptiles, and thus, in some manner, account for the great respect and veneration in which the ibis was held by the ancient Egyptians; but M. Savigny† has endeavoured to prove that this bird did not feed upon such animals, and he grounds his conjecture against this commonly-received opinion from the structure of the beak and the tongue and other parts, and the known food of other birds of a similar nature, such as the curlews, who subsist upon small shell-fish, worms, little fish, and aquatic insects. The white ibis is now very rare in Egypt. M. Savigny saw some in descending the Nile in his way to Rosetta; but he was not able to follow them; and he could only obtain an examination of the bird three months afterwards, whilst in the environs of Damietta and Menzalé.

The black ibis was frequently brought to him, but the white only once. He thus describes the manners of these birds:—"Ces oiseaux apparemment fatigués m'ont alors paru tristes et peu disposés à prendre de la nourriture. Ils se tenoient haut sur jambes, le corps presque horisontal, le cou fléchi, la tête inclinée, et ils dirigeoient celle-ci, tantôt à droite, tantôt à gauche, tantôt la portoient en avant, ou la ramenoient, en frappant la terre du bout du bec. Quelquefois, ils ne posoient que sur une patte. Ils n'étoient que peu sauvages; ils ouvroient pourtant le bec, dès qu'on en approchoit le doigt, comme pour se défendre; mais, ainsi que je l'ai dit, ce bec est beaucoup trop foible pour pincer, et il l'est sur-tout dans l'ibis noir."‡ M. Savigny then goes on to state that the black ibis is ordinarily seen in troops, but the white solitary, or in groups of not more than eight or ten individuals.

These birds are now not resident in Egypt. They appear as soon as the Nile begins to rise, and as it advances their numbers also increase, and as it sinks they also diminish; their migration is complete when the inundation has passed. Connecting the appearance of the ibis with the rise of the Nile and the consequent fecundity of the earth, M. Savigny conceives the first motives to the veneration of this bird by the Egyptians to have arisen, and not to any power exercised by it in the destruction of the serpents. The ibis is never found in the neighbourhood of salt water. M. Savigny sought for it in vain even at the Lake Menzalé, which, receiving the water of the Nile, is rendered scarcely saline.

At Medinet-Abou there is a temple especially dedicated to Thoth, the Protector of the Sciences, the inventor of writing and of all the useful arts, and, in short, the organizer of human society. In this temple he is represented with the face of an ibis, and ornamented with varied head-dresses. The Ibéum or city of the ibis, wherein those sacred birds were generally buried, is a little north of Minyeh and Oshmúneïn, and is now called Tahà-el-âmúdeïn (Taha of the Two columns). At Memphis there are thousands of the embalmed ibis,* but they are generally very badly preserved. They appear to have been made with great heat, for, of one hundred drawn from the pits at Saccara, Jomard says hardly one was found perfect or entire. They were either prepared with bitumen or natron; the latter were in a very bad condition. I have a specimen in which the plumage is very fairly preserved. As to the position of these birds in their embalmed state, the wings are placed in their natural situation along the sides of the body; the head and neck beneath the left wing, and the beak extends the whole length

---

* M. Denon says, " On trouvé, dans le désert de Saccara, un grand nombre de grottes souterraines, où étaient déposées des momies d'hommes, et particulièrement un grand nombre de momies d'ibis. Ces souterrains consistent en une longue galerie divisée en plusieurs embranchemens, des deux côtés desquels sont des réduits de huit pieds de haut sur dix de large. C'est là que sont les pots qui renferment les momies d'ibis : leur disposition est celle de bouteilles dans les caves. Il est probable que Memphis était la sépulture de tous les ibis morts dans les temples, ou trouvés dans les différentes parties de l'Egypte."—*Voyage*, II. 40.

of the body; the leg is drawn upon the thigh, and the thigh lies upon the body. In this manner the bird assumes a somewhat conical shape. M. Savigny reports that M. Olivier found in the mummy pits of birds at the plain of Saccara an embalmed ibis not done up in the usual form, and in the interior of this mummy there were shells of the eggs of the bird, small quadrupeds of different kinds, some entire, but of others only portions. This shows that the respect entertained by the Egyptians for the bodies of animals was so great as to extend itself to the preservation of even the fragments of their bodies. The eggs of the ibis have been found preserved in the tombs dedicated to this bird.* It has been said to be the only animal enclosed in a case when embalmed. This, however, is not the fact, but it is excessively rare for any other animal to be so arrangèd. At Memphis the bird is deposited in a vase; at Hermopolis in small oblong cases of wood or stone; and at Thebes only in its envelopes.† M. Passalacqua met with a specimen of this bird with the human form. I am happy in acknowledging my obligation to this distinguished traveller for a drawing of this specimen. See Plate XIII. *fig.* 6.

In Plate LXI. *fig.* 3, of "Monumens Egyptiens," published in folio at Rome in 1791, there is a representation of the mummy of an ibis in the human form; and Count De Caylus has figured in the sixth volume of his Recueil d'Antiquités (Plate XI. *fig.* 1) another specimen of mummied ibis in human form. The bandages are very neatly applied, and folded with great precision. This specimen was in the possession of the Duc de Sully; it was not opened. It measured one foot seven inches and four lines, and nowhere was the circumference greater than five inches and a half.

The mummy pots are either of common stone or blue ware, or a hard polished stone, and are of a lengthened conical figure.‡

ANAS NILOTICA—TURKEY GOOSE.

BELZONI has figured § for an ibis that which appears to me to have been a goose. This bird we know constantly occurs as an hieroglyphical emblem, and I have a small but exceedingly perfect specimen which had been pre-

---

* Passalacqua, 347. I have a well preserved specimen of this kind.

† See Plate XIII. *fig,* 7, 8,   ‡ See Plate XIII. *fig. 5,* and vol. V. d'Antiq. Descr. de l'Egypte.

§ See Plate XIII. *fig.* 9.

served by embalming.   It is represented in Plate XIII. *fig.* 10.   Browne
mentions* the *Anas Nilotica* of Linnæus (the turkey goose) as a large fowl,
the flesh of which is palatable and salubrious food.

* Travels, p. 65.

CHAPTER XV.

ON THE SACRED ANIMALS—AMPHIBIA—PISCES—INSECTA.

The crocodile typical of Typhon—principally worshipped at Arsinoe—mode of feeding the consecrated crocodile—used as food at Elephantis, Tentyris, Heracleopolis, and Apollono-polis—crocodiles embalmed and placed in catacombs expressly excavated for them—serpents—the god Cneph worshipped in Thebais—the worship of serpents common throughout Egypt—the adder—the uræus—the asp—the coluber—the ophiophagi—lizard—toad—fishes : lepidotus a species of carp—oxyrhynchus—mæotis forbidden at Elephantis—Variole—probably the perch held in veneration at Latopolis—the eel—doubtful whether to be considered as a sacred animal—sir—found embalmed according to Abd'Allatif—Insects. The Scarabæus—synopsis of the genera and species—Buprestis—probably the Œstrus—Cantharis—squill or sea-onion.

THE CROCODILE.

IT was at Crocodilopolis, or the City of Crocodiles, a town of Egypt, S. E. of the Lake Moeris, afterwards called Arsinoë, in honour of the wife and sister of Ptolemy Philadelphus, that the worship of this animal was particularly practised. The crocodile was held sacred at Thebes, Ombos, in the environs of Lake Moeris, and in other parts of Egypt.

At Arsinoë the priests nourished one to which the name of Suchus was given ; it was fed upon bread, flesh, and wine offered to it by strangers; it was preserved in a particular lake, and, whilst reposing, the priests approached the animal, opened his mouth, and put the food within its jaws; after its repast it usually descended into the water and swam away, but it would suffer itself to be handled, and pendants of gold and precious stones were placed about it.*   Strabo relates that his host, a man of consideration,

---

* Mem. de l'Acad. des Inscript., tom. IX. p. 25.

conducted him and his companions to the lake, and that he there saw the crocodile at the border of it; that one of the priests to whom was entrusted the care of the animal opened his mouth and placed within it a cake, another a portion of flesh, and a third poured in some wine. The repast thus made, the animal passed over to the other side, to receive from other hands similar marks of attention.

Diodorus Siculus* says that the Egyptians reverenced the crocodile on account of their king Menes, whose life was said to have been preserved when in danger of drowning, by being floated to land upon the back of one of these animals.

Between Essouan and Thebes is the scite of the Ombite nome. The temple of Ombos, which from its Greek inscription † first gave rise to the conjecture that, perhaps, many of the Egyptian temples may be attributed to the Ptolemies, was dedicated to the worship of the crocodile. In Elephantis, the crocodile was called campsa, which signifies an ark or receptacle, and the people of this city are said to have eaten its flesh.

Herodotus tells us that in visiting the Labyrinth he was not permitted to descend into the subterranean apartments, because they were strictly guarded, and were the places of interment for the sacred crocodiles, and the sepulchres of the kings under whose care they had been constructed. Mr. Hamilton observed two long narrow subterraneous galleries immediately under the temple of Isis, near the level of the water at Ombos, and he says that they are constructed of very strong masonry, in the rustic manner, and have every appearance of being continued as far as the great temple, serving perhaps as secret passages for the priests in their mysterious ceremonies, or more probably for the convenience of conducting the sacred crocodiles into the adytum of the temple.‡ M. de Pauw states§ that in the year 1770, having been particularly engaged in studying the topography of Egypt, it first occurred to him that Coptos, Arsinoë, and Crocodilopolis the second, the towns most remarkable for the adoration of crocodiles, were all situated on canals at some distance from the Nile. Thus, by the least negligence in allowing the ditches to be filled up, those animals, from being

* Lib. i.   † Hamilton's Egyptiaca, p. 75.   ‡ Egyptiaca, p. 80.
§ Philos. Dissert. II. 100.

incapable of going far on dry land, could never have arrived at those three places, where they were considered as the symbols of water fit for drinking and watering the fields, as we learn from Ælian, and more particularly in a passage of Eusebius.* As long as this worship was in vogue, the government might remain assured that the superstitious would not neglect to repair the canals with the greatest exactness.

At Ombos, the remains only of two temples are now to be found. Denon and Hamilton have remarked upon the peculiarity of the larger temple in having two entrances. The greatest part of the paintings within relate to the adoration of the crocodile, and every where, according to Denon,† offerings are addressed to the figure of a deity (Sabak) in human form, but with the head of this animal. In the second temple, especially dedicated to Typhon, the figure of the evil genius is also represented with the head of a crocodile, but with the body of a bear. And at Taud Denon‡ saw another temple dedicated to the crocodile, where the animal was frequently represented with the head of a hawk; and to the south of this temple he found the ruins of a large pond which he presumes served either for the keeping of the crocodiles or the sacred fishes; however, it appears that they were not peculiar to temples where the crocodile was adored, but were merely tanks for religious use.

Although the flesh of this animal has a musky flavour, it was used as food at Elephantis, Tentyris, Heracleopolis, and Apollonopolis, which latter city, according to Strabo, was remarkable for making war against the crocodiles, and Mr. Hamilton observed in the large temple at Edfou the representation of a priest, over whose head a hawk is flying with the *crux ansata* in his claws, piercing the head of a crocodile with a spear. At Apollonopolis, all except the priests, who considered it as fish, were obliged to taste of the flesh of this animal. Strabo speaks§ largely of the aversion of the Tentyrites for the crocodile. The inhabitants of Tentyris, he says, abhor the crocodile, and make continual war against it as an animal of the most dangerous character. Others, regarding it as pernicious, avoid it; the Tentyrites, on the contrary, seek it out, and destroy it, if possible. The

* Præparat. Evangel. lib. iii. c. 11.   † Voyage, tom. II. p. 16.   ‡ Ibid. tom. II. p. 21.
§ Lib. xvii.

Psylla of Cyrene have been supposed to be endowed with supernatural powers over the serpents; the Tentyrites, in like manner, have been said to have no less dominion over the crocodile; in short, they boldly plunge into the midst of the Nile, and are not known to receive any injury from the attempt. In the spectacles at Rome, several crocodiles were placed in a basin of water, which, having an opening in one of the sides, admitted of their coming out. The Tentyrites threw themselves into the water amidst these animals, bound them with fillets, and dragged them out. Having exposed them to the gaze of the spectators, they, in the most intrepid manner, returned them into the basin. It is also said that they were so bold and dexterous in hunting these animals that they would leap on their backs, and placing a stick across their mouths as they opened them to bite, managed them as with a bridle, and brought them to land.*

The crocodiles were embalmed and deposited in catacombs purposely excavated for them. Mr. Hamilton visited one of these situated about a mile from Ombos; it was on the side of a light sandy bank, and the entrance was very low. The natives who showed it said it went to a great distance under ground, and they brought out many skulls, jaw-bones, spines, tails, &c., of these animals, on which were still to be seen the bitumen which preserved them, and the cotton cloth in which they were wrapped.† Belzoni speaks of having only seen the head of this animal embalmed, which was probably the case when they had attained any considerable size. The collection of M. Passalacqua contains eleven specimens of small crocodile, six of which have been unrolled. I owe to my learned friend Mr. Douce, in company with my friend Dr. Richardson, the opportunity of examining one of this kind of mummies, and to his kindness I am indebted for the specimen figured in Plate XII. *fig.* 8, 9, now in my collection. The bandage, or rather envelope in immediate contact with the body of the animal, was of a very coarse texture. Jomard says that he never met with an entire crocodile embalmed; it was only the head, the remainder of the animal being represented by stalks of palm-trees, bandages, &c. At Eleithia the crocodile was mostly found. He saw also false

* Univ. Hist. I. 500. Pliny, lib. viii. c. 45.   † Egyptiaca, p. 79.

mummies of the crocodile.* Two of the mummies in M. Passalacqua's collection (Nos. 351 and 354) are enveloped in bandages of different colours. Mr. Wilkinson acquaints me that mummied crocodiles are found in the caves of Maabdeh, opposite Manfaloot, perfectly preserved, and of the largest size.

Serpents.

"THE Egyptians (according to Porphyry) acknowledged one intellectual Author or Creator of the world, under the name of Cneph; and that they worshipped him in a statue of human form, and dark-blue complexion, holding in his hand a girdle and a sceptre, wearing upon his head a royal plume, and thrusting forth an egg out of his mouth. By the egg thrust out of the mouth of this god was meant the world, and from this Cneph was said to be generated, or produced, another god, whom the Egyptians call Phtha, and the Greeks Vulcan."

According to Plutarch Cneph was worshipped by the inhabitants of Thebaid, who refused to contribute any part towards the maintenance of the sacred animals, because they acknowledged no mortal god, and adored none but him whom they called Cneph, an uncreated and immortal being.

Strabo says the temple of Cnuphis, or Cneph, was in the island of Elephantine, at the confines of Egypt and Ethiopia. Cneph is often alluded to as the Phœnician Agathodæmon, or the good genius.†

The worship of serpents is said to have been common in all the temples of Egypt.‡ An innocent adder represented Cneph as the divine goodness. Strength and power were personified by an asp. The priests of Ethiopia and Egypt wore the latter coiled up in their bonnets of ceremony,§ and the diadem of the Pharaohs was ornamented with this emblem. It is the same as the urœus, which, bending its bosom forward, is represented on the front of the door of the Monolithe temple at Memphis. The serpent with his tail in his mouth has been supposed to be an Egyptian emblem, and to denote time and eternity, but it is not to be found in any sculptured mythological representation of an early epoch.

* p. 46.   † See Manethon. lib. i.; also, Euseb. Præp. Evang.

‡ Ælian, lib. x. c. 31.   § Diod. Sic. lib. iv.

Under various appellations and characters the serpent is to be found an object of adoration and worship.* In Egypt there was a serpent named *Thermuthis*, regarded as sacred, and statues of Isis have been found in which the tiara of the goddess has been made up of the representations of this reptile. This serpent *Thermuthis* is no other than the basilisk or royal serpent, figures of which are so common in the tombs, and may be seen by referring to the plates which accompany the travels of Belzoni.

" What the priests of Egypt have related," says de Pauw,† " concerning the *basilisk*, the *aspic*, and the *thermuthis*, is merely allegorical. This deceived the greater part of ancient authors, and particularly Ælian. The serpent *tebham-nasser*, easily known among the hieroglyphics, by the veil under its neck, which it puffs out at will, was the reptile generally taken for the aspic of Egypt, as we find from the words of Pliny and Lucian. Yet nothing is more certain than that the *tebham-nasser* has no venomous qualities, any more than the *ceraste*,‡ concerning which so many fables have been published. The Egyptian viper was the *aspic* employed by Cleopatra; and the same reptile occasioned the death of the learned Demetrius Phalareus, whose catastrophe is attributed by Cicero to the infamous dynasty of the Ptolemies."

The cerastes is very common in Egypt, but is never used as food as some have erroneously supposed.

Shaw says that more than 40,000 persons in Cairo and the neighbouring villages lived upon no other food than lizards and serpents. These people were called Ophiophagi (Eaters of serpents),‖ and among other religious

---

* M. Larcher quotes from Ælian (lib. xvii. cap. 5), that Phylarchus relates that great honours are rendered in Egypt to the asp, and that by these honours, and the food that is given to them, they become tame, and live amongst the children without doing them any harm. They come from their holes when called, by a noise made with the fingers. The Egyptians, after their dinner, place on the table meal moistened with wine and honey, and call to the asps, which come and take their food. This kind of asp is called " Thermouthis."

† Note, vol. I. p. 114.

‡ On the contrary the cerastes and the asp are decidedly, the most venomous of the serpents of Egypt. The asp is not the viper, but a species of cobra.

‖ It is scarcely necessary to observe that this is not true. The sect who perform the ceremony of tearing the snakes with their teeth in the religious processions of the pilgrimage, and

privileges they were entitled to the honour of attending more immediately upon the embroidered hangings of black silk, which are made every year for the *Kaaba* of *Mecca*, and conducted with great pomp and ceremony from the castle through the streets of Cairo. Upon these occasions numbers of this order sing and dance before it, and throw their bodies into a variety of enthusiastic gestures. These acts of devotion, however ludicrous they may appear to us, have been always looked upon with reverence by the Eastern nations.*

The sacred *cerastes* were embalmed and buried in the temple of Jupiter. They are frequent about Thebes. It is, therefore, not a little surprising that the French Commission in Egypt should not have obtained a better specimen than that which is figured in the Description de l'Egypte, and which is the only fragment of the kind seen by the naturalists and antiquarians engaged in this expedition. I have examined several and found them in various states of preparation. There were generally five or six or more enclosed in one envelope. In some instances the bandaging was very carefully arranged, and the cloth was of a red colour, in addition to the usually yellow stained linen. Mr. Davidson has also opened some mummies of snakes and his observations coincide with mine. In Plate XII., *fig.* 1, I have shown the case containing an embalmed serpent. From the figure of the animal which is carved upon the case, we may presume that it is the asp. The case is, Mr. Wilkinson thinks, made of tamarisk, extremely hard and dense; the whole has been plastered over and the serpent gilt. The embalmed contents are exceedingly hard, consisting of cloth that has been dipped into heated bitumen. I have not yet attempted to unroll it. I know of no other specimen of the kind, nor have I yet met with any traveller who has seen a similar one.

M. Passalacqua's collection contains two specimens only of embalmed serpent, and M. Geoffroy St. Hilaire was unable to determine their particular species.

the prophet's birthday, are the Saâdeh; but they do not eat them as food. The snake they use is generally the asp.

* Shaw's Travels, p. 430. See also Psal. cxlix. 3. Psal cl. 4. Exod. xv. 20. 2 Sam. vi. 14.

LIZARD.

ABD'ALLATIF speaks of a lizard of the species called sohliyya enclosed in bandages and embalmed with care. He heard of its being found upon opening a sarcophagus of stone in which also another was embalmed.

TOAD.

M. PASSALACQUA obtained four specimens of toad embalmed at Thebes.* M. Geoffroy St. Hilaire describes them thus:—" Batraciens, d'espèce voisine du crapaud."

PISCES.

LEPIDOTUS—OXYRHYNCHUS—MÆOTIS—VARIOLE—SPARUS—ANGUILLA—
SIR.

VARIOUS species of fish have been held sacred in different parts of Egypt. The carp at Lepidotum, a town of Thebais ; the mizdeh at Oxyrhynchus ; the Mæotis at Elephantis ; the variole at Latopolis ; the sparus at Syene.

According to Larcher the word LEPIDOTUS signifies scaled, but he is at a loss to conjecture the particular kind of fish. Linnæus thought it the red carp of the Nile (Cyprinus rubescens Niloticus). The Abbé Sicard, in his Memoirs of the Levantine Missions, asserts that it is the fish known at Cairo by the name of " bunni," which weighs from twenty to thirty pounds; and Maillet says that at Cairo there is a species of fish called " boulti," which greatly resembles the carp. Larcher remarks that if this be the " bunni" of Sicard it cannot be the same that Herodotus calls lepidotus, because, according to Macrisi, it was not always known in Egypt. Passalacqua states it to be the Cyprinus lepidotus, the binny, a small carp, and the fish that has given rise to the proverb, " If you can find a better eat me not." De Pauw states that at Lepidotum, a town situated on the right bank of the Nile, in the

* Catal. 422 to 425.

district of Thebais, a fish was prohibited as food. This he conceives, from a passage in Athenæus must have been a carp, yet its history is extremely doubtful. It has been taken for the *dorado*, consecrated among the Greeks to Cytherean Venus, the same with the Nephthys of Egypt, or the wife of Typhon; but the latter fish, he thinks, was too remarkable to be mistaken by the Greeks in changing the term *crysophrys*, used among them, to *lepidotos*, which expression was already employed in the Orphies.*

M. Passalacqua collected several specimens of embalmed fish enclosed within cases representing the form of the animal. Some of them were enveloped in bandages, others without. M. Geoffroy St. Hilaire examined them, and declared them to be of the species named by him in the Description de l'Egypte as the Cyprinus lepidotus.

The Egyptians were obliged by law to eat a fried fish on one day only in the whole year. This was the 9th of the month Thoth.

The OXYRHYNCHUS, doubtless, received as much honour at Oxyrhynchus as the lepidotus did at Lepidotum, and it is probable that this was confined to their cities, for Plutarch tells us that the Egyptians held in abomination the fishes lepidotus, phagrus, and oxyrhynchus, from their having devoured one of the fourteen portions of the body of Osiris, separated and scattered abroad by Typhon. Father Sicard calls the oxyrhynchus " quechoué," and describes it as of the size of the shad, and as having a pointed snout.† The disputes and wars between the Oxyrhynchites and Cynopolitans have already been adverted to.

The character of the MÆOTIS is unknown; it was forbidden at Elephantis.

The VARIOLE, de Pauw says, was the perch, and held in great veneration at Latopolis.

ANGUILLA. De Pauw denies to the eel the character of sacred; but the Greeks have ridiculed the Egyptians for their worship of this fish. I have already quoted the comic poet of Rhodes on this subject :—

> " You fancy in the little eel some power
> Of dæmon huge and terrible; within
> We stew it for our daintiest appetite."

* I. 129.

† A representation of the fish oxyrhynchus is given in Plate XLV. *fig. 5*, of the Monumens Egyptiens, Roma 1791, folio. The oxyrhynchus has been conjectured to be the pike,

And Antiphanes,* in his Lycon, also says that "the Egyptians, so wise in other things, are still more so in regarding the eel as the equal of the gods. It is of more consequence than they are. Our prayers suffice to obtain from the gods what we require of them; but we must spend a dozen drachmas to get a smell only at the eels, so perfectly holy is that animal." Larcher defends the Egyptians from the ridicule of the Greeks. "The flesh of this and of some other fish," says he, "having a tendency to thicken the blood and diminish perspiration, brings on those diseases that resemble elephantiasis. The priests forbade the people to eat them, and, in order to secure obedience, caused them to be held sacred."

Sir. Abd'Allatif relates that an emir, a man worthy of confidence, reported to him that, whilst at Kous, some persons came to him and announced that they had made an entry into an excavation where much treasure was supposed to be deposited. He accompanied them with a troop of soldiers, and there found a large vessel, of which the orifice was firmly closely with plaster. It was with much difficulty opened, and its contents were found to consist of a great number of packets about the size of a finger surrounded with bandages. Upon being unrolled, they were found to be embalmed fishes of the species named *sir*. They were reduced to dust; the vessel containing them was removed to Kous, and deposited in the hands of the prefect. The whole of the packets were unrolled in the presence of more than one hundred persons, but nothing else was discovered.

This little fish is the μαινὶς of Dioscorides. De Sacy has given the following translation of the Arabic text of this author: "*Mainous*, autrement *manidous*: c'est un petit poisson que les habitans de la Syrie nomment *sir;* sa tête, brûlée, pulvérisée, et saupoudrée sur les gercures qui surviennent au siège, les guérit : la saumure faite de ce poisson, prise en gargarisme, guérit les mauvais ulcères, corrompus et fétides, qui viennent dans la bouche."† According to M. Geoffroy St. Hilaire, the *sir* is the joël (*athe-*

---

but that fish was never known in Egypt. Mr. Wilkinson believes it to have been the mizzeh or mizdeh, a species of mormyras.

  * Athenæi Deipnosoph. lib. vii. cap. 13.

  † Manuscrit Arab. de Dioscoride, à la Bibl. Imp. trad. par De Sacy.

rina hepsetus). At certain seasons this fish is exceedingly abundant in the Nile, and a source of considerable traffic.*

INSECTS.

Scarabæus.—Beetle.

The high veneration in which this insect was held by the Egyptians is matter of notoriety, and the representation of it is one of the most commonly met with among antiquities. The regard which has been paid to this insect has been attributed to its power of sustaining life for an extraordinary length of time without food. It has arisen more probably from the fact of the beetle being the first living animal observed upon the subsidence of the waters of the Nile, and hence has been regarded as the emblem of regeneration or reproduction.

The antiquity of the worship of the scarabæus is very great. From the account of De Pauw,† it would appear to have been common to the Ethiopians, and other inhabitants of Africa, even before Egypt was inhabited. Traces of the same worship are found, according to this author, in the holy cricket of Madagascar, and even among the Hottentots, who look with veneration on the persons over whom the scarabæus with golden rays, or the horn beetle of the Cape, chances to pass.

The scarabæus has been regarded as emblematical of the sun. It is generally represented with its ball, and according to Plutarch these insects, casting the seed of generation into round balls of dung, as a genial nidus, and rolling them backward with their feet, while they themselves look directly forward, are considered solar emblems. As the sun appears to proceed through the heavens in a course contrary to the signs, thus those scarabæi turn their balls toward the west, while they themselves continue creeping toward the east; by the first of those motions exhibiting the diurnal, by the second the annual motion of the earth and the planets. It is also a type of spring, of fecundity, and of the Egyptian month anterior to the rising of the Nile, as it appears in that season of the year which immediately precedes the inundation. ‡

* The reader is referred to a very copious note on this subject by De Sacy, in his Translation of Abd'Allatif, pp. 278—288. Also, pp. 321—324.　　† II. 104.　　‡ See Psammis, p. 9.

Mr. Hamilton describes* the ruins of a magnificent temple marking the site of the ancient Ombite nome. Some of the hieroglyphics of this interesting monument serve to explain the deities which were worshipped within its walls—the crocodile and the sun; or, more properly speaking, the sun under the mysterious emblems of the crocodile and the beetle. This latter animal, with the ball or circle within its claws, is frequently represented on the most conspicuous part of the building, and the former is generally seen *couchant* on an altar or table, receiving the adorations and offerings of his votaries. The same author tells us also that in the most conspicuous part of the great temple, priests are paying divine honours to the scarabæus or beetle, which is placed upon an altar; and, that it might have a character of more mysterious sanctity, it is generally represented with two mitred heads : that of the common hawk, and that of the ram with the horn of Ammon. This insect is said to have been typical of the sun, because it changes its appearance and place of abode every six months, or because it is wonderfully productive.† Montfaucon and Count Caylus have described monuments in which Egyptian women are seen feeding the scarabæi on altars.

As the scarabæus has always been considered a symbol of the Egyptian Minerva, it is constantly found upon military rings. The Egyptian militia (the Calasires and Hermotybes) were established principally in Sais, where a temple was erected to Minerva, who was considered by the soldiers as their guardian. The scarabæus was their amulet. Arnobius states‡ that some chapels were entirely dedicated to the scarabæus.

The beetles in the zodiac of Dendera have, according to Dr. Young,§ much more of a mythological than of an astronomical nature. The beetle near the beginning of the zodiac is the well-known symbol of generation, and he is in the act of depositing his globe : on the opposite side, at the end of the zodiac, is the head of Isis, with her name as newly born ; both the long female figures are appropriate representations of the mother ; and the zodiac between them expresses the "revolving year" which elapsed between the two periods. This explanation Dr. Young conceives to be completely con-

* Egyptiaca. chap. V. On the Antiquities between Es-Souan and Thebes.
† p. 88. ‡ Adversus Gent. lib. i. § Suppl. to Ency. Brit. Art. *Egypt*, p. 51.

fined by a similar representation of two female figures on the ceiling of the first tomb of the kings at Biban-el-Molouk; one with the beetle, the other with the name of the personage just born: between them, instead of the zodiac, are two tablets, divided into 270 squares, or rectangles, corresponding to the number of days in nine Egyptian months, with ten circles placed at equal distances, probably intended to represent full moons, and relating to the ten incomplete lunations to which those days must belong. The number 270 is too remarkable to be supposed to have been introduced by mere accident; and, when the argument is considered as a confirmation of other evidence in itself sufficiently convincing, the whole must be allowed to be fully conclusive. Dr. Young has remarked that all the inscriptions on the scarabæi run from right to left, so that if they were used as seals the impression must have assumed the form which is somewhat less usual in other cases.

M. Passalacqua found an embalmed scarabæus at Thebes.* M. Latreille states this to be the *copris sabæus* of Fabricius.†

* Catal. No. 441.

† The Rev. F. W. Hope has obligingly favoured me with a short tabular synopsis of the genera and species said by the best writers on entomology to belong to the *scarabæus sacer*.

Sacred Genera.	Species of Ateuchus.(a)	Species of Copris.
1. ⎰Heliocantharus of the Egyptians. Cantharus of the Greeks. Scarabæus of the Latins. Ateuchus of Weber and Fabricius.⎱ 2. Copris, Fab. 3. Onitis.§	1. A. Egyptiorum, Lat. 2. A. Sacer, Fab. 3. A. Sanctus, Fab. 4. A. Pillularius, Fab. 5. A. Puncticollis, Lat. 6. A. Flagellatus	1. Copris(b) Isidis, Savigny. 2. ——— Paniscus, Fab. 3. ——— Sabæus, (c) Fab. 4. ——— Lunaris, Fab. 5. ——— Mimas, Millin.

§ From the temple at Karnac, probably a Maris or Calcaratus.

(a) According to Mr. Mac Leay, good representations of the following species of Ateuchus may be traced in the sculpture and drawings from Egypt: viz. 1. A. semipunctatus, Fab. 2. A. laticollis, Linn. 3. A. morbillosus, Fab. 4. A. puncticollis, Lat.

(b) Mons. Latreille states that a Copris, somewhat allied to Midas and Hamadryas (both Indian species) was worshipped at Heliopolis. Fabricius describes two species from tropical Africa (Giganteus and Antenor), and from the same country the following seven undescribed

Buprestis.

This genus of insects is remarkable for its rich metallic colours, frequently having the appearance of the most higly polished gold or copper.   Latreille supposes their fine green colour have given to these insects their consecration to religious ceremonies.   It may also have arisen from some transformation of the animal.   The buprestis gibbosa has been found embalmed by Passalacqua and is common in Sennaar, Nubia, and the Cape of Good Hope.

Although the above species of buprestis has been found embalmed, there are great doubts whether the insect so named is the buprestis of the Greeks. The derivation of the word implies insects, which produce inflammation in oxen, &c.   These insects, if swallowed by cattle when grazing, are said to produce a disease called Tympanites, and this induces Mr. Hope to believe buprestis a lytta, mylabris, or meloë, all which are vesicatory insects, and, if swallowed, would probably have the effect described.   Mouffet, however, thinks buprestis was a carabus; the former opinion is more likely to be accurate, as the carabidæ are chiefly ground beetles, while the former are found on grass and other herbage.   Mr. Hope thinks it not unlikely that buprestis was the same as œstrus of the Greeks.   The œstrus bovis deposits its eggs on the back of cattle; when hatched the grubs work their way into the skin, forming at length tumors and abscess, they live on the juices of

insects, allied to Copris Isidis in form, are in Mr. Hope's collection, viz. C. Osiris, C. Apis, C. Memnon, C. Sesostris, C. Mœris, C. Shishaek.

(c) An insect closely allied to this species was found embalmed by Passalacqua.   Mr. Hope doubts whether C. sabæus, Fab., is ever found in Egypt.   The C. pithecius closely resembles it, and has probably been mistaken for it.   Latreille's remark, " Variété et femelle du bousier sabeen," seems also to express a doubt.   Other insects, and even crustacea, are found inscribed or engraved on the temples and monumental needles of Egypt.   Among the former we discover an Apis, Sphex, and Pompilus.   Among the Arachnidæ, Galeodes, and Scorpio, and under the sign of Cancer, there are good representations of Leucosia, Pinnotheres, Portunus, and Astacus.

the animal till fully grown, then work their way out, and drop to the earth, in which they change into the pupa state. Mouffet gives us the following signs of an animal having swallowed a buprestis :—" Si quis Buprestem intus hauserit, eadem fere patitur quæ a Cantharide: Corpus in tumorem attolitur ac si tympanite laboraret, flatuum copia inter cutem et carnem valde multiplacata." This passage agreeing altogether with the Natural History of the Œstrus would incline one to think buprestis the same insect. As the god Apis was worshipped under the form of an ox, it is not likely the Egyptians could have failed to observe the *œstrus*, particularly as they discovered a small mark on the tongue resembling a cantharis. The effect produced on the sacred oxen being found not ultimately injurious to their health (as the œstri always attack the healthiest beasts), they became objects of veneration. As the Greeks derived their notions of heliocantharus, cantharus, or sacred beetle from the Egyptians, so also it is highly probable they did the same respecting buprestis.

CANTHARIS.

AN embalmed specimen of one of the species of this rapacious genus of insects, a genus which *preys not only on other insects, but also on its own tribe*, is mentioned as being in the collection of M. Passalacqua (No. 442) ; he obtained it at Thebes.

From the above description the cantharis seems to belong to the carabidæ family. Mr. Hope is not aware, however, that any true carabus has hitherto been recorded as Egyptian. It may, therefore, belong to Scarites, Anthia, or Siagona. It is rather singular that Monsieur Passalacqua has not given us Latreille's opinion on cantharis, as he has on the rest of the embalmed insects.

SCILLA—SQUILL, SEA ONION.

DIODORUS SICULUS tells us that different kinds of leguminous and bulbous plants were permitted as food in particular provinces and prohibited in others. M. De Pauw says* that "on the eastern bank of the Pelusian

* I. 130.

mouth, in a canton never formed into a prefecture, but dependent apparently on the Sethroite nome, stood a temple where the sea-leek was worshipped, and probably the kind with red roots." The sea-leek or squill* is an article of medicine much esteemed in the present day, and the reason of the strange worship of it may, perhaps, be found in the virtues it possesses of relieving disorders of obstruction and consequent effusion with which it appears the inhabitants of Pelusium were particularly affected. The tympany of Pelusium is represented in several small Egyptian figures said to have been made at Pelusium, and represent dæmons rather than human beings, with their bodies immoderately distended. The disorder appears to have been produced by a marshy soil in which Pelusium was situated, and it was also exposed to the wind blowing from the east and carrying thither the vapours of the Lake Sirbon, impregnated with bitumen and sulphur.

The Egyptian onions, Browne tells us,† are remarkably mild, more so than the Spanish, but not so large. They are of the purest white, and the *lamina* are of a softer and looser contexture than those of any other species. They deteriorate by transplantation, so that much must depend on the soil and climate. They remain a favourite article of food with all classes, and it is usual to put a layer or two of them, and of meat, on a spit or skewer, and thus roast them over a charcoal fire. The desire of the Israelites for the onions of Egypt, Mr. Browne says, is not to be wondered at.

* Mr. Wilkinson found the squill in the desert of Egypt on both sides of the Nile; it is an indigenous plant of the country.

† Travels, p. 127.

CHAPTER XVI.

ON DECEPTIVE SPECIMENS OF MUMMIES.

*Deceptive specimens of frequent occurrence—Mr. Madden's description of the frauds prac-
tised by the Arabs at Gournah—Blumenbach's examination of several fictitious mummies.*

FREQUENT deceptions have been practised in the manufacture of mummies,
as we have seen in a previous chapter. I purchased three mummies at the
sale of the museum of the late Mr. Heaviside, to whom they had been presented as Egyptian. I have opened two of them, one apparently that of an
infant of very tender age, the other that of a child about six or seven years.
The former consisted literally of saw-dust, bundles of rags of various
descriptions, and a portion of stick to serve the place of the spine. There
were some of the vertebræ of a cat mixed up with the dust. The bandages
enclosing this rubbish were of the true Egyptian character, and had, doubtless, been taken off from other and real mummies in the country. The face
was formed of linen covered with plaster of Paris, and carefully made out.
The second specimen was of a similar manufacture, the face of the same
description, but the contents of the head consisted of the bones of a human
skull about the age of eight years, which led me in the first instance to
think that it had been a genuine mummy; but, upon examination, I found
three temporal bones, which was conclusive on the matter. Around the
body of this figure were the proper kind of bandages, and some linen with
hieroglyphics painted upon it. The contents consisted of bones of various
kinds, some belonging to a human fœtus, others of a more advanced age,
and some bones of the monkey, and the entire hand of a small species of
this animal. M. Jomard mentions the making up of mummies similar to
these.*

* Descr. des Hypogeés, p. 41.

M. de Maillet says that in some of the chambers of the tombs heaps of bones and pieces of linen, such as I have described, may be seen; and that the outer bandages of genuine mummies had been removed to cover fictitious ones. Among other travellers Mr. Madden bears his testimony to the frauds practised by the Arabs of Gournah. Having cured one of these old inhabitants of the tombs of a fever, he was permitted to penetrate further into the habitation of the troglodyte than customary, and he gives the following as the description of his visit: " His dwelling was in the most spacious chamber of a superb sepulchre, the walls were covered with paintings, the roof was supported by four magnificent pillars, his divan was formed of an inverted coffin, and the lamp, which feebly illumined this gloomy chamber, was made of the cover of an alabaster vase. Various antique utensils furnished his cupboard, and the screen which separated the women's alcove from the common chamber was formed principally of the cloth torn from the mummies. It was with great difficulty I could prevail on him to let me visit the interior of the tomb; I did so, however, on the condition of not telling any thing of what I saw to the Franks at Gournah, and, to my utter surprise, the first thing I observed, at the extremity of the gallery, was a manufacture of mummies. Three beautiful mummy-cases were laid open, an ordinary mummy was placed in the last, the original one having been previously pillaged; and what convinced me of the fraud was several new wooden pegs lying on the cover of the large case, undoubtedly intended as substitutes to the old ones, which had been broken in bursting open the external case. There are generally three cases, and the nails which join them are made of hard wood. I asked no questions: I knew it would be useless; but my eye was inquisitive for the few moments I remained, and some red paint in a coffee-cup beside the coffins left me no doubt of the justice of my first suspicion. I proceeded through a narrow passage into another cave, which was literally crammed with mummies, placed in horizontal layers, as they had been, in all probability, deposited some thousands of years ago. Not one was upright, as Herodotus describes them to have been. I never found a mummy in a standing posture."*

* Travels, II. 79.

In 1792 Professor Blumenbach was in this country, and opened several mummies belonging to private individuals, and in the collection of the British Museum. Some of these were fictitious, and he has given an account of them in the Philosophical Transactions for 1794. A mummy not above one foot in length, of the usual form of a swathed puppet, wrapped up in cotton bandages, painted and gilt on its front part, and placed in a small sarcophagus of sycamore wood, into which it fitted exactly, was permitted by its owner, Dr. Garthshore, to be opened by the Professor. The mask of the face was of a gypseous plaster, similar to the infant one I have mentioned, but which here and there showed some signs of having been once gilt. Some fragments of a semicircular breast-plate were found. The lower part of the covering was divided into regular compartments like to the larger mummies, and on it were painted two standing figures, *Anubis* with the jackal's head on the right, and *Osiris* with the hawk's head on the left. Twenty circumvolutions of bandages enveloped the body, which, when displayed, was found to consist of a portion of the integuments of a larger mummy, eight inches long and two inches in circumference. This mass was strongly impregnated with a resinous substance, and appeared to have been purposely shaped into its present form.

Another specimen which belonged to my late friend Dr. Lettsom rather larger than the preceding, but resembling it in many particulars, was also opened, and was found to consist of a great number of detached bones of the skeleton of an ibis, here and there impregnated with resin. Professor Blumenbach was permitted by the trustees of the British Museum to examine among other mummies a specimen from the Sloanian collection. This was also small in size, and the mass was found to have for its centre a human *os humeri*, being part of the mummy of a young person, perhaps about eight years old, who had been embalmed with resin, and some of the integuments impregnated with this matter were found in it. The head of the bone formed the caput of the mummy, and the condyles the feet. Disappointed in the three preceding instances, the Professor was permitted to examine another specimen in the Museum. It appeared by its stature to be that of a person about fourteen years of age. This proved to be a real mummy; but not in a good state of preservation, for little remained beyond the naked bones. One circumstance in the examination of this mummy is remarkable, and has not been noticed by any other author: there were two artificial external ears made of cotton cloth and resin, and applied on each side of the head. The right one was prominent; the left had been displaced from its proper situation, and was much compressed and disfigured. The cavity of the trunk was filled with bundled rags and dark brown vegetable mould intermixed with portions of resin. In the examination of another and a larger mummy measuring five feet five inches, deposited in the British Museum, the Professor was not more fortunate than in the previous instance, for no trace of the soft parts was to be found—the naked bones alone remained.

Professor Blumenbach has described the mask of a mummy which belonged to Mr. Symmons, which he says interested him much. The inner part of this mask was of sycamore wood, and the outer surface was shaped by means of a thick coat of plaster in *bas-relief* into the form of a face, the surface of which seemed to have been stained with natural colours, but which time had now considerably blended and obscured. Upon steeping this mask in warm water he was enabled to separate all the parts of it, and he thus discovered the fraudulent artifices that had been practised in the construction of it. The wooden part was evidently a piece of the front of the sarcophagus of the mummy of a young person, and, in order to convert its *alto-relievo* into the *basso relievo* of the usual linen mask of a mummy, plaster had been applied on each side of the nose, after which paper had been ingeniously pasted over the whole face, and the paper then stained with the colours generally observed on mummies.

The sculpture and paintings of the cases and sarcophagi in which mummies have been transported into this country one might expect would enable us to form something like a judgment of the period at which the mummy was made; but it is well known, and it is well supported by the evidence of travellers whose veracity may be depended on, that the Arabs have been in the practice of breaking in pieces the mummies contained in the tombs and enclosed within the most ornamented sarcophagi, to abstract from them idols, jewels, &c., which are known to have been frequently placed within them. Fictitious mummies have then been substituted for the originals.

CHAPTER XVII.

ON THE GUANCHES—THE MUMMIES OF PERU—THE DESICCATED BODIES AT PALERMO—THE BURMAN EMBALMINGS.

Modes of preserving the dead adopted by many nations—the bodies at Toulouse—in St. Michael's vaults—the Guanches—mode of embalming—specimens of this description—Blumenbach's account of the skull of a Guanche—the peculiarity of the teeth—mummies of the ancient Peruvians—their position and appearance—specimens of this kind of desiccated bodies—Captain Basil Hall's account of a Peruvian mummy—desiccated bodies at Palermo —description of the Cadavery by Captain Smyth, Captain Sutherland, and Sonnini— embalmed Burman priests—Captain Coke's account of the mode of embalming a Burman priest—the ceremony of its destruction.

HAVING treated of the methods of embalming adopted by the Egyptians, it is proper to notice the practices which have been resorted to by other nations for the preservation of their dead. The principal of these deserving of notice are—

I. The mummies of the Canary Islands, commonly called the Guanches.

II. The mummies of the ancient Peruvians.

III. The desiccated bodies at Palermo.

IV. The embalmed Burman priests.

In dry, and particularly in calcareous vaults, bodies may be preserved for a great length of time. In Toulouse bodies are to be seen quite perfect although buried two centuries ago. In the vaults of St. Michael's church, Dublin, the same effect is produced, and Mr. Madden says he there saw the body of Henry Shears, who was hanged in 1798, in a state of preservation equal to that of any Egyptian mummy. The dryness of the air of Upper Egypt principally tended to prevent decomposition. In Lower Egypt the mummies go to pieces on exposure to the external air, and in Alexandria, where the atmosphere is exceedingly moist, Mr. Madden saw several mummies melt away in a damp storehouse where he kept them, and decomposition take place after an exposure of forty hours to the humid air, though the same bodies had resisted corruption in a dry air for perhaps forty centuries.*

I. The Guanches.

In the Atlantic Ocean about four degrees south of the Madeiras, on the coast of Africa, there is a cluster of thirteen islands known by the appellation of the Canary Islands. Of these, Teneriffe is the principal. In 1344, these islands were bestowed by the court of Rome on Luis de la Cerda, the Infanta of Spain; but the inhabitants repulsed, for nearly half a century, the expeditions which were sent to enforce the claims of the Infanta. Nor were these islands subdued until the latter part of the fifteenth century, when nearly all the original inhabitants of the country were destroyed. These people, now believed to be quite extinct, were called the Guanches,† and from the accounts of early historians it would appear that they were not only a valiant people, but also considerably advanced in civilization. It would be out of place here to do more than allude to one of their most remarkable customs, which approaches, in some manner, to that of the ancient Egyptians, and relates to their embalming of the dead.

In Glass's History of the Canary islands,‡ there is a translation from an ancient Spanish MS. found in the island of Palma, one of the thirteen I have above alluded to, and from this curious document we learn that when any person died they preserved the body in this manner: " First, they carried it to a case, and stretched it on a flat stone, where they opened it, and took out the bowels; then twice a day they washed the porous parts of the body, viz. the arm-pits, behind the ears, the groin, between the fingers, and the neck with cold water: after washing it sufficiently, they anointed

* Travels, II. 76.

† Jos. de Viera (y Clavijo) Noticias de las Islas de Canaria. This author says the word GUAN, from which Guanche is derived, signifies MAN. The Guanches have been said to be the remains of the primitive people of the Atlantis, alluded to by Plato in his Timæus.

‡ 4to. Lond. 1764.

those parts with sheep's butter, and sprinkled them with a powder made of the dust of decayed pine-trees, and a sort of brush-wood, which the Spaniards call Bressos, together with the powder of pumice-stone; then they let the body remain till it was perfectly dry, when the relations of the deceased came and swaddled it in sheep or goats'-skins* dressed, girding all tight with long leather thongs; they put it in the cave which had been set apart by the deceased for his burying-place, without any covering. The king could be buried only in the cave of his ancestors, in which the bodies were so disposed as to be known again.† There were particular persons set apart for this office of embalming, each sex performing it for those of their own. During the process, they watched the bodies very strictly, to prevent the ravens from devouring them, the wife or husband of the deceased bringing them victuals, and waiting on them during the time of their watching."†

M. Bory de St. Vincent, in his Essay on the Fortunate Islands, a title by which they were sometimes called and well known, also treats of the mode of the preservation of their dead, and from him we learn that it was done by removing the intestines, washing the body with salt water, filling the large cavities with aromatic plants, and then drying the body either in the sun or by means of a stove. In some cases it is stated that corrosive liquids were merely poured down the throat prior to the process of desiccation. This process is said to require fifteen or sixteen days, at the expiration of which time the body was folded in goats'-skins, and then put in a kind of coffin, made out of one solid piece of wood, and this was deposited in a grotto excavated in the solid rock. In caverns of this description, which are met with on the eastern slope of the peak between Arico and Guimar, these mummies or xaxos, as they are called, are found in an upright position. A few of these specimens have been brought to this country, and I have seen

* The inhabitants of the Island of Teneriffe wore garments composed of dressed goats'-skins.

† " Not many years ago two of those embalmed bodies were taken out of a cave: they were entire, and as light as cork; but quite fresh, and without any disagreeable smell. Their hair, teeth, and garments, were all found fresh. About two years ago I employed some of the natives of Teneriffe to go into one of these caves (which are almost inaccessible) to try if they could find any of those bodies; they brought me some bones, pieces of goat-skin garments, &c., and a skull with some hair upon it, which was black and lank; the garments were quite fresh, and had the hair upon them."   ‡ p. 151.

2 H

five.   One of these is in my own possession: it formerly belonged to Dr. Lettsom, who obtained it, and another from Teneriffe, which he gave to the British Museum, but which has since been transferred to the Museum of the Royal College of Surgeons.   Neither of these is furnished with hair.   The upper part of the head of my specimen has, from long exposure, suffered injury even to the bones; the lower part of the face with the remainder of the body is quite perfect.   The skin has the appearance of having been tanned and is quite elastic; it preserves its follicular structure, and all the nails are perfect.   It is a female, and the teeth and other parts denote it an aged subject.   There are the remains of a slight beard on the chin distinctly to be felt at this day.   The specimen at the Museum of the College is that of a male; the figure is diminutive; it is very much distorted, and of a very disagreeable appearance.   Two very good specimens were shown privately in London a few years since, and were intended to be disposed of.   I do not know what has become of them; but they were well worthy of attention.   One of these, a male, had been deprived of its covering of goats'-skins, in the expectation of finding some treasure concealed within it; but the other, a female, was perfect and in good condition.   In Trinity College, Cambridge, there is also a specimen, the hair of which is abundant and in good preservation.   Its aspect is disagreeable; but an examination of it shows somewhat the manner in which it had been prepared.   Each finger and toe is separately bound by strips of leather.

In Dodsley's Annual Register,* I find the following notice:—

"Cadiz, August 10, 1764.

"A few days ago a dead body was landed here, enclosed in a long skin nearly resembling that of a bear.   It was found, with several others of the same kind, in some caverns in the Canary Islands, where they are supposed to have been buried before the conquest of those islands by John de Betancourt, a Norman, in 1417, or by Peter de Vera, a Spaniard, in 1483. The flesh of this body is perfectly preserved, but is dry, inflexible, and hard as wood, so that to the touch it seems petrified, though it is not. The features of the face are very perfect, and appear to be those of a very young man; nor is that or any other part of the body decayed; the body

* VII. 95.

is no more shrunk than if the person had not been dead above two or three days, only the skin appears a little shrivelled. This body is sent to Madrid to be deposited in the Royal Academy of Surgery. The case in which it was placed had another small case within it, containing two or three vases, and a hand-mill, which were found in the same cavern."

In the same work* is another notice of a specimen of Guanche:— "Captain Young having touched at Teneriffe, in his return from the coast of Guinea, had the curiosity to ascend the Peak with a guide; whereon in a cave (the burying-place of the ancient pagan inhabitants) he discovered several dead bodies, sewed up in goats'-skins, one of which he opened, and discovered a body perfect, fresh, and the features not in the least mutilated: some were seven feet long, and others five feet three inches. He expressed a great desire to obtain one of these bodies; but the Romish priest made many objections. These, however, a little gold removed, and he procured him a female mummy. The body is perfect in every particular, the bowels are extracted, and the skin appears of a deep tanned copper colour. The hair is long and black, and retains the curl, and the teeth and nails of the toes and fingers are fresh. According to the tradition of the priest, and the extinction of the ancient inhabitants, it cannot be less than 500 years since the decease of this body. Indeed it may be as probably 1000, for, according to its appearance, it may as well continue *ad infinitum* as remain one year in its present condition. It looks like a tanned hide, and consists of bone and skin; the nerves, tendons, veins, and arteries, appear distinctly like strings."

Baron Humboldt has noticed the subject of the Guanches. "The Guanches," says he,† "famed for their tall stature, were the Patagonians of the Old World; and historians exaggerated the muscular force of the Guanches, as, previously to the voyage of Bougainville and Corboda, a colossal force was conferred on the tribe that inhabited the southern extremity of America. I never saw Guanche mummies but in the cabinets of Europe; at the period of my journey they were very scarce. A considerable number, however, might be found, if miners were employed to open the sepulchral caverns which are cut in the rock on the eastern slope of the Peak between Arico and Guimar. Those mummies are in a state of desic-

* Dodsley's Annual Register, XVI. 66. An. 1773.   † Personal Narrative, I. 278.

cation so singular, that whole bodies with their integuments frequently do not weigh above six or seven pounds, or a third less than the skeleton of an individual of the same size recently stripped of the muscular flesh. The conformation of the skull has some slight resemblance to that of the white race of the ancient Egyptians, and the incisive teeth of the Guanches are blunted like those in the mummies found on the banks of the Nile. But this form of the teeth is owing to art alone;* and, on examining more carefully the physiognomy of the ancient Canarians, able anatomists have recognized in the cheek-bones and the lower jaw perceptible differences from the Egyptian mummies. On opening those of the Guanches remains of aromatic plants are discovered, among which the *chenopodium ambro-sioides* is constantly perceived. The corpses are often decorated with small laces, to which are hung little disks of baked earth that appear to have served as numerical signs, and resemble the *quippoes* of the Peruvians, the Mexicans, and the Chinese." In the fifth Decade of Professor Blumenbach's Collection of Skulls he has figured (Tab. XLII.) the head of a Guanche, which he thinks to be that of a female. It was brought from Teneriffe to London, sewed up in goats'-skins, and was so perfectly desiccated that the entire body weighed only seven pounds and a half, although, according to the Professor, the skeleton belonging to a female of the same size would be found in its ordinary state of dryness to weigh not less than ten pounds. The skull is described as belonging to the Caucasian variety, and therefore in the same class as the Egyptian mummies, which it resembles in many respects. The facial part is, however, broader, the cheek-bones standing out. The top of the head is depressed; the occiput projects out. The forehead is spacious. The brim of the superciliary arch greatly projects out to the external orbitar or malar process; the lower part of the face, from the nostrils to the chin short, the curvature of the lower jaw more bowed than elliptic and the chin rounded. But what is most singular, the crowns of the lower incisor teeth (the top ones had fallen out) were not lancet shaped, but obtuse, almost cylindrical, the outer superficies rubbed away; in a word, such as are noted in various Egyptian mummies.†

* This is not possible: the formation of the teeth is peculiar, but quite natural, as will be seen by reference to Blumenbach's Decades Cranior. Dec. V. p. 7. Tab. 42.

" † Coronæ vero dentium primorum inferiorum neutiquam scalpriformes ad demordendum

That the inhabitants of the Canary Islands should have adopted a practice of embalming in some measure similar to that of the Egyptians is rather singular, seeing that they were separated from each other by the entire breadth of Northern Africa ; and it is not a little surprising that Mr. Marsden should have traced an affinity between the language of the Berbers or Numidians, where the remains of the Guanche tongue are to be found, and the language of the Tuariks, near Egypt, as shown in a vocabulary collected by M. Hornemann.

Blumenbach states that the viscera of the body of his Guanche had been preserved within it.   This does not appear to have been the case with mine, for through two large openings, one above the clavicle on the right side, the other below the clavicle on the left, the several organs I should conceive had been extracted.

My female Guanche measures four feet eleven inches, and that in the Museum of the Royal College of Surgeons five feet.

II. The Mummies of the ancient Peruvians.

Mr. Fryer * has given an account of some articles taken from the graves of the ancient Peruvians in the neighbourhood of Arica, on the west coast of South America.   In a grave which he caused to be opened in a place that appeared to have been a fishing village, and not to have been used as a burial-place since the conquest of Peru by the Spaniards, he found several articles of much interest.   The graves extend for a mile along the coast.   Mr. Fryer found a tumulus, consisting entirely of graves in three courses, one above the other.   The space occupied by these graves did not exceed a cube of two feet square, being formed either of pieces of wood, apparently the masts and paddles of their boats, or of thin pieces of sandstone.   The bottom he found invariably covered with a considerable quantity

aptæ, verum obtusæ, fere cylindricæ, extima superficie plana detrita, verbo tales quales pridem ab aliis et a me ipso in variis mumiis Ægyptiacis annotatæ sunt." The incisor teeth of my specimen, and also of that in the Museum of the Royal College of Surgeons, are wanting.

* Archæologia Æliana, or Miscellaneous Tracts relating to Antiquity, published by the Society of Antiquaries of Newcastle-upon-Tyne. Vol II. p. 248.

of shell-fish, placed there, as he supposes, from religious motives, either for the food for the person interred, or to serve for bait to his fishing-hook, which occur in every grave. A straw mat was placed upon this bed of shells, on which the body was found. The body (he says) was in a sitting posture, the knees bent up close to the sides, the hands crossed over the breast; in this position it was enveloped in a woollen cloth, which, in its manufacture, resembled an extremely coarse crape, over which the poncho was put, wrapped round the whole and tightly secured, and covered by a neat net-work of well-made cordage, with large meshes. The head was enveloped in the same crape-like cloth, with a closely-woven cap, or surrounded by a wreath of feathers. The bodies were in a perfect state of preservation, dry, hard, and brown (like an Egyptian mummy, says Mr. Fryer), but soon mouldered away upon exposure to the air. Their state of preservation he attributes not to any mode of embalming that had been adopted; but solely to the perfect dryness of the atmosphere, and the sand and salt in which the bodies are deposited. On the breast, underneath the poncho, was a small bag, which contained *coco*, the leaf of a plant very much used by the Peruvians for chewing, being mixed with wood, ashes, and lime, in the same manner as the betel nut is used in the East Indies. In the joint of the elbow, on each side, were found some vessels of pottery, which, together with other earthen vessels found upon the floor of the grave, a model of a boat, baskets, &c., is figured in the work from which this account is collected. In the graves of the females a bag of cotton and a spindle were found in addition to those articles already mentioned.

In the British Museum there is a small specimen of Peruvian mummy sent to this country by Lord Colchester. It is wrapped up in a crimson-coloured cloth, which I am assured by Mr Brookes, who dug up this specimen, is always the colour of the envelope in which the bodies are found, and was in a pit between two and three feet in depth. The pits are very numerous, and found chiefly at Arica; the bodies are always wrapped up and tied, and the pits are never of any considerable depth. The saline nature of the earth, and the dryness of it, appear to be quite sufficient for the purpose of embalming; for animals of all kinds, thrown loosely into the earth, are, with great certainty, preserved. By the permission of the Board of Curators of the Museum of the Royal College of Surgeons, I am enabled to present to the reader the representation of an adult Peruvian mummy presented to the College by King George IV.*

* The following account is extracted from the Catalogue of the Museum, Part VI. No. 742. 'The body of a Peruvian, which was found in one of the native sepulchres, or guacas, in some calcareous hills in the district of Caxamarca, in Peru. Tradition, preserved among the inhabitants of the country, stated the spot in which the body was found buried to have been the site of a voluntary sacrifice of the life of a Curaca, one of an order of nobles, immediately following in dignity the members of the blood royal. Colonel Thomas Heres, at that time (1821) Governor of the province of Caxamarca, hearing of this tradition, and knowing it to have been the custom of the ancient Peruvians to bury with their dead whatever household goods or implements they had, during life, been possessed of, ordered these guacas to be opened. As he expected, he found therein various objects of interest, which he remitted to the Museum of Lima. He also found, at about ten or twelve feet below the surface, three human bodies, viz. the above specimen, which is a male, another of a female, which crumbled to dust when exposed to the air, and a third of a young child about a year old, which latter was presented by Colonel Heres to General Don Juan Gregorio las Heras, and is preserved in the Museum of Buenos Ayres. Tradition also places the period of interment a very short time previous to the arrival of Pizarro at Rimac, or Lima, somewhere between 1530 and 1540. The only weapon found with the bodies was an axe, or bludgeon, of green jade-stone, very similar in shape to those brought from New Holland. Under the arm of the child was a ball, of two or three inches diameter, of very fine thread or worsted, of Vicugna wool. The bodies were merely placed in an excavation in the earth of about ten feet deep. The soil is calcareous; and perhaps to this circumstance, as well as the dryness of the air, is to be attributed the preservation of the bodies in an undecomposed state. Indeed, throughout the highlands of Peru, the desiccating process goes on so fast as to arrest the putrefactive process very much; animal substances will be completely dried up by mere exposure to the air. The bodies are not found wrapped up in linen, as amongst the Egyptians, but they are sometimes covered with the skin of the Vicugna or Peruvian camel, bound closely to the body with ligatures. The poorer classes were generally buried on the eastern aspect of mountains, while the richer were entombed in their own dwellings; the bodies being clothed in their accustomed garments, and the weapons, utensils, &c., they had used during life were buried with them; the house was then forsaken by the rest of the family, and the interior of its walls filled up with earth, so as to become quite solid. The bodies are generally found extended and lying on the back. The above specimen was brought to England by the late General Paroissien, deputy from the government of Peru, as a present from General San Martin to his late majesty King George the Fourth, by whom it was presented to the Museum in 1823."

This figure* represents very accurately the position in which those dried (for it is really not proper to call them embalmed) bodies are met with. There is no hair upon this specimen; but, three or four years ago, a very fine example of the kind, with the hair very abundant, finely preserved, and ingeniously plaited, and lying over the shoulders, was exhibited in London. With the body was also found a kind of float, formerly used by the natives in ferrying across rivers; it consisted of three pieces of wood firmly lashed together. The paddle to propel it, a peculiarly-shaped earthen vessel containing a fishing-line, a comb, and some decayed grains of Indian corn, was also discovered in the pit. The position of the body corresponded perfectly with that in the College of Surgeons.

In the Museum of the London University are two heads of Peruvians, taken also from the mummy-pits, and presented to the University by Captain Waldegrave, R.N.; one of these has also the hair plaited, and a comb is attached to it. The hair of this is black, and appears coarser than that generally found on these heads. In the other specimen the hair is of a lighter colour, fine and lank, as in most of the instances I have seen. A small portion of the skin only remains upon these specimens. Captain Basil Hall has favoured the public with an account of a Peruvian mummy. The following is taken from his "Extracts from a Journal written on the coasts of Chili, Peru, and Mexico." 12mo. Edinb. 1824.

" 13th of Dec.—I went this morning to the palace to breakfast with the Protector, and to see a curious mummy, or preserved figure, which had been brought the day before from a Peruvian village to the northward of Lima. The figure was that of a man seated on the ground, with the knees almost touching his chin, the elbows pressed to the sides, and the hands clasping his cheek bones. The mouth was half open, exposing a double row of fine teeth. The body, though shrivelled up in a remarkable manner, had all the appearance of a man, the skin being entire, except on one shoulder. In the countenance there was an expression of agony very distinctly marked. The tradition with respect to this and other similar bodies is, that, at the time of the conquest, many of the Incas and their families

* Plate VI. *fig.* 5.

were persecuted to such a degree that they actually allowed themselves to be buried alive rather than submit to the fate with which the Spaniards threatened them.

They have generally been found in the posture above described, in pits dug more than twelve feet deep in the sand; whereas the bodies of persons known to have died a natural death are invariably discovered in the regular burying-places of the Indians, stretched out at full length. There was seated near the same spot a female figure with a child in her arms. The female had crumbled into dust, on exposure to the air; but the child, which was shown to us, was entire. It was wrapped in a cotton cloth woven very neatly, and composed of a variety of brilliant colours and quite fresh. Parts of the clothes also which the female figure had worn were equally perfect, and the fibres quite strong. These bodies were dug up in a part of the country where rain never falls, and where the sand, consequently, is so perfectly dry as to cause an absorption of moisture so rapid that putrefaction does not take place. The male figure was sent to England in the Conway, and is now in the British Museum."*

Garcillasso de la Vega, who wrote a History of Peru and the Incas, is said to have been allowed, before he left his country in 1579, to see the bodies of his royal ancestors who were placed in a sitting posture with their hands crossed upon their breasts.†

III. THE DESICCATED BODIES AT PALERMO.

ABOUT a mile from the city of Palermo is the famous burial place belonging to the convent of the Capuchins. It is a subterraneous apartment, divided into four galleries, in the walls of which there are niches containing dead bodies of all the Capuchins who have died in the convent since its foundation, as well as the bodies of several persons from the city, all standing

---

* pp. 72, 73. I believe this is the mummy preserved at the Museum of the Royal College of Surgeons.

† Art. Mummy, Ency. Metrop.

in an upright posture and habited in the clothes they usually wore. The skin and flesh have, by a process of preparation, been rendered quite hard and resist putrefaction. It is said that some of them have been preserved in their recesses 250 years, and no decay has taken place. This burial-place also contains the bodies of some of the nobility and more opulent people; but they are confined in chests locked up, and of which the nearest relations hold the keys.

Captain Smyth visited this cemetery, and he says* that, upon descending it, it is difficult to express the disgust arising from seeing the human form so degradingly caricatured, in the ridiculous assemblage of distorted mummies that are here hung by the neck in hundreds, with aspects, features, and proportions, so strangely altered by the operation of drying, as hardly to bear a resemblance to human beings. From their curious attitudes (he observes), they are rather calculated to excite derision than the awful emotions arising from the sight of 2000 decayed mortals. There are four long galleries with their niches filled, besides many coffins containing noble-men in their court-dresses; and among the principal personages is a king of Tunis, who died in 1620. At the end of the great corridor there is an altar, the front of which is formed of human teeth, skulls, &c., and inlaid like mosaic work. There is also an apartment at the end of one of the galleries in which the bodies in various states of putrescence were undergoing the operation of drying, which is effected by means of an oven. It has been said that they were thus prepared by being gradually dried before a slow fire. Captain Smyth has given a representation of this cadavery in his Memoir on Sicily.

In a tour to Constantinople by Captain Sutherland, a description of the Palermo cadavery is given. After the funeral service is performed, he says, the bodies are dried in a stove, heated by a composition of lime, which makes the skin adhere to the bones. The following is the account given by this gentleman of his visit to this celebrated repository. " It was nearly dusk when we arrived at the convent. We passed the chapel, where one of

* Memoir of Sicily and its Islands, 4to. Lond. 1824, p. 88.

the order had just finished saying vespers, by the gloomy glimmering of a dying lamp. We were then conducted through a garden, where the yew, the cypress, and the barren orange, obscured the remaining light; and where melancholy silence is disturbed only by the hollow murmuring of a feeble water-fall. All these circumstances prepared our minds for the dismal scene which we were going to behold; but we had still to descend a flight of steps impervious to the sun; and these, at last, conveyed us to the dreary mansion of the dead. But notwithstanding the chilling scene through which we had passed, notwithstanding our being in the midst of more than a thousand lifeless bodies, neither our respect for the dead, nor for the holy fathers who conducted us, could prevent our smiling. The physiognomies of the deceased are so ludicrously mutilated, and their muscles are so contracted and distorted in the drying, that no French mimic could equal their grimaces. Most of the corpses have lost the lower part of the nose; their necks are generally a little twisted; their mouths drawn awry in one direction, their noses in another; their eyes sunk and pointed different ways; one was perhaps turned up, the other drawn down. The friars soon observed the mirth which these unexpected visages occasioned; and one of them, as a kind of *memento*, pointed out to me a captain of cavalry, who had just been cut off in the pride of his youth: but three months ago he was the minion of a king—the favourite of a princess—alas! how changed! even on earth there is no distinction between him and the meanest beggar. This idea in a moment restored my reflection; and I felt with full force the folly of human vanity."

Sonnini also describes this lugubrious mansion, and remarks that " a preservation like this is horrid." The skin discoloured, dry, and as if it had been tanned, nay, torn in some places, is glued close to the bone. It is easy to imagine, from the different grimaces of this numerous assemblage of fleshless figures, rendered still more frightful by a long beard on the chin, what a hideous spectacle this must exhibit; and whoever has seen a Capuchin alive may form an idea of this singular repository of dead friars.*

The relations of the deceased are said to be obliged to send two wax tapers

* Travels I. 47.

every year for the use of the convent, in default of which the body is taken down and thrown into a charnel-house. But for the vacancies occasioned by non-payment of this condition, niches could not be found sufficient for the dead.

In the cathedral of Palermo there are several magnificent sarcophagi of fine red porphyry, the workmanship of which, according to Captain Smyth,* attests great age, it being much too good for the date of the Sicilian sovereigns whose remains are enclosed within them. In 1781, the sarcophagus containing the body of Frederic was opened, and it was found that although a period of 444 years had elapsed since his entombment the corpse was perfect and entire. It was clothed in a triple imperial dress, the alba, dalmatica, and pluviale, all highly ornamented with embroidery, gold, and pearls.

IV. EMBALMED BURMAN PRIESTS.

I AM much indebted to my friend Captain Coke for an account of the modes of embalming practised in the Burman empire. This gentleman was attached to the 45th regiment, engaged in the late war, and was an eyewitness of the curious and interesting circumstance he relates respecting the disposal of the remains of a Burman phongyee, or priest. During his stay in this country Captain Coke had frequent opportunities of witnessing this extraordinary funeral ceremony, and the following is the account given to me by this intelligent officer :—

" The first body of a phongyee I saw prepared for the above public exhibition was a few months after our regiment had left Rangoon, and retired to the eastern bank of the Saluein River, which divides the Burman territories from those districts ceded to the British on the Tenasserim coast. We were at that time busily employed in housing ourselves against the fury of the approaching monsoon, from whose first blast our canvas dwellings would be a poor protection. Every day was an object of importance to us, and every workman was easily grasped at, though demanding three times the usual wages of an Indian labourer : judge, then,

* Memoir, p. 76.

of my dismay and astonishment at finding myself one morning deserted, without any previous warning, by my whole host of bamboo splitters, rattan peelers, cadjan carriers, and bungalow builders. I had invariably made a point of treating them kindly; so thinking that the urgency of the case must be great, which compelled them to leave me in such a helpless state, I for that day was content to put up with the uninteresting spectacle of my house *in statu quo.* The next day coming, and bringing with it no change, my stock of patience was exhausted, and I sallied forth fully resolved upon solving the mystery in person. Walking down to my *architect's* or building factotum's house, in the village of Obo, I found him with several of his fellow-labourers set hand and heart at work in the construction of a huge elephant of wood, some eighteen or twenty feet in height, at whose feet lay a rude warlike-looking gun, resembling a long twenty-four pounder in size and shape; round about which a covey of naked young brats were assembled, at one time attempting in high glee to creep within the bore of the cannon, at another viewing the fast increasing monster with mingled feelings of awe and delight. After much significant shaking of heads, and flourishing of hands, with very few words of speech, I was made to understand that, the time being near at hand when a phongyee's body was to be burnt with unusual pomp, the natives were engaged in the necessary preparations, and that if I had any wish to see this dignitary of their church lying in state my master builder would be happy to accompany me to the kioum, or convent, in which the deceased had resided. Upon our arrival there we found the body lying exposed to public view upon a stage constructed of bamboos, gaudily but rather tastefully decorated, with tinsel and coloured paper. The entrails of the deceased (who had been dead upwards of a month) had been taken out a few hours after death by means of an incision in the stomach, and the vacuum being filled with honey and spices the opening was sewed up. The whole body was then covered over with a slight coating of resinous substance called *dhamma,* and wax, to preserve it from the air, after which it was richly overlaid with gold leaf, thus giving the body the appearance of one of the finely moulded images so common in the temples of the worshippers of Boodh.

" Another method which I have known to be practised, but not as common as the one above detailed, of embalming bodies in the Burman country, is by forcing two hollow bamboos through the soles of the feet, up the legs, and into the body of the deceased; then by dint of pressing and squeezing the fluid (if I may so call it) is carried off through the bamboos into the ground, the other end of them being fixed into it for that purpose. The necessary ingredients for the preservation of the body are then passed up into it by the same tubes. The body of the deceased afterwards lies in state for several weeks, the exact period, if there be a limited one, I do not know; but the impression upon my mind is that the time varies from seven or eight weeks to three months; in some very rare instances bodies have not been destroyed until a year after death, which circumstance rather strengthens my opinion that there is no limited period for the preservation of a body.

" A few days after we had visited the kioum there was a grand procession of all the monstrous representations of animals that Burman ingenuity had devised, through the principal streets of the town, and along the lines of the cantonment. These animals were elevated on a low stage with wheels, and were drawn by the retainers of the petty chieftains, who had each constructed a huge rocket of timber, well secured by belts of iron, and then strongly lashed with green rattan between the legs of the beast which each had chosen to construct. Bodies of the natives, too, who lived independently, and owned no chief's supremacy, had associated themselves together for the purpose of sending delegates to this strange assembly. The procession was headed by a long single file of women bearing flags in their hands, and highly lackered vessels filled with flowers and fruits upon their heads; these were followed by a band of music, consisting of shrill clarionets, cymbals, drums, gongs, and fiddles, playing a favourite selection of Burman melodies. Numerous dancing-women, and chorus-singers followed; the latter, as they approached the English lines, striking up the complimentary air of "Ta boung ta gar," beating time with their hands at intervals of the tune, or with a kind of castanet formed of two pieces of split bamboo; while here and there moved on a steady old fellow whom one might have supposed to have been born both deaf and dumb, so sedately did they view the noise and confusion around them. Then came the monsters! the aforementioned elephant and formidable rocket in the van; next approached an unwieldy rhinoceros, then boars with bristly backs, camels whose heads overtopped the loftiest of our mansions, bisons who were all neck and eyes, tigers with tails borne aloft, buffalos with crimson eyes and vermilion nostrils, bears with shaggy skins, horses equalling the famed one of Ulysses in dimension, and one *par eminence* surmounted by a figure in due proportion of an English sergeant brandishing a halbert of the size of a weaver's beam. The rear of the lengthened array was brought up by representatives of most of the natives of the field, the forest, and the flood, and finally closed by a vast concourse of chorussingers and standard-bearers. In the evening some of the principal chiefs kept open house, and gave a 'pwa,' not as the term would signify 'a feast' for the body, but rather a musical soirée, where the ears were regaled with a second edition of singing, dancing, and the acting of some pathetic tale of love; the performers at times being singing boys and girls; at others, as if in keeping with the principal personages of the morning's parade, they were relieved by large puppets excellently manœuvred by some simple machinery. To these parties we were invited by a card, in the shape of a *paun* leaf filled with pickled tea,—not the most savoury dish in the world, being left at our houses. They were usually kept up to a late hour, and often, when I have returned home at midnight, the throng appeared as great as ever.

"Wrestling and boxing formed also one of the amusements by day, when hard cuffs and heavy falls were dealt about with no unsparing hand, the combatants being invariably separated when either began to lose his temper, and the prize being awarded to him who first drew blood.

"About the middle of April, the beginning of the new year, and two months after the phongyee's decease, the body was brought out of the kioum, and placed upon a lofty stage on wheels, from twenty to twenty-five feet in height, formed of open fretted bamboo work, with a profusion of small flags and pinnacles highly decorated with paint, tinsel, and gold leaf. The body was about twenty feet from the ground, with an open canopy above, about which much ingenuity had been called into action, and no expense spared to render it imposing in the eyes of the multitude. Several huge creepers which entwine and strangle the forest trees of the east, and of the thickness of a ship's cable, were spliced together and attached to opposite extremities of the car, which was drawn out to an open plain in the vicinity of the kioum. Here from ten to twelve thousand people were assembled, as many of whom as could possibly find room for their hands linked themselves to the wooden cables, and each party raising a tumultuous shout strove to drag the car in contrary directions.* At the first heave of the vast multitude, I expected to see the car rent into a thousand pieces; but it stood firm against the efforts of both parties. For a length of time neither party gained the ascendancy; sometimes one would be dragged bodily a few feet to the rear; but rallying again, and by a desperate effort, they would soon recover the lost ground, and by the exertion gain somewhat of their adversary, holding it in turn but for a moment. At last a cable snapped, and away whirled the car at the full speed of 1500 devotees, now worked up to an enthusiastic phrensy by the joyous exclamations of the assembled host of idle but not uninterested spectators. Their triumph was, however, of short duration, part of their opponents clinging to the car and clambering on the stage impeded its progress, while the remainder pursued with the broken cable borne aloft on their shoulders; in a few minutes the disjointed part was again lashed to the car, and a check and again a struggle took place. This laborious contest continued for two or three days, when the time had arrived that the body was ultimately to be destroyed. By early morn the town was emptied of its inhabitants, who had assembled at the kioum, and every street was deserted except by a few half-starved Pariah dogs which rushed yelping under the elevated floors of the houses, as soon as the patroles of English, to prevent plundering, came in sight. People flocked in from the surrounding villages and across the Burman frontier in such quantities that it was deemed probable they might embrace the opportunity of coming prepared for other enterprises than the destruction of an old phongyee. Patroles of our troops were accordingly ordered through the streets, and several officers' guards upon the ground where the last

---

* Captain C. tells me that these parties represent the worshippers of water and of fire, and that according to the success of the one or the other the body of the priest is to be consumed.

solemnity was performed. It was well known that the Burmans had not yet forgiven the Peguers for their three months' blockade of the town of Rangoon after our departure from it; and that they were still burning with an anxiety to wipe off the disgrace which had stained their arms upon that occasion. The Peguers had ultimately (for want of ammunition) raised the siege, and, with their king, throwing themselves under the British protection, had been received as subjects, and allotted lands on the Tenasserim coast. At mid-day the car, with its numerous attachès of miniature pagodas, wooden monsters, and their rockets, was drawn out along a road cut expressly for the purpose through the dense jungle which enclosed the village on the land side, into a small plain about a mile distant. The scene now became of the greatest interest, and one of the finest that could be imagined ; the gracefully shaped car was placed in the centre of the plain, which was girt on three sides by an amphitheatrical range of low hills, which run in a parallel line to the Saluein River. The fanciful figures of the beasts were drawn up in a kind of battle array, at some short distance upon every side of the stage upon which lay the Phongyee's body. Round about them not fewer than 30,000 people were assembled, who, unshackled by castes, were dressed in brilliant, and many-coloured costumes, that were well relieved by the dark mass of the foliage which enriched the plain, and connected the rugged sides of the hills, whose loftier eminences were crowned with the light taper- ing spires of pagodas, and temples of GUADMA.

The unfortunate ex-king of Pegu, with his golden chattah,* and sur- rounded by his mimic court, took a prominent part in the proceedings of the day. The ascent of a few rockets was the signal for the commencement of a general attack upon the Phongyee's car by the surrounding monsters. The rocket between the legs of each being lighted, the animals were pro- pelled by the force of the powder in the direction towards which they were pointed : so from every side they were seen bearing down upon the car, vomiting forth a long train of fire and smoke, and (to make a simile) like so many line-of-battle ships firing their bow-guns in full chase. Some indeed deviated a little from the line intended, and, charging the crowd on the

* None but the king and royal family are allowed to bear umbrellas covered with gold leaf.

2 K

opposite side of the circle, trampled down all before them. Two or three people were crushed to death by this 'untoward event,' and the shaft of a sky-rocket descending through an unfortunate boy's head, killed him on the spot. One *poor* representative of a pig (the cunning construction of some Shans who had possessed sufficient interest to procure English powder for the loading of their rocket), true to its nature, would not advance a single step. It retrograded, obliqued to the right and left, made a dead halt, and blazed away; but no efforts could induce it to come to the charge. The Shans smote their breasts in dismay, and, dancing about like so many maniacs, poured in volleys of oaths and abuse, while the shrill 'ahma ta ma-koung-boo' of their wives could be distinguished amidst the uproarious peals of laughter which rose from the assembled multitude, and seemed to shake the very ground on which we stood. The *vis à tergo* in vain was tried; a chosen few of the tribe, with their brawny shoulders, gave an impulse *à posteriori*, to no avail; the rocket expired, and the pig had not advanced ten paces from the starting place. His assistance, however (had not the honour of the Shans been touched), to complete the work of destruction, might have well been dispensed with : the combustible materials of the car were soon ignited, and, when the dense cloud of smoke had swept away to leeward, all that was mortal of the Phongyee had disappeared, and not a vestige of the car remained."

CHAPTER XVIII.

ON MODERN EMBALMINGS.

The practice of embalming royal personages of an early date—Edward IV.—Henry VIII. —Charles I.—Sir Henry Halford's account of the examination—remarkable mummy at Auvergne—modern methods of embalming very similar to each other—methods of De Bils — Clauderus — Paré — Guillemeau—Guybert — Charas—Penicher—Sue—Hunter— Cruikshank—Sheldon—Baillie—Brookes—Madden.

THE practice of embalming kings, princes, and nobles, is of very early date, and probably was introduced from the East even while the Egyptian embalmings were employed. Its introduction may perhaps be dated as far back as the fourth century; but the embalming of the middle ages does not from any of the specimens that have been discovered appear to have been attended with any great degree of preservation. The coffin of Edward IV., who died in 1483, was opened in 1789, and little more than the skeleton was discovered. There was a little brown hair, and a small quantity of fluid arising from decomposition. The body of Henry VIII. scarcely presented any thing beyond this; but the body of Charles I. appears to have been more perfectly preserved.

Sir Henry Halford has published an exceedingly interesting account of what appeared on opening the coffin of King Charles I., in the vault of King Henry VIII. in St. George's Chapel, Windsor, on the 1st of April, 1813. It is inserted in a volume of Essays and Orations, read and delivered at the Royal College of Physicians : *—

" On removing the pall (of black velvet) a plain leaden coffin, with no appearance of ever having been enclosed in wood, and bearing an inscrip-

---

* 12mo. London, 1831.

tion, ' KING CHARLES, 1648,' in large, legible characters, on a scroll of lead encircling it, immediately presented itself to the view.   A square opening was then made in the upper part of the lid, of such dimensions as to admit a clear insight into its contents.   These were an internal wooden coffin, very much decayed, and the body carefully wrapped up in cere-cloth, into the folds of which a quantity of unctuous or greasy matter, mixed with resin, as it seemed, had been melted, so as to exclude as effectually as possible the external air.   The coffin was completely full ; and, from the tenacity of the cere-cloth, great difficulty was experienced in detaching it successfully from the parts which it enveloped.   Wherever the unctuous matter had insinuated itself, the separation of the cere-cloth was easy ; and when it came off a correct impression of the features to which it had been applied was observed in the unctuous substance.   At length the whole face was disengaged from its covering.   The complexion of the skin of it was dark and discoloured.   The forehead and temples had lost little or nothing of their muscular substance ; the cartilage of the nose was gone ; but the left eye, in the first moment of exposure, was open and full, though it vanished almost immediately : and the pointed beard, so characteristic of the period of the reign of King Charles, was perfect.   The shape of the face was a long oval ; many of the teeth remained ; and the left ear, in consequence of the interposition of the unctuous matter between it and the cere-cloth, was found entire.

" When the head had been entirely disengaged from the attachments which confined it, it was found to be loose, and without any difficulty was taken up and held to view.   It was quite wet, and gave a greenish-red tinge to paper and to linen which touched it.*   The back part of the scalp was entirely perfect, and had a remarkably fresh appearance ; the pores of the skin being more distinct, as they usually are when soaked in moisture; and the tendons and ligaments of the neck were of considerable substance and firmness.   The hair was thick at the back part of the head, and in appearance nearly black.   A portion of it, which has since been cleaned and dried, is of a beautiful dark-brown colour.   That of the beard was a

* Sir Henry conjectures this fluid to have been blood discharged from the large blood-vessels after decapitation.

redder brown. On the back part of the head it was not more than an inch in length, and had probably been cut so short for the convenience of the executioner, or perhaps by the piety of friends soon after death, in order to furnish memorials of the unhappy king. On holding up the head, to examine the place of separation from the body, the muscles of the neck had evidently retracted themselves considerably; and the fourth cervical vertebra was found to be cut through its substance transversely, leaving the surfaces of the divided portions perfectly smooth and even, an appearance which could have been produced only by a heavy blow, inflicted with a very sharp instrument, and which furnished the last proof wanting to identify King Charles I."

After this examination of the head it was restored to its situation, the coffin soldered up, and the vault closed.

This account is deposited in the British Museum, and its accuracy authenticated by the signature of his Royal Highness the Prince Regent, who was present at the examination.

In the Memoirs of the Royal Academy of Sciences at Paris, for the year 1756, there is an account of a remarkable mummy.

" Some peasants being at work in a field belonging to the village of Martres-d'Artier, near Riom in Auvergne, found a kind of trough, seven feet long and five feet high, cut out of a stone which seemed to be a granite, and covered with another stone of the same kind. In this trough was a leaden coffin, which contained the body of a lad about ten or twelve, so well embalmed, that the flesh was still flexible and supple. The arms were covered with bands twisted round them from the wrist to the top of the shoulders, and the legs in the same manner from the ancles to the top of the thighs: a kind of shirt covered the breast and belly, and over all was a winding sheet. All these linens were imbibed with a balm of such a strong smell that the stone trough retained it, and communicated it to those who came near it, long after the coffin was taken out of it. This mummy was carried first to the curate's of the parish: it had at that time on its head a wooden cap, lined with an aromatic paste, which had the same smell as the balm in which the linen had been dipped. It had also in its hands balls of the same paste, which were kept on by little bags, which covered the hands, and were tied to the wrists; and the arms, thighs, and legs were covered with the same paste. But, being removed soon after to Riom, by order of the intendant of that place all the coverings were taken away; and the colour of the skin, which was at first very clear, changed to a dark brown. The drug employed in embalming had very much diminished the bulk of the fleshy parts; but had preserved their suppleness so well that a surgeon making an incision in the stomach, one of the by-standers put in his finger, and could feel the diaphragm, the great lobe of the liver, and the spleen; but these last two had lost much of their bulk. A part of the epiploon, about three inches in length, being extracted at this opening, was found to be quite sound, and as flexible as in its natural state. About twelve inches of the jejunum being likewise extracted, and tied at one end, it was inflated by blowing in it, as readily as if it had been that of an animal just killed. In short, the body seemed to be embalmed in a quite different manner from that of the Egyptians, whose mummies are dry and brittle."*

" No inscription on the coffin or linen, no medal, nor any symbol whatever, was found, that might discover the time when it was deposited in this place; and the peasants affirmed, with oaths, that they had not removed or embezzled any thing."

The modes of embalming practised by the moderns vary very little from each other. Some few have proposed to preserve the body without removing the viscera; but the greater number have recommended evis-

---

* This opinion we have seen is not correct; the best specimens of Egyptian embalming are perfectly soft and flexible. The account of the mummy of Auvergne must be regarded with suspicion after reading such a passage as the following:—" On ne lui avait enlevé, comme on le faisait en Egypte, ni la cervelle, ni les intestins : son corps était entier, sans mutilation aucune, et par conséquent avec tous ses principes de corruption; et cependant il avait un air de vie qui paraissait tenir du prodige. Ni les oreilles, ni les dents, ni la langue, non plus que les différentes parties du visage, n'avaient subi la moindre altération. Les lèvres étaient fraîches et vermeilles; les mains blanches et potelées; les yeux enfin, chose plus étonnante encore! les yeux, qu'on aurait cru devoir être éteints et oblitérés, conservaient, dit-on, le brillant et la vivacité qu'ils ont dans l'homme vivant. Enfin, toutes les articulations étaient flexibles, et elles obéissaient au mouvement qu'on voulait leur imprimer; les doigts avaient même, lorsqu'on les pliait, assez de ressort pour se restituer dans leur position."—*Roquefort des Sépultures Nationales,* p. 116.

ceration. In the removal of the organs contained within the cavities of the skull and body, in the injection of saline and spirituous fluids, and in the insertion of aromatic powders into the body, and into the flesh of the limbs, consist the principal points of modern embalming. To these the application of cloths dipped in oil and wax to exclude the external air, have been added, prior to depositing the body in its cases or coffins. Little else has been done.

M. Rouelle* gives an account of the methods employed by two writers on the Art of Embalming, Lewis de Bils, a Flamand, a very learned anatomist who lived in the middle of the seventeenth century, and Gabriel Clauderus, an eminent physician, who published a work entitled "Methodus Balsamandi Corpora Humana, aliaque majora sine evisceratione et sectione hucusque solita" at Altenburg in 1769. The works of both these authors are now before me, and from them it would appear that De Bils had devoted much time to arrive at a good method of preserving anatomical preparations; that he was largely engaged in disputes with the anatomists of his time in consequence of his assertion that he had found out a means of drying bodies dissected, at the same time preserving the muscles, vessels, viscera, and other parts all in their natural situation, having deprived them of their moisture and fat. De Bils denies having used any balsamic matter in his preparations. Clauderus is elaborate on this subject; his work extends to 216 pages in quarto. He reviews the statements made by De Bils, and contends that he did not employ any balsamic materials in his mode of preparation. He admits that aromatics were diffused in the cabinet of preparations, which might give rise to the opinion generally entertained of their having been employed in his process. Clauderus states that he had seen the preparations and had wetted his finger and tasted them; that they were not balsamic but saline, and hence he was induced to employ saline substances in his own method, and ultimately came to use the alkaline salts, without however appearing to be aware of their true nature and adaptation in the process of embalming. The method of Clauderus was to macerate or saturate in a liquor made of the ashes of tartar, dissolved in

* Mem. de l'Acad. des Sciences pour l'An. 1750.

water in the proportion of one pound of the former to six pounds of the latter. To this solution he added half a pound of sal ammoniac. The liquor was then filtered; he denominated it his Balsamic Spirit. This liquor he injected into the different cavities of the chest and abdomen, and then placed the body in the fluid. It was allowed to remain six or eight weeks; but, in order to shorten the process, at the expiration of a fortnight the liquor was either renewed or renovated by the addition of some volatile alkali. The body when taken out was dried either in the sun or in a stove. The cabinet of Ruysch, the celebrated Dutch anatomist, which was sold to the Czar Peter, has always been much extolled for the manner in which preparations of the human body had been rendered capable of resisting putrefaction. The method adopted by this anatomist is unknown. The dead bodies prepared by him were said to have rather resembled persons asleep than devoid of life.

The methods recommended by Paré, by Guillemeau, Guybert, Charas, Penicher, Sue, and others, differ little from each other, and are scarcely deserving of notice; and the manner in which a body was mutilated, by the various openings and incisions made into it, is a subject calculated rather to excite disgust than admiration.

Louis Penicher, a celebrated apothecary at Paris, published in 1699 a small work entitled, "Traité des Embaumemens selon les Anciens et les Modernes." This work contains the description of a variety of balsamic compositions intended for the preservation of bodies, and gives a very circumstantial account of the mode adopted in the embalming of Madame la Dauphine. The balm used on this occasion consisted of upwards of sixty articles, which are enumerated by M. Penicher. In the journal book of the Royal Society for December 1, 1686, I find the following notice:—"Dr. Sloane said that formerly he with some others made a muscular dissection of a human body at Montpellier, and that, to preserve the body from putrefaction, the bowels being taken out, they infused a tincture of myrrh and aloes drawn with spirit of wine; and kept it covered with fir shavings in a coffin, whereby it was preserved three months in the middle of summer. The same said that cedar dust is affirmed the best preservative in this case, but that was not procurable at Montpellier."

M. Sue in his " Anthropotomie, ou l'Art de Dissequer," 12mo. Paris, 1750, devotes a considerable portion of the second volume of his work to a description of the manner of preparing and preserving the different parts of the human body, and treats also of embalming in general, in which he considers those substances which are best adapted to resist putrefaction, and the mode of employing them. He gives an immensely lengthy list of aromatics of all kinds, consisting of different kinds of flowers, fruits, leaves, barks, woods, roots, gums, resins, and other juices of plants, essences, spirits, tinctures, &c., too numerous to be noticed here. He is equally elaborate in his enumeration of the instruments, bandages, &c., with which an embalmer ought to be furnished, and he concludes by directing the manner in which the various incisions into the body are to be made, the mode of extracting several of the viscera, removing all humidity, &c., and the immediate application of the numerous medicaments he recommends should be employed.

Dr. William Hunter was in the habit of delivering, at the close of his course of anatomical lectures, an account of the manner of making anatomical preparations, and on this occasion he advanced a method of embalming, as being in some measure connected with the subject of his lectures. The method he proposed was to throw into the blood-vessels, in the most minute manner he was able, an injection composed of essential oil of turpentine, in which a small proportion of Venice turpentine had been dissolved. To this he added different proportions of oil of camomile and oil of lavender, and coloured the whole with vermilion. This fluid having been forced into the large arteries with such power and continuance that even the skin exhibited a red appearance, the body was allowed to remain some hours undisturbed, to admit of the mixture thoroughly impregnating it. The next step was to open the cavities of the chest and belly, to remove the viscera and squeeze out the fluid contained in them. The vessels of these parts were to be again injected, ligatures put upon them, and well bathed in camphorated spirits of wine. The vessels of the body were then again to be injected from the large artery (the aorta) rising from the heart, and the cavities of the chest and belly well washed with the camphorated spirit. All the spaces between the viscera were now to be filled up with a powder composed of camphor, resin, and nitre. This powder was also to be put into the eyes, nostrils, ears, and other cavities, the whole body to be rubbed over with the essential oils of rosemary and lavender, and the body then placed upon a bed of plaster of Paris, by which all moisture would be absorbed. The coffin was to be closed up, and at the expiration of four years opened, and, should the desiccation of the body be imperfect, another bed of gypsum was to be added to complete the process. A body prepared according to this manner by Dr. Hunter is preserved in the museum of the Royal College of Surgeons. It is the body of the wife of a well-known eccentric character, the late Martin Van Butchell.* It re-

* I am happy to be able to lay before the reader the following verbatim copy of a paper in Van Butchell's own writing, preserved at the Royal College of Surgeons :—

"14 Jan. 1775. At ½ past 2 this morning my wife died. At 8 this morning the statuary took off her face in plaster.

" At ½ past 2 this afternoon Mr. Cruikshanks injected at the crural arteries 5 pints of oil turpentine mixed with — of Venice turpentine, and — of vermilion.

" 15. At 9 this morning Dr. Hunter and Mr. C. began to open and embalm the body of my wife: her diseases were a large empyema in the left lung (which would not receive any air), accompanied with pleuro-pneumony, and much adhesion; the right lung was also beginning to decay, and had some pus in it. The spleen hard and much contracted; the liver diseased, called rata malpigi. The stomach very sound. The kidneys, uterus, bladder, and intestines in good order. Injected at the large arteries oil of turpentine mixed with camphored spirits, i. e. 10 oz. camphor to a quart sp^{ts}, so as to make the whole vascular system turgid: put into the belly part 6 lb. rosin powder, 3 lb. camphor powder, and 3 lb. nitre powder mixed with rec. sp^{ts}.

" 17. I opened the abdomen to put in the remainder of powders, and added 4 lb. rosin, 3 lb. nitre, and 1 lb. camphor. In all there were 10 lb. rosin, 6 lb. nitre, and 4 lb. camphor, i. e. 20 lb. of powders mixed with spirits of wine.

" 18. Dr. Hunter and Mr. Cruikshanks came at 9 this morning and put my wife into the box on and in 130 lb. w^t of Paris plaster at 18d. a bag: I put between the thighs 3 arquebusade bottles, one full of camphored spirits very rich of the gum, one containing 8 oz. oil of rosemary, and in the other 2 oz. of lavender.

" 19. I closed up the joints of the box lid and glasses with Paris plaster mixed with gum water and spirits of wine.

" 25. Dr. Hunter came with Sir Thos. Wynn and his lady.

" Feb. 5. Dr. Hunter came with two ladies at 10 this evening.

" 7. Dr. Hunter came with Sir John Pringle, Dr. Heberden, Dr. Watson, and about 12 more Fellows of the Royal Society.

" 11. Dr. Hunter came with Dr. Solander, Dr. ——, Mr. Banks, and another gentleman.

sembles a Guanche or Peruvian, rather than an Egyptian mummy, and is, properly speaking, a desiccated, rather than an embalmed body.

In the same museum is also an embalmed body of a female, aged twenty-four, of the name of Johnson, who died of phthisis in the Lock Hospital about the year 1775, and who left her body for dissection to Mr. Sheldon. No account of the method employed has been preserved, but it is presumed to have been similar to that adopted by Dr. Hunter in the preceding instance, as a letter which accompanied the specimen when it was sent to the College of Surgeons stated that "much camphor was used, that all the arteries and veins were filled with injection, and that spirit of wine was used as well as camphor; that the heart and intestines were taken out and injected, and replaced, as was also the brain."

The late Dr. Baillie published a Paper on the Embalming of Dead Bodies,* the object of which was to describe a method to preserve them from decay, and to be more easy of execution than any previously employed by modern anatomists. He made an experiment of embalming upon the bodies of three children, and in these his process answered perfectly. His method varies little from that of Dr. Hunter. Instead of removing the viscera, he injects into the stomach and bowels, and into the wind-pipe and lungs, the same fluid as that proposed by Dr. Hunter, and thus simplifies the process by not having recourse to the removal of the contents of the several cavities of the body, and in having only one injection of the blood-vessels.

The late Mr. Joshua Brookes prepared the body of a boy after this manner. It was disposed of at the sale of his museum by public auction.

Mr. Madden employed common tar as an embalming ingredient. In 1823 he accompanied an invalid from Naples, by sea, to London; the

---

" I unlocked the glasses to clean the face and legs with spirits of wine and oil of lavender.

" 12. Dr. Hunter came to look at the neck and shoulders.

" 13. I put 4 oz. of camphored spirits into the box, on sides of neck, and 6 lb. of plaster.

" 16. I put 4 oz. oil of lavender, 4 oz. oil of rosemary, and ½ oz. of oil of camomile flowers (the last cost 4 sh.) on sides of the face, and 3 oz. of very dry powder of camomile flowers on the breast, neck, and shoulders."

* Transactions of a Society for the Improvement of Medical and Chirurgical Knowledge, III. 7.

voyage was long and perilous, the provisions were expended, and the privations were such that his companion died thirty days previously to the arrival of the vessel at Plymouth. Believing that the friends of the deceased would be glad to have his remains brought home, Mr. Madden turned his attention to the preservation of the body; but on board there were neither spirits nor spices. He determined on employing common tar, and having removed the intestines he applied the tar both within and without, and then enveloped the body in a well-tarred sheet; by this means he completely excluded the air, and was enabled to bring home the body after a voyage of no less than seventy-two days.

EXPLANATION OF THE PLATES.

———

PLATE   I. FRONTISPIECE. Whole-length view of the Græco-Egyptian mummy, showing the colour of the same and the appearance of the gilding on different parts of the body. From the Author's collection.

II. Profile of the same mummy, natural size.

III. The Sacred Barge for conveying the mummies to the tombs. Drawn from a model in the collection of Mons. Passalacqua at Berlin (see page 33). *Fig.* 1, 2, 3, 4. Representations of the Four Deities of the Amenti, Netsonof or Kebhnsnof, Smof, Hapee, and Amset (see page 58). *Fig.* 5. represents a box in which twenty-four figures of mummies carved in wood, were found deposited. These are regarded as donatives to the deceased by those who assisted at the funeral. On the box, which measured 18½ inches in length and 17 inches in height, are representations of the Four Genii of the Amenti, and also of the Sacred Eye of Osiris (see page 110.)

IV. *Fig.* 1. Case to contain Fœtal mummy. *Fig.* 2. Fœtal mummy in the bandages (see page 73). *Fig.* 3. The substance of the heart found in the Græco-Egyptian mummy (see page 60). *Fig.* 4. The leathern Amulet found in Dr. Lee's mummy (see page 96). *Fig.* 5. Representation of Fingers found in a mummy. Taken from M. Passalacqua's collection (see page 96). *Fig.* 6, 7, 8. Knives of Silex found in a box near to a mummy by M. Passalacqua (see pages 57 and 112). *Fig.* 9, 10. Bronze Crotchets for the extraction of the brain. From the collection at Berlin (see page 53).

V. Insects found in the heads of mummies (see page 53, et seq.) *Fig.* 1, 2. Necrobia mumiarum, natural size. *Fig.* 3. magnified. *a, b, c, d,* anatomical sections of the same. *Fig.* 4, 5. Dermestes pollinctus, natural size. *Fig.* 6, 7, magnified. *Fig* 8. Larva of the same magnified. *Fig.* 9. Larva, natural size. *e, f, g, h, i, j, k,* anatomical sections of the Dermestes pollinctus. *l.* ova of the same.

VI. *Fig.* 1. Gold plate found upon the tongue of a mummy (see page 63). *Fig.* 2. The outer bandages as they appeared in Dr. Lee's mummy, showing also the position of the leathern Amulet over the heart (see page 95). *Fig.* 3. The second layer of bandages (see page 95).

Fig. 4. Sycamore Sarcophagus which contained Dr. Perry's mummy (see page 122). *Fig.* 5. Peruvian mummy at the Museum of the Royal College of Surgeons (see page 239).

PLATE VII. Copy of the portrait upon an Egyptian mummy in the British Museum (see page 101).

VIII. *Fig.* 1, 2. Representations of a Funereal Tablet in the possession of Samuel Rogers, Esq. *Fig.* 3. Another Tablet from the same collection (see page 108). *Fig.* 4. Representation of the breast-plate of a King (see page 109). *Fig.* 5. The Sacred Eye of Osiris from Dr. Lee's collection (see page 109). *Fig.* 6. Representation of Osiris in bronze, from Kárnak, in the Author's collection (see page 110). *Fig.* 7. Isis and the Infant Horus, from the collection of Samuel Rogers, Esq. Many fabulous accounts have been transmitted to us by the Greeks concerning the son of Isis and Osiris, but we are still ignorant of the real meaning of this mytho-logical subject, which, though generally supposed to be the most intel-ligible part of the Egyptian Pantheon, is in reality the most difficult and obscure ; nor can we expect to unravel the great mystery con-cerning Osiris, Isis, and Horus, till our acquaintance with the Egyptian language and religion becomes more extensive.

It will probably be found that Osiris, in one of his characters at least, was the greatest of the Egyptian deities, that neither he nor Isis was ever supposed by the Egyptians to have been mortals deified, and that Horus, the avenger of his father, will prove to be of much more consequence in their Pantheon than any thing the Greeks have told us could lead any one to suppose ; though at the same time it is highly probable that many other allegories may be traced, in the story of these personages, which have a physical as well as a moral signification.

IX. Inner case of Dr. Lee's mummy. *Fig.* 1. Representing the mytho-logical emblems painted upon it. The ornamental details on the upper side of the figure are arranged in compartments with a line of hieroglyphics down the centre. On the breast immediately below the necklace are the winged globe and asps, the emblems of the god Hat or Agathodæmon. The upper compartments contain, on the right, two of the genii of Amenti, Hapi, and Smof, standing before an asp, crowned with the cap of the upper country, and on the opposite side the other two, Amset and the hawk-headed

Kebhnsnof. In the next are represented two winged asps; and in the lowest is on one side a jackal-headed, and in the other a hawk-headed figure with the ostrich feather of Truth. The line of hieroglyphics contains the usual formula of funereal inscriptions, and, as far as the sense can be ascertained, it signifies, "This is a (royal?) chosen gift to Re Atmoo, Lord of the two regions of Phut (or the Libyan side of the Nile), Pthah Sokari Osiris, Lord of the sacred place, the manifester of good, king of the gods, the great Re, Lord of heaven. Give chosen offerings of incense for Osiris, the lady of the house, priestess of the (sacred abode?) TAN'NOFRE, deceased." *Fig. 2.* Showing the manner in which the cartonage is secured (see page 116).

PLATE X. Outer case of Dr. Lee's mummy. *Fig. 1.* Front view, representing a line of hieroglyphics down the centre, which contains the usual funereal ritual, thus: "This is a (royal?) chosen gift to Osiris, dominator or president of the west, the good God, lord of the land of (Abydus?). Give chosen offerings of oxen and geese incense and libation for Osiris, the lady of the house, priestess of the (sacred abode?) TAN'NOFRE . . . . *Fig. 2.* Inner part of the case, representing a figure of the goddess Netphé, the wife of Seb and mother of Osiris, who held one of the principal offices in the regions of the dead, and is frequently represented in this form and position in Egyptian sarcophagi (see page 123).

XI. *Fig.* 1, 2. Brass coin of one of the Ptolemies, the reverse of which is almost entirely obscured by a portion of the bandage of a mummy adhering to it. In the possession of Mr. Kirkmann (see page 111). *Fig.* 3. The leaden seals attached to the bandages of a Greek mummy. From the two impressions the name of ΚΟΠΡΗC may be distinctly made out. From Mr. Burgon's collection (see pages 111 and 113). *Fig.* 4. Line of hieroglyphics from the Rosetta Stone, with a translation of the same. *Fig.* 5. The same written in the Hieratic character, to show the similarity of form. *Fig.* 6 is the same in the Enchorial character, taken from the Rosetta Stone. *Fig.* 7, 8, 9, illustrate the manner in which dates are expressed in the Hieroglyphic, Hieratic, and Enchorial characters.

XII. Sacred animals. *Fig.* 1. Embalmed Asp in a case, upon which a representation of the animal is carved. From the author's collection (see page 217). *Fig.* 2. Unrolled snake. From the author's collection (see page 217). *Fig.* 3. Head of an embalmed Ram in the bandages. From the collection at Berlin (see page 193). *Fig.* 4. Embalmed Fox. From Belzoni (see page 191). *Fig.* 5. Embalmed Cat. From ditto (see page 189). *Fig.* 6. Embalmed Bull. From ditto (see page 202). *Fig.* 7. Embalmed Cynocephalus. From the same (see page 183). *Fig.* 8, 9. The Crocodile in the bandages and unrolled. From the Author's collection (see page 214).

XIII.   Sacred Animals. *Fig.* 1. Embalmed Hawk. From the Author's collection (see page 204). *Fig.* 2. Embalmed Hawk in human form. From the collection at Berlin (see page 204). *Fig.* 3. Embalmed Owl. From the same (see page 204). *Fig.* 4. Unrolled Ibis. From the Author's collection (see page 209). *Fig.* 5. Ibis Pot. *Fig.* 6. Embalmed Ibis in human form. From the collection at Berlin (see page 209). *Fig.* 7, 8. Embalmed Ibis in bandages (see page 209). *Fig.* 9. Embalmed Goose. From Belzoni (see page 209). *Fig.* 10. Embalmed Goose. From the Author's collection (see page 210).

Thoms, Printer and Stereotyper, 12, Warwick Square.

ERRATA ET CORRIGENDA.

Page 14. Line 6   for *ὕστερον*   read   *ὕστερον.*

16. Note *   for *Σκόθης*   read   *Σκύθης.*

17. †   for *Chap. i.*   read   *Chap. l.*

18. *   for *Theseus*   read   *Adrastus.*

     γη   read   *γᾷ.*

     εκασον   read   *εκαστον.* Mr. Long tells me that these last lines of Euripides are an imitation of a beautiful passage by Empedocles.

25. Line 20   for *Memnonuim*   read   *Memnonium.*

28. 11   for *Damies*   read   *Damis.*

35. Note †   for *θημας*   read   *θηκας.*

45. Line 2   for *εἷλο*   read   *εἷλον.*

     25   for *ὁμότεκνον*   read   *ὁμότεχνον*

51. 22   dele the *κατέαται.* The original passage does not say that they were specially appointed for the purpose; it merely means that there were individuals who made it a profession.

69. Line 15   *συρμαίη.* This is not the name of a liquor; it means a purge generally, and nothing more. It is, however, spoken of as *Potus ex Aqua et Sale, purgatione serviens.*

74. Line 15   for *three*   read   *four.*

84. 12   for *Necropolis*   read   *Necropolies.*

95. 6   for *cotton*   read   *linen.*

     7   for *linen*   read   *cotton.*

124. 6   I believe the great temple of Diana at Ephesus was of stone.

125. 18   for *pietro*   read   *pietra.*

146. Note *   for *lenity*   read   *unity.*

151. Line 1   for AUTOGRAPH   read   ANTIGRAPH.

157. 10   *μελάχροες και ουλότριχες.* Black in complexion and *woolly* headed will perhaps be more correctly rendered by *curly* headed.

162. Line 6   for *Seommering*   read   *Soemmering.*

169. 3   for *faturum*   read   *saturam.*

193. Note ‖   for *hippopotamus*   read   *crocodile.*

     Line 18   for *Apollonopolis*   read   *Apollinopolis.*

196. 7   for *under*   read   *on.* See Herod. III. 29.

197. 8   Epaphus. See Æschyli Prometheus, where the name Epaphus first occurs :

     ἐπώνυμον δέ τῶν Διὸς θιγημάτων (γεννημάτων)

     τέξεις κελαινὸν Ἔπαφον. See Æsch. Prom. 875.

198. Line 10   for *aversatis*   read   *aversatus.*

200. 9   Basis at Hermonthis. According to Ammianus, Porphyry, and Ælian, Apis was sacred to the moon, Mnevis to the sun. Jablonski mentions Basis or Pasis as the bull of Hermonthis. At this place Cleopatra is seen worshipping a bull, but it is not certain that the hieroglyphics over it present the name of Basis. Mr. Wilkinson tells me that it seems to be the emblem of the god Mandoo, who was particularly adored in this town.

214. Line 1   for *Psylla*   read   *Psylli.*

215. 28   for *Monolithe*   read   *Monolith.*

219. 7   for *Orphies*   read   *Orphics.*

222. 21   for *Calasires & Hermotybes*   read   *Calasiries and Hermotybies.*

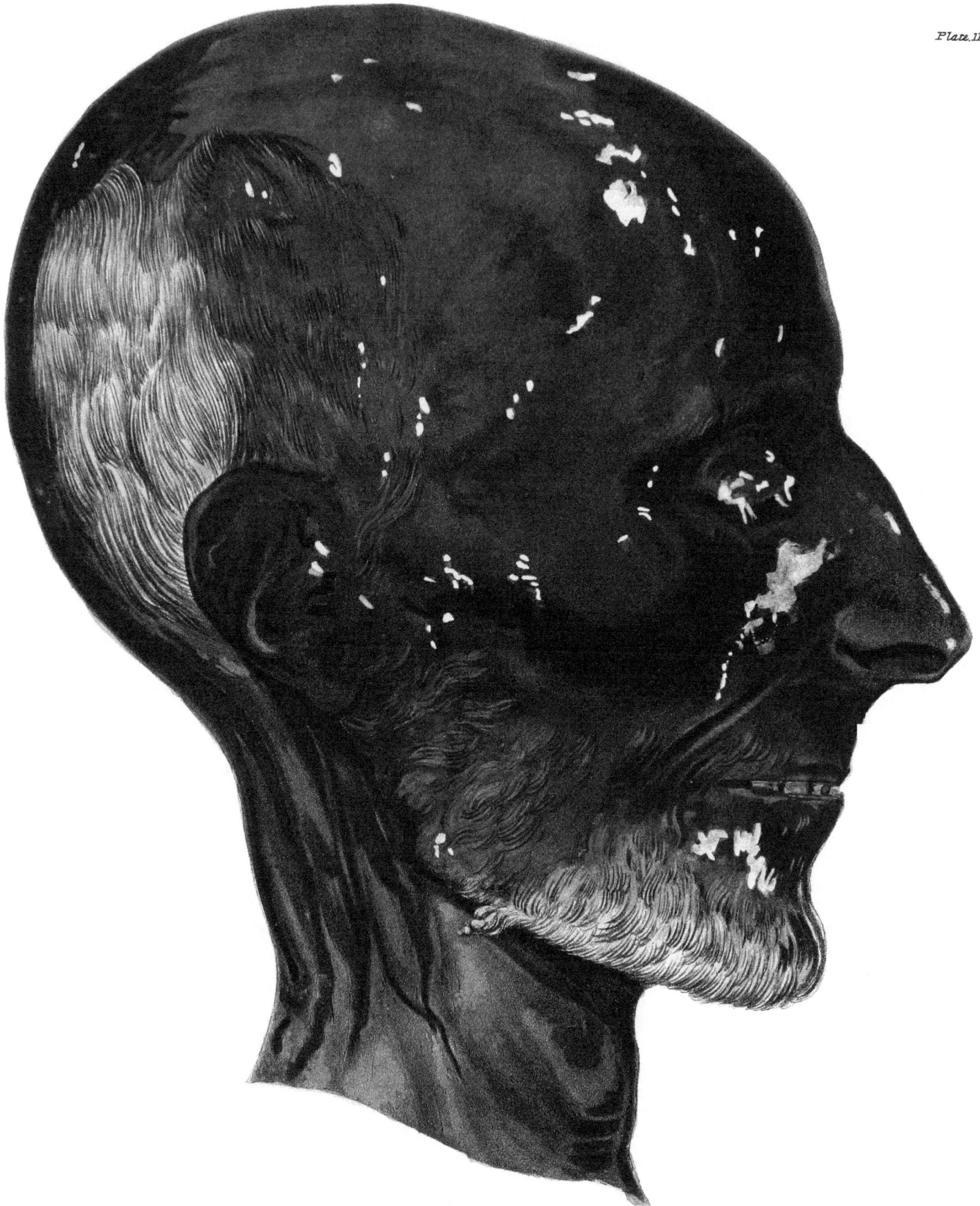

Geo Cruikshank. delt.

Published by Md.rs Longman&Co March.1.1834

Plate III.

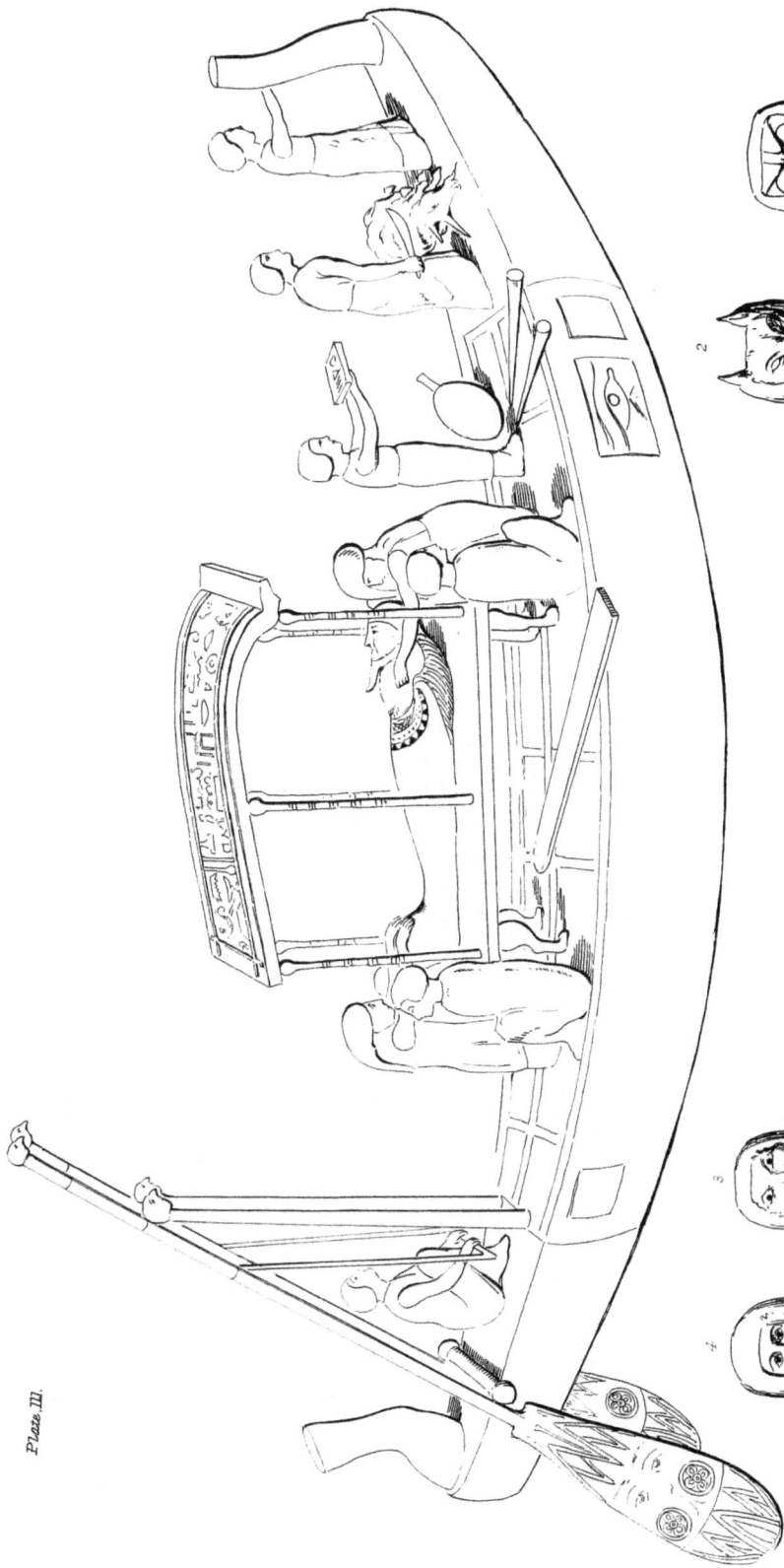

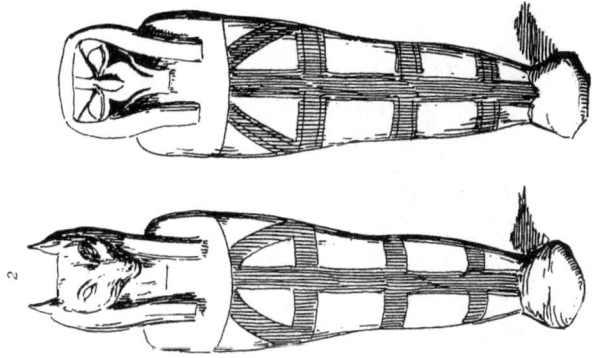

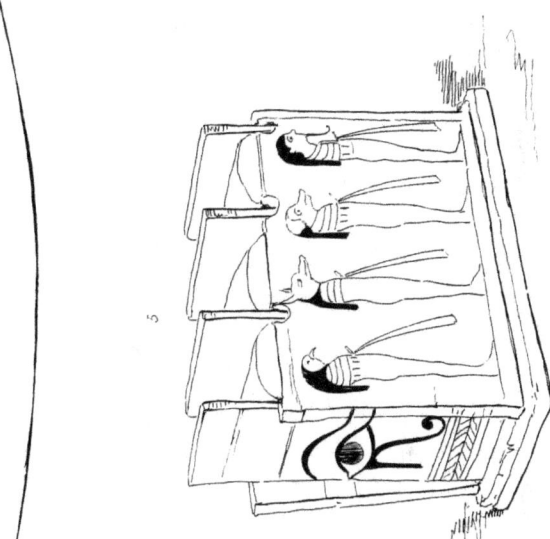

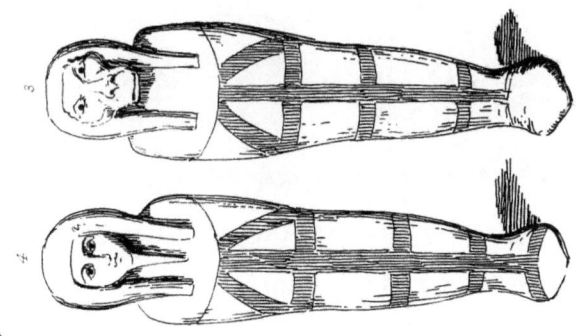

Published by Mess.rs Longman &c.t March. 1.1834.

Geo Cruikshank. del.t

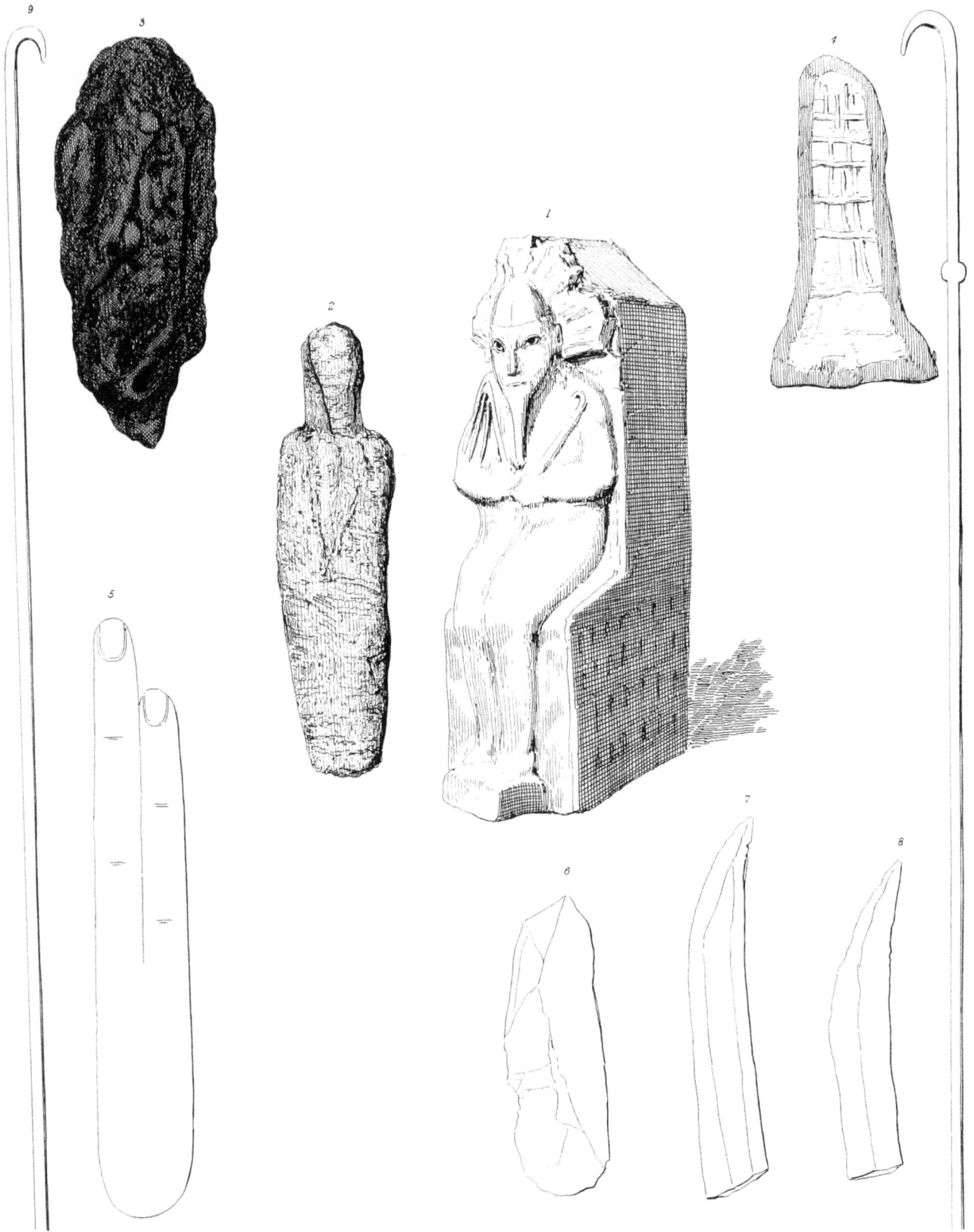

Plate IV

Geo. Cruikshank del.t

Published by Mef.r.s Longman & C.o March 1.1834.

Plate. V.

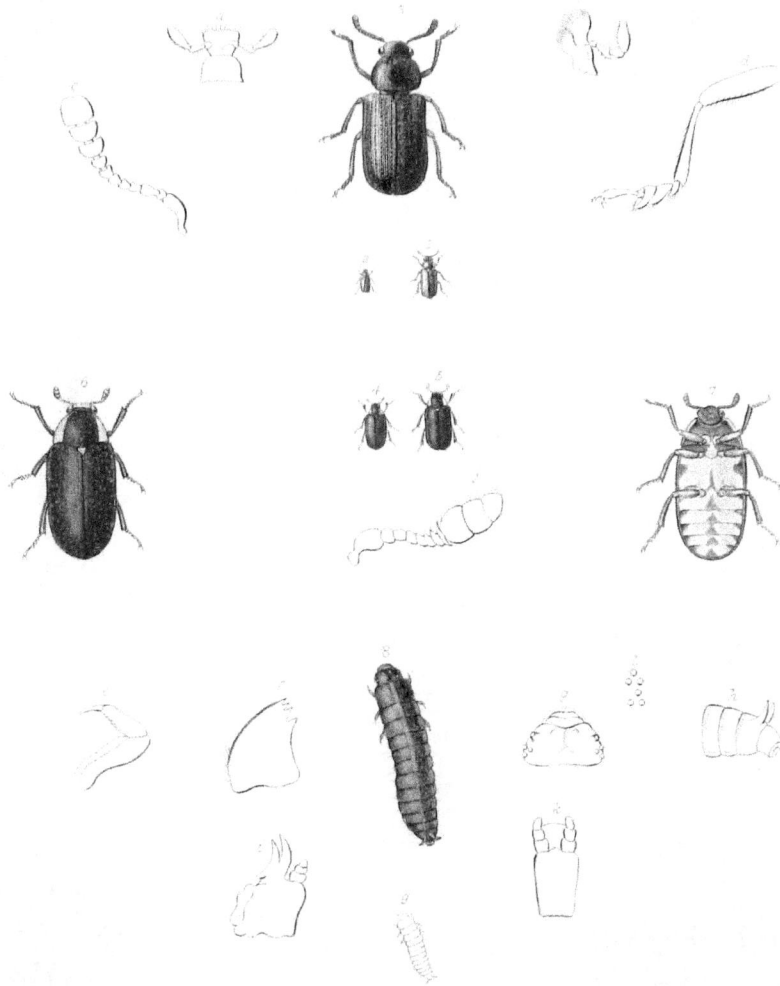

J.O.Westwood, F.L.S. delin.t

Published. by Mers Longman & Co March. 1 1834.

Plate. VI.

1

2

3

4

5

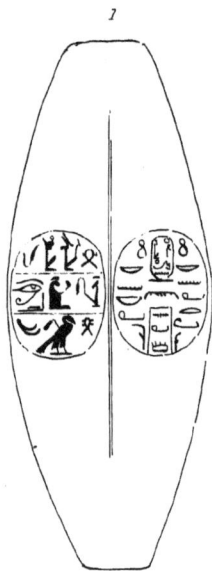

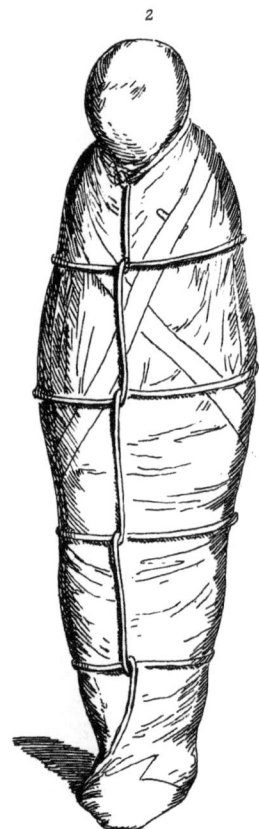

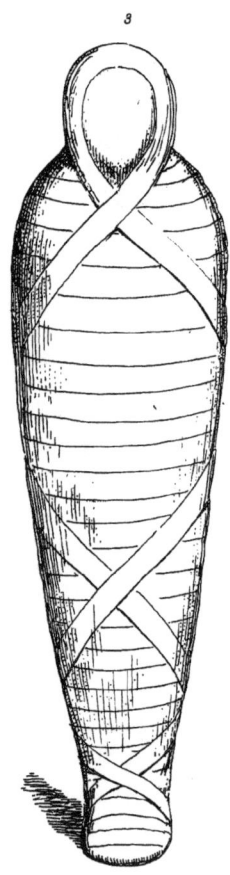

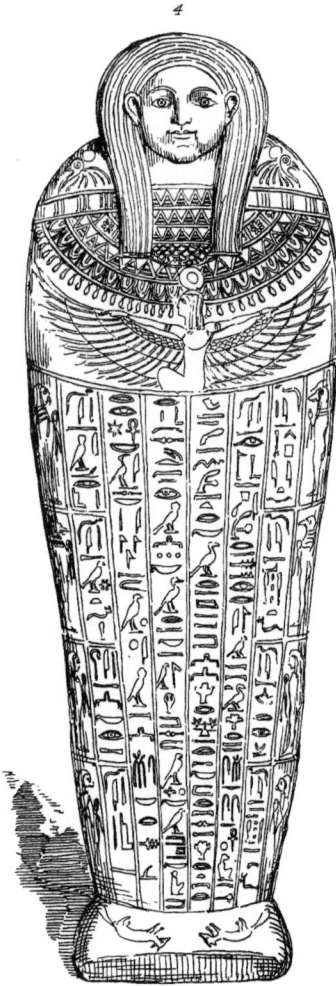

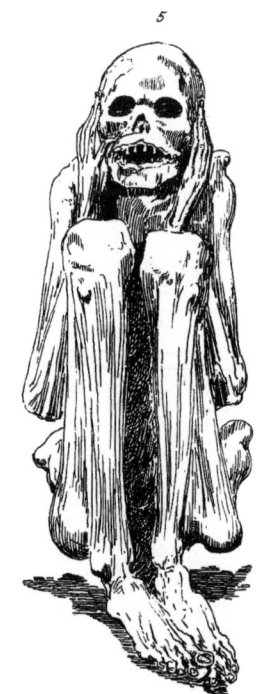

Geo Cruikshank. del.ᵗ

Published by Mesᵗˢ Longman &Cᵒ March 1.1834.

Plate. VII.

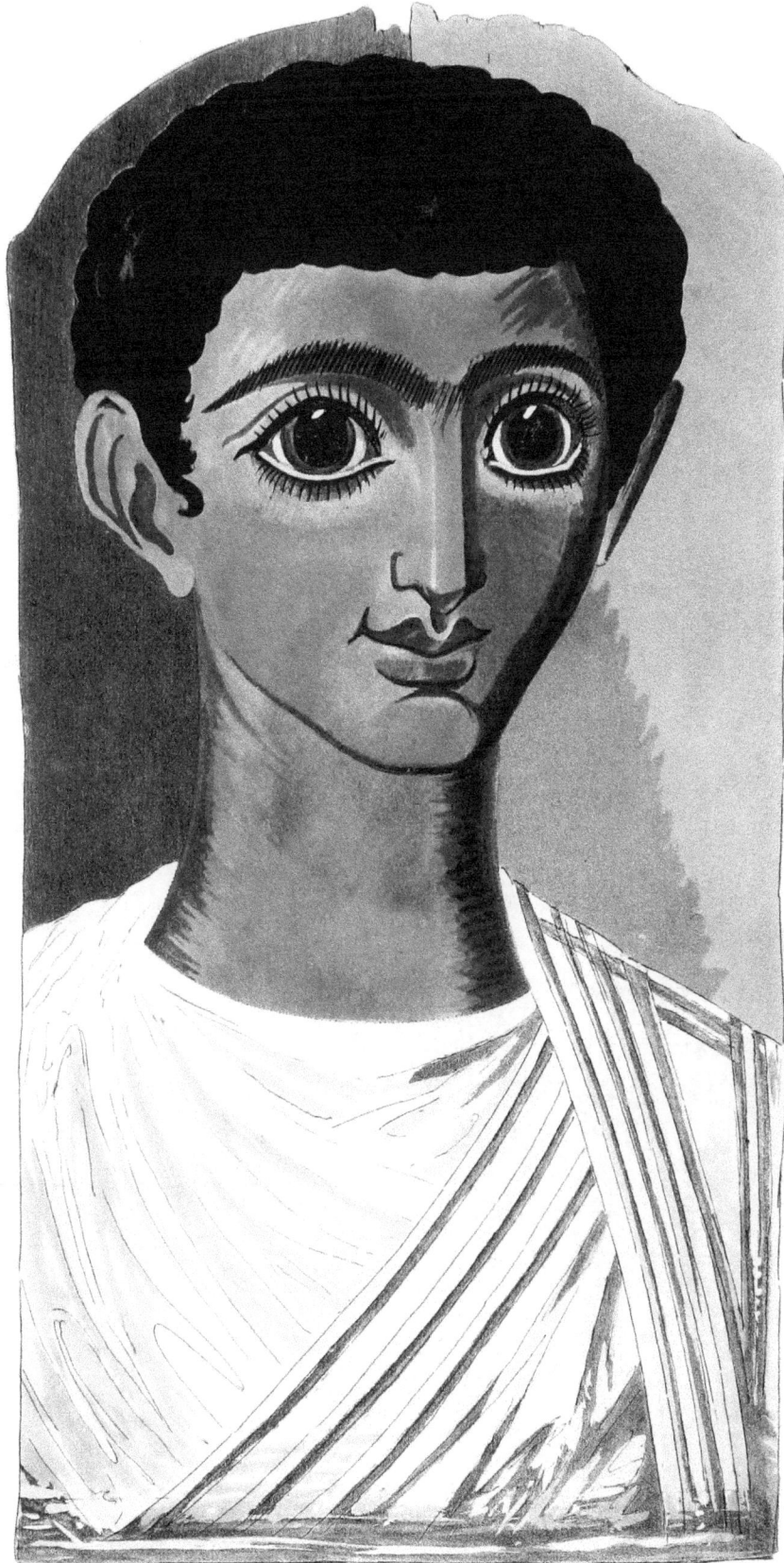

Geo Cruikshank. del.

Published. by Mes.rs Longman & C.o March. 1 1834.

Plate VIII.

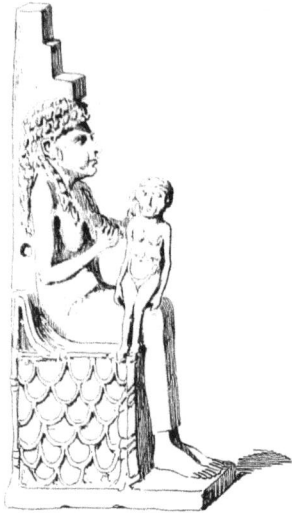

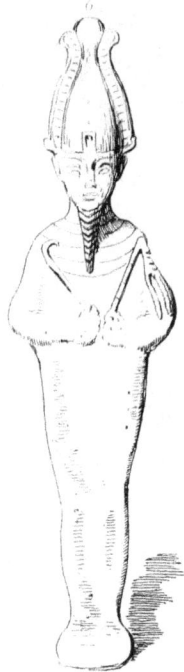

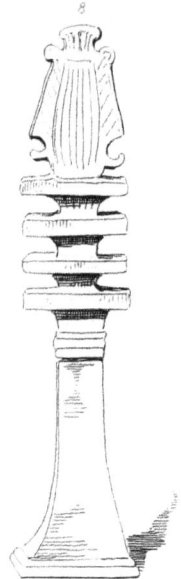

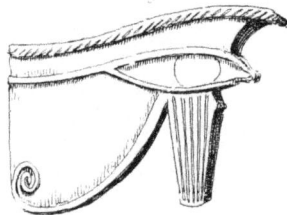

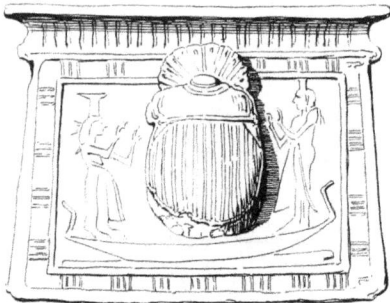

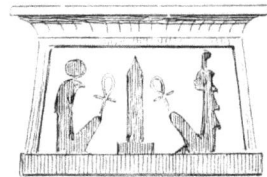

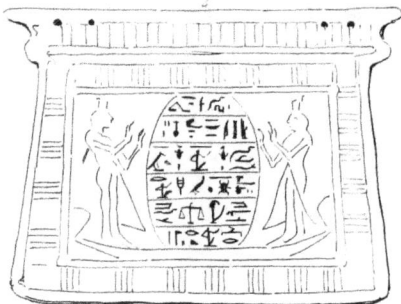

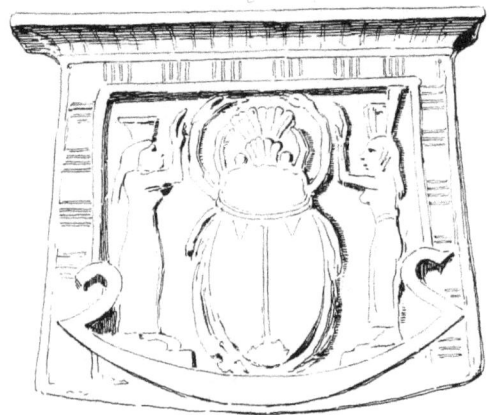

Pl. IX.

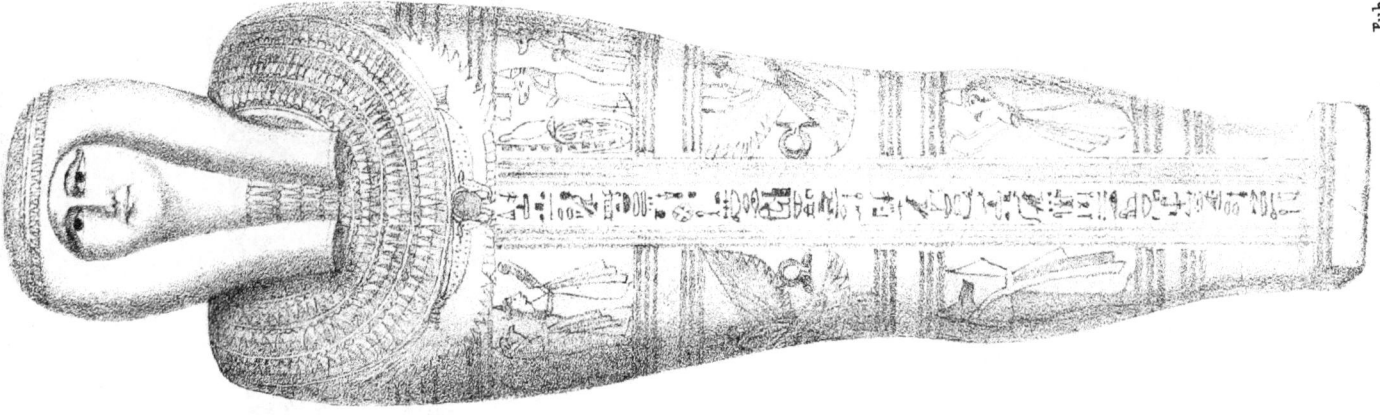

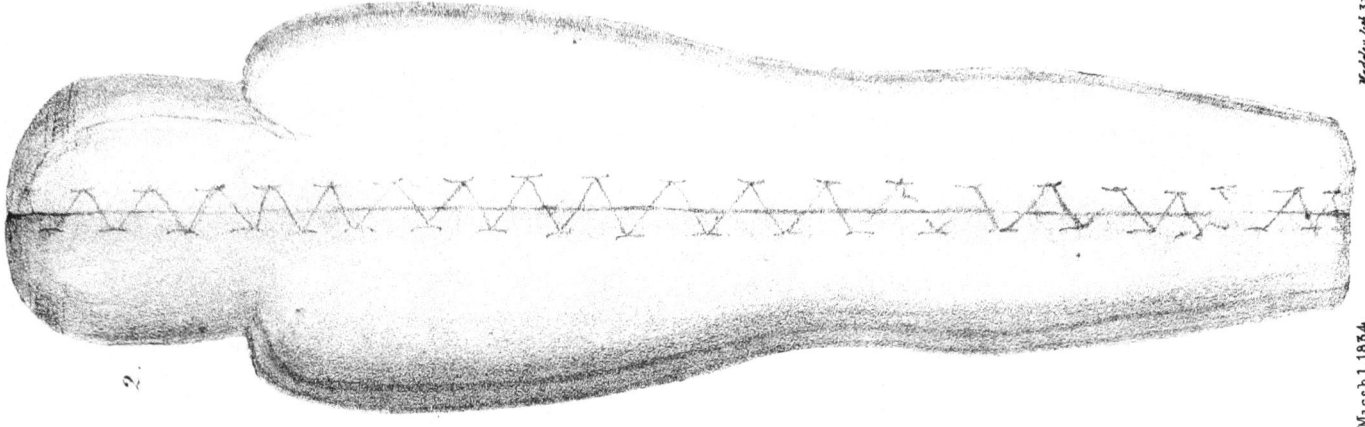

Madeley, lith.3.Wellington.N.Strand.

Pub: by Longman & Cº. Paternoster Row. March 1. 1834.

Pl. X.

2.

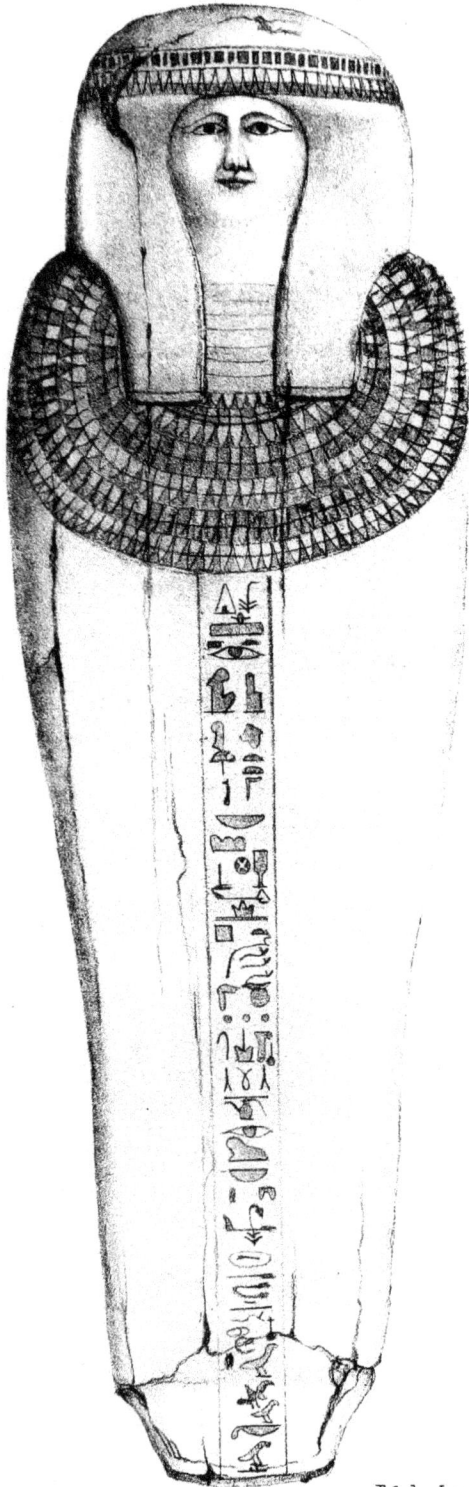

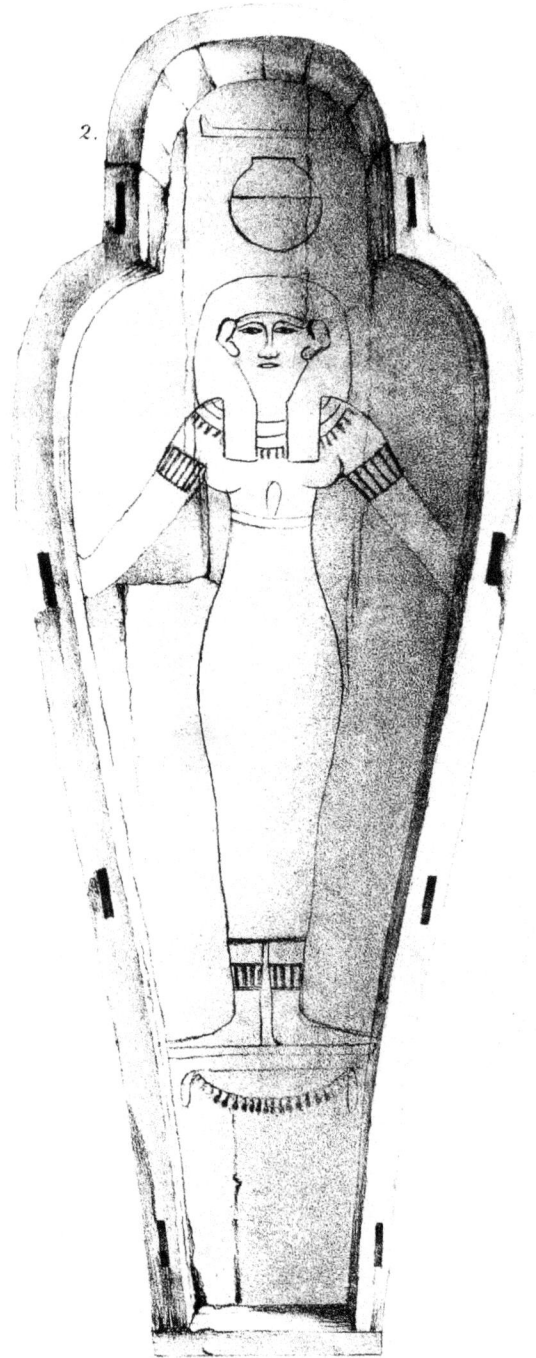

Pub. by Longman & Cº Paternoster Row. Mar. 1. 1834.

Madeley Lith 3 Wellington St

Plate. XI

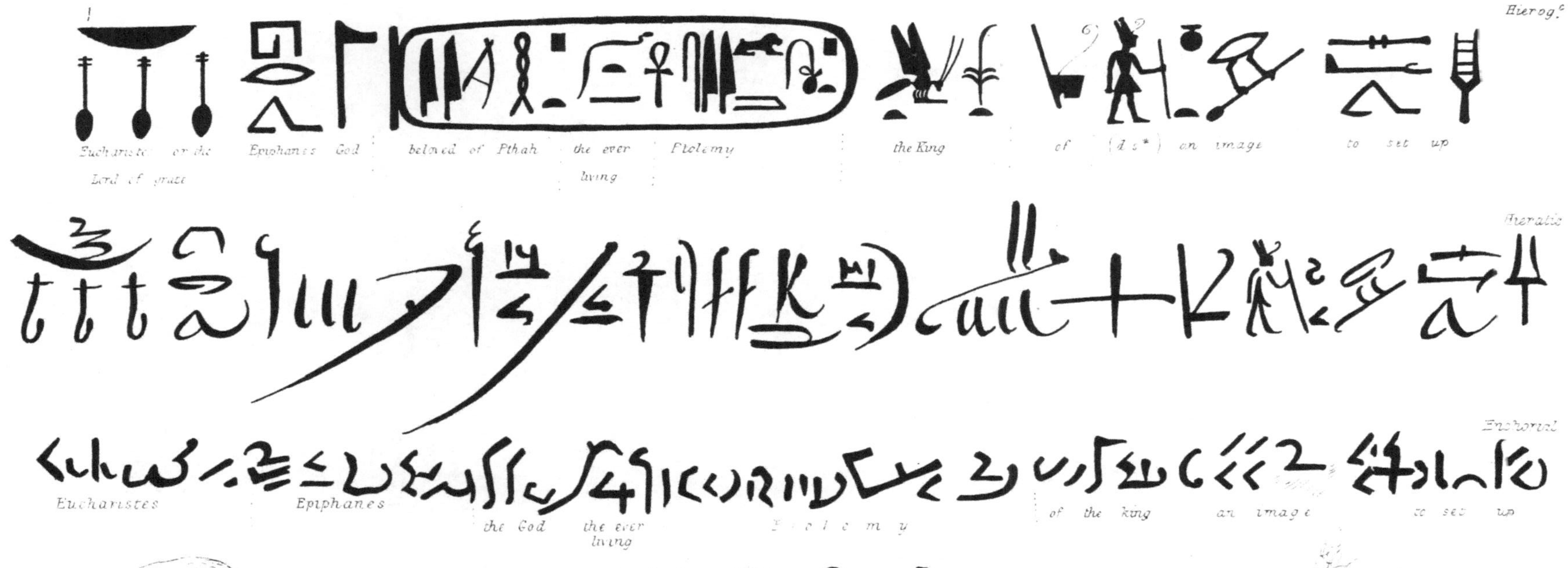

Hierog.c
1
Eucharistes or the Lord of grace
Epiphanes God
beloved of Pthah
the ever living
Ptolemy
the King
of (d. s.*) an image
to set up
Hieratic
Enchorial
Eucharistes
Epiphanes
the God
the ever living
P t o l e m y
of the king
an image
to set up

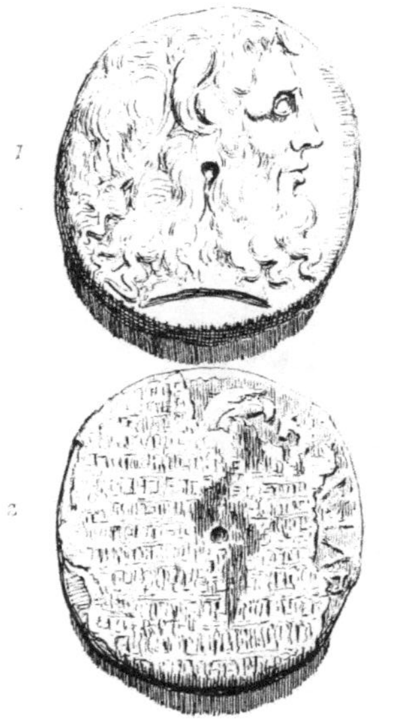

7

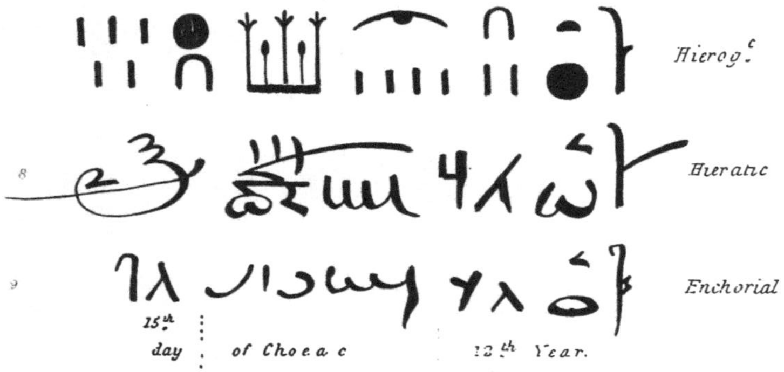

Hierog.c
8
Hieratic
9
Enchorial
15th day
of Choeac
12th Year.

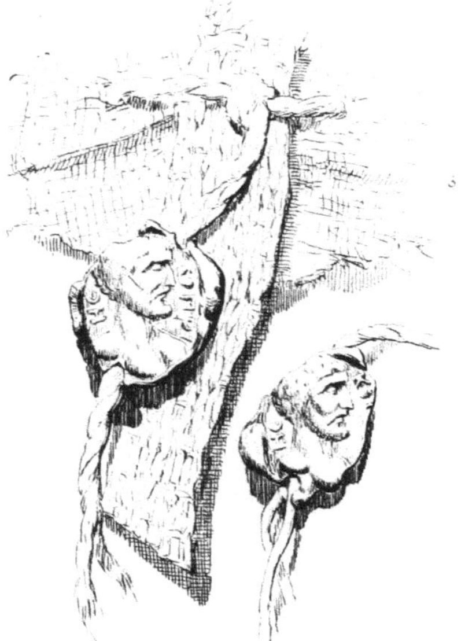

* The demonstrative sign, being a figure of the object which immediately precedes it & is expressed alphabetically.

Geo Cruikshank. del.t

Published by Mess.rs Longman & C.o March 1. 1834.

Plate XII.

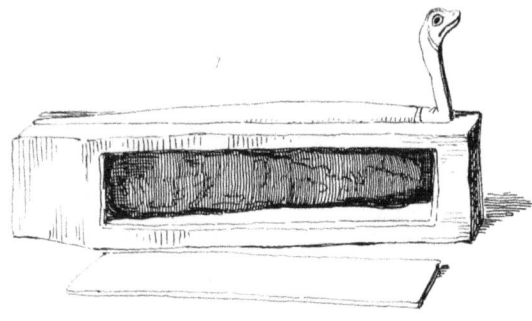

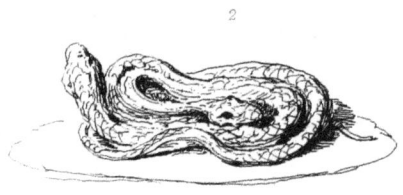

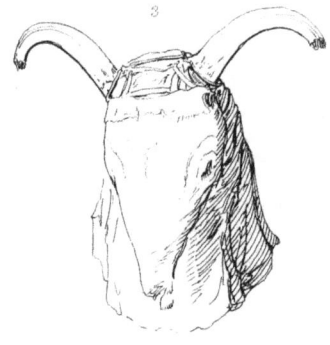

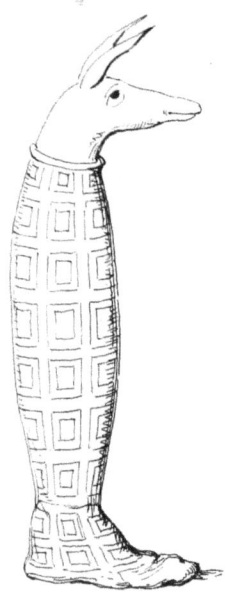

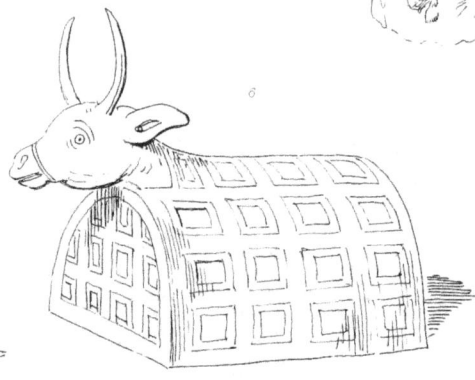

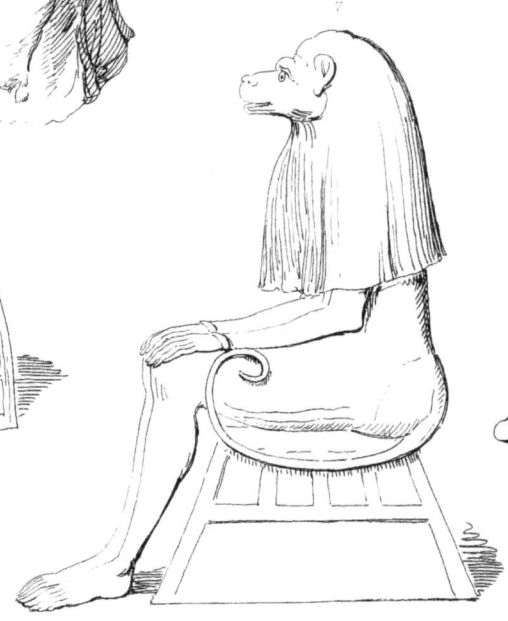

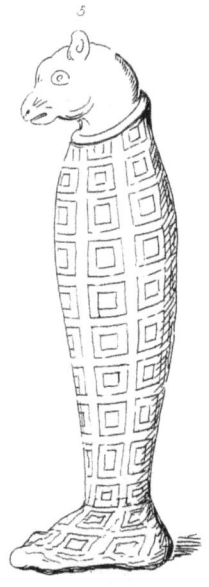

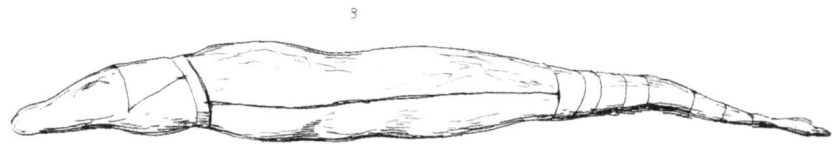

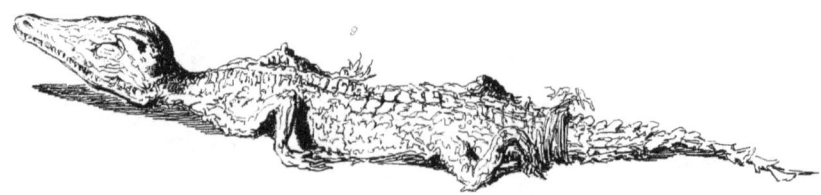

Published by Mefs.rs Longman&Co. March.1.1834.

Plate XIII.

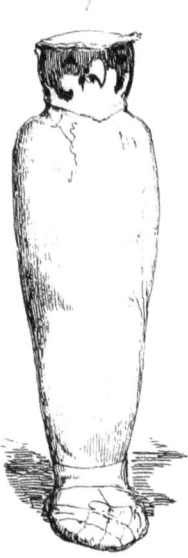

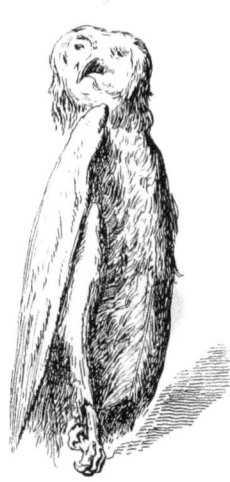

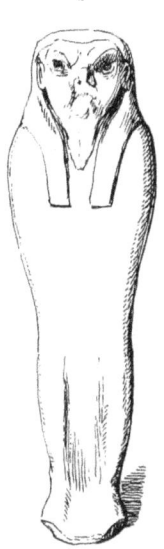

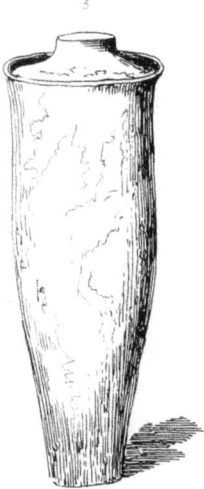

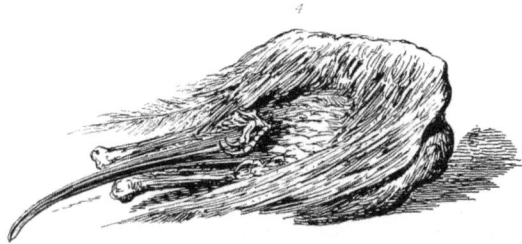

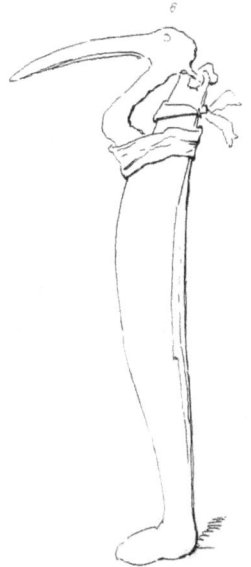

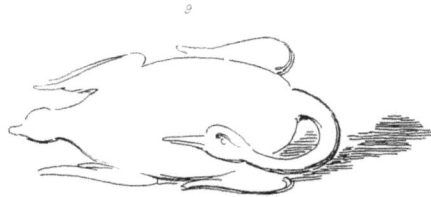

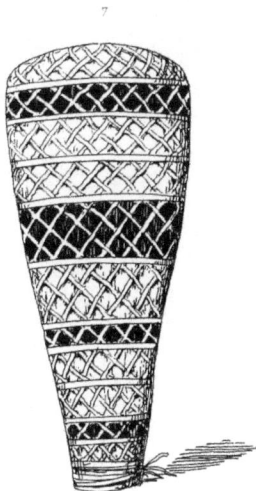

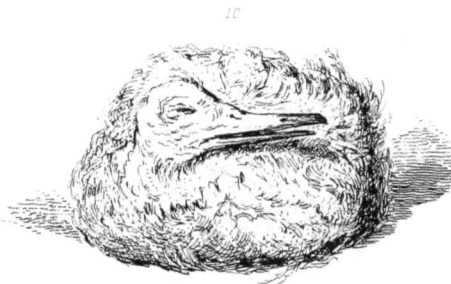

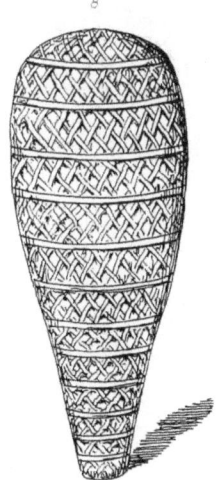

Geo. Cruikshank. del.

Published by Mel.rs Longman & Co. March.1.1834.

Lightning Source UK Ltd.
Milton Keynes UK
UKHW051952291120
374189UK00015B/417